Common Hand Problems in Primary Care

Common Hand Problems in Primary Care

Matthew J. Concannon, MD
Director, Hand and Microsurgery Unit
Division of Plastic and Reconstructive Surgery
University of Missouri Health Sciences Center
Columbia, Missouri

HANLEY & BELFUS, INC. / Philadelphia

Publisher: HANLEY & BELFUS, INC.
             Medical Publishers
             210 S. 13th Street
             Philadelphia, PA 19107
             (215) 546-7293, 800-962-1892
             FAX (215) 790-9330
             Website: http://www.hanleyandbelfus.com

Library of Congress Cataloging-in-Publication Data

Common hand problems in primary care / Matthew J. Concannon.
        p.   cm.
     Includes bibliographical references and index.
     ISBN 1-56053-209-2 (alk. paper)
        1. Hand—Wounds and injuries—Atlases.   2. Hand—Surgery—Atlases.
     3. Hand—Diseases—Atlases.   4. Primary care (Medicine)—Atlases.
     I. Concannon, Matthew J., 1962–
        [DNLM: 1. Hand Injuries—diagnosis atlases.   2. Hand Injuries—
     therapy atlases.   3. Primary Health Care atlases.   WE 17C734 1998]
     RD559.C65   1999
     617.5′75—dc21
     DNLM/DLC
     for Library of Congress   98-37041
                                                                    CIP

COMMON HAND PROBLEMS IN PRIMARY CARE   ISBN 1-56053-209-2

Last digit is the print number: 9 8 7 6 5 4 3 2 1

Dedication

This book is dedicated to my wife and best friend, Kathy. Without her constant support and encouragement, this work never could have been finished. She is responsible for most of my accomplishments, and I cherish her.

Table of Contents

		Page
Chapter 1:	Hand Anatomy	1
Chapter 2:	Examination of the Hand	27
Chapter 3:	Anesthetic Techniques	57
Chapter 4:	Treatment of Lacerations	65
Chapter 5:	Soft Tissue Loss and Amputation	77
Chapter 6:	Fractures and Dislocations	99
Chapter 7:	Infections of the Hand	127
Chapter 8:	Common Hand Problems	133
Index		165

Preface

Hand injuries currently account for 1 in 10 of all emergency room visits. In our modern era of managed care, primary care physicians are under increasing pressure to limit specialist referral in virtually all clinical situations. This book was written to serve as a "curbside consultant" for these physicians in the diagnosis and treatment of hand injuries.

A straightforward, clear format facilitates accurate diagnosis of injuries, outlines treatment options for the various hand injuries that present in the emergency room, and provides step-by-step technical instructions. "Tricks of the trade" and common pitfalls to avoid are included. Clinical examples and more than 400 photographs supplement the text.

Despite external pressures to limit specialist referral, there *are* certain situations that require the consultation of a hand surgeon. Guidelines for specialist referral, to help the physician decide on the appropriate course of action, are provided in every chapter.

Finally, note that traumatic hand injuries—which have such enormous potential for both physical and emotional debilitation in the patient—also are addressed.

I hope this book is helpful to you in caring for your patients.

Matthew J. Concannon, MD

Acknowledgments

There are many individuals, mostly teachers and mentors, that I would like to gratefully acknowledge for their assistance and guidance through the years. Foremost among these role models are my parents, Jerry and Jackie Concannon. Others that have motivated and inspired me (whether they know it or not) include Ben Asen, Erwin Montgomery, M.D., W. Kirt Nichols, M.D., and James W. May, Jr., M.D. In particular, C. Lin Puckett, M.D. has evolved (in my eyes) from a mentor to an instructor and, most recently, to a friend and partner. He is a consummate hand surgeon and an exemplary leader and teacher. Most of the facts and pearls that appear in this work I originally learned from him.

I would like to thank the following individuals for their "volunteer" work as hand models (despite the occasional anomaly, Mark): Stefan Craig, M.D., Mark Boschert, M.D., Patricia Arledge, M.D., Matthew Ragsdell, and Brad Medling. Thanks also to Ms. Denise Boland for her help in manuscript preparation.

The anatomic line drawings were done by Arlene Priest: her ability to translate difficult anatomic concepts into straightforward images has strengthened this work a great deal.

Special thanks are in order to Linda Belfus of Hanley & Belfus, Inc. for her support and guidance, particularly in the early, formative stages of this project. Jacqueline Mahon has performed miracles in translating my original manuscript into readable text.

Finally, I would like to acknowledge and thank my family—Kathy, Meghan, Chaeleigh, Ryan, Bridget, and Erin—for their never-wavering support throughout this process.

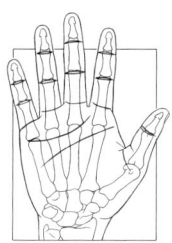

1 Hand Anatomy

A basic understanding of hand anatomy is crucial to adequately diagnosis and treat chronic or acute hand injuries. Form follows function very closely in the hand, and any injury or derangement of the underlying bones, tendons, nerves, or arteries is likely to produce an unwelcome limitation in function. The purpose of this chapter is not to provide an exhaustive encyclopedia of hand anatomy, but rather to provide the reader with basic hand anatomy and function to facilitate examination and diagnosis of hand injuries.

Terminology

There are certain terms that are relatively unique to this field. These descriptors of movement and position are used throughout this book and are defined here for your convenience.

Abduction is defined as movement away from the axial line of the limb. The central axis of the hand is the third metacarpal (supporting the long, or middle, finger). Therefore, spreading the fingers apart (away from the long finger) is abduction (Figure 1A). **Adduction** of the fingers brings them back together toward the long finger (Figure 1B). Confusing matters is abduction of the thumb: while it can be abducted radially (see Figure 1A), it also can be abducted from the palmar axis of the hand (Figure 2).

Pronation is defined as the act of assuming the prone position. Applied to the hand, the act of pronation involves turning the palm backward (or posteriorly) so that the thumb is pointed towards the body. **Supination** is the op-

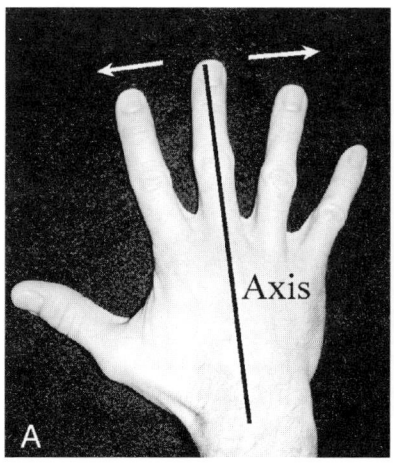

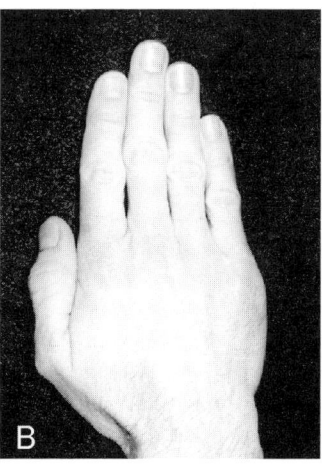

Axis

A   B

FIGURE 1. **A,** Abduction of the fingers is defined as movement *away from* the axial line of the limb. In the hand, the long finger metacarpal serves as the central axis. **B,** Adduction of the fingers is defined as movement *toward* the central axis of the hand (the long finger).

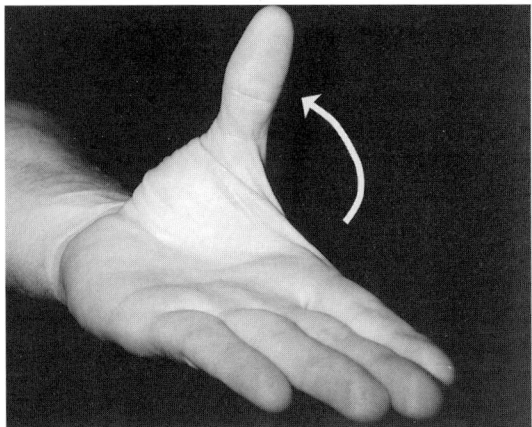

FIGURE 2. Due to its unique range of motion, the thumb also can be abducted from the palmar plane of the hand.

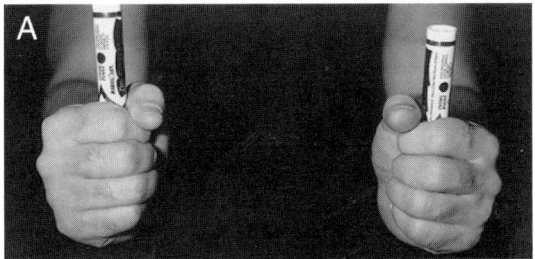

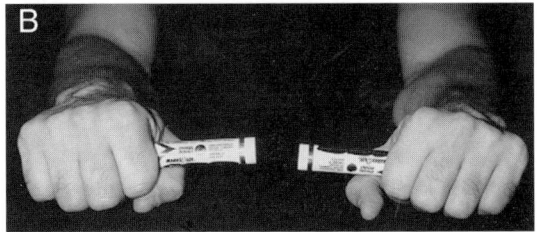

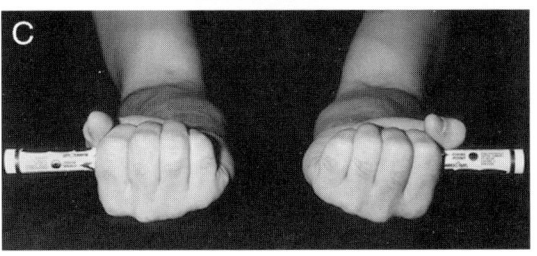

posite motion, involving outward rotation of the hand such that the thumb is pointing away from the body (Figure 3).

Opposition of the thumb is the combination of movements which brings the thumb away from the plane of the palm and pronates it, allowing pulp-to-pulp pinch between the thumb and the other fingers (Figure 4). Thumb opposition is a critical component of hand function, and its loss can be very disabling.

The palmar aspect of the hand and fingers is

FIGURE 3. **A,** The hands in neutral position. **B,** Pronation involves turning the palm so that the thumb is pointed *toward* the body. **C,** Supination is outer rotation of the hand so that the thumb is pointed *away from* the body.

FIGURE 4. Opposition of the thumb is the combination of movements that abducts the thumb from the plane of the palm and pronates it, allowing pulp-to-pulp pinch between the thumb and the other fingers.

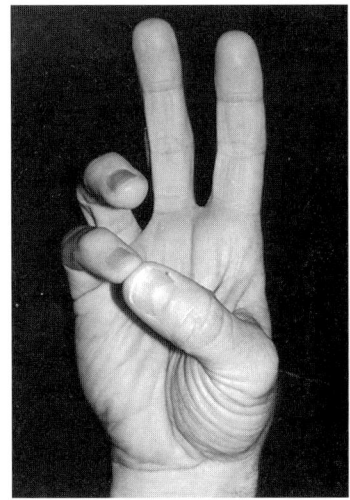

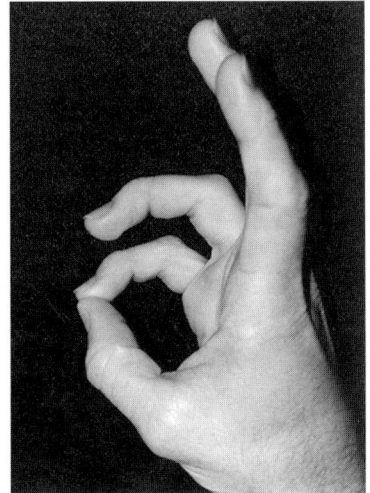

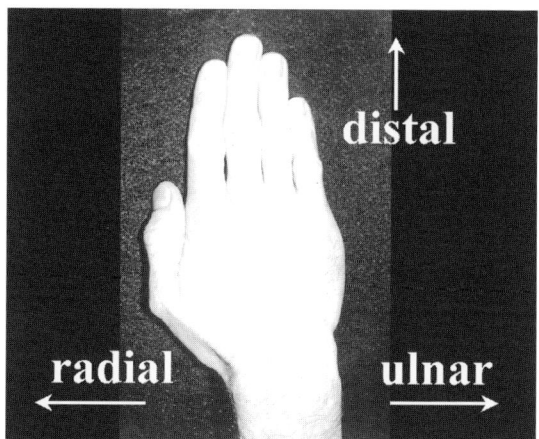

FIGURE 5. Dorsum of the hand. The terms radial and ulnar are used to describe relative position. For example, the thumb lies radial to the index finger. A distal position refers to a location farther away from the body; proximal means nearer to the body.

termed the **volar** aspect, while the dorsal aspect is simply referred to as the **dorsum** of the hand. In addition, it is helpful to use the terms **radial** (toward the radius) and **ulnar** (toward the ulna) when describing the hand (Figure 5). The palmar surface of the hand is lined with flexion creases that correspond to the underlying joints (Figure 6). The exception is the proximal digital crease, which lies at the mid-portion of the proximal phalanx.

A few words concerning the nomenclature of the digits: the metacarpal of the thumb is the **first metacarpal,** the metacarpal of the index finger is the **second metacarpal,** and so on in an ulnar direction (Figure 7). However, to avoid confusion, it is best to refer to the digits as the index, long, ring, and small fingers instead of referring to them by number.

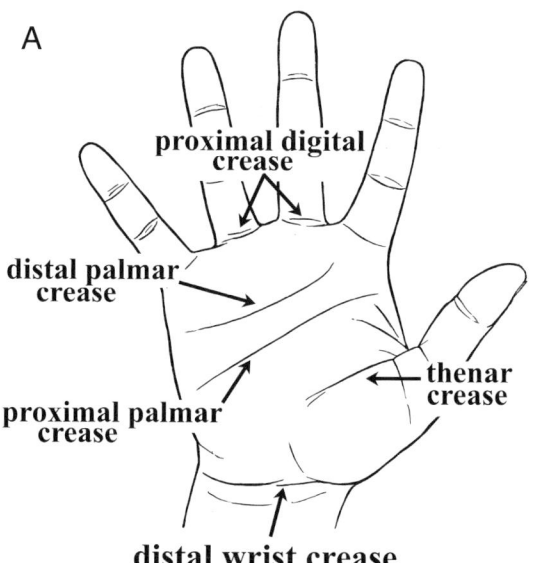

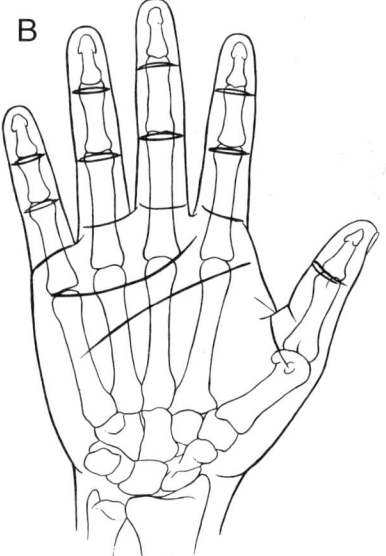

FIGURE 6. **A,** Certain constant creases on the volar aspect of the hand can assist in describing locations of lesions or lacerations on the palmar surface. The thenar crease separates the thenar mass from the mid-palm. The distal and proximal palmar creases correspond roughly to the positions of the MCP joints. The proximal digital crease lies at approximately the mid-portion of the proximal phalanx. The distal wrist crease marks the boundary between the distal forearm and the hand. **B,** The bony anatomy of the hand is demonstrated in relationship to the volar creases of the hand. Note that the distal and proximal palmar creases correspond roughly to the level of the MCP joints. The proximal digital crease is the only crease not associated with an underlying joint. The other creases of the fingers correspond almost exactly with the underlying DIP or PIP joints.

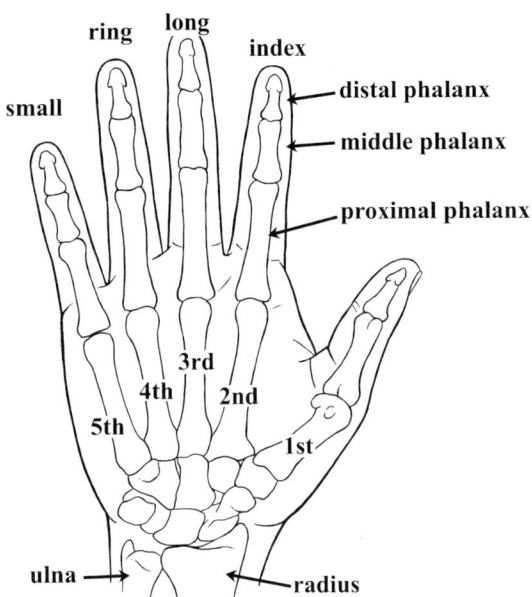

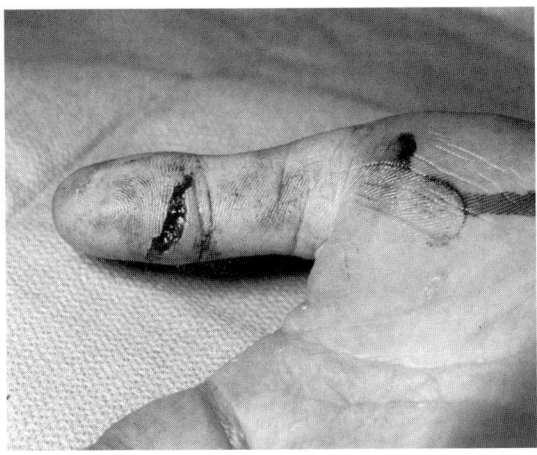

FIGURE 8. A two-centimeter, transversely oriented laceration of the volar aspect of the thumb, immediately distal to the interphalangeal crease.

FIGURE 7. Bony anatomy of the hand. There are three phalanges in each of the four fingers: proximal, middle, and distal. There are only two phalanges at the thumb: distal and proximal. The thumb metacarpal is the first metacarpal, the index metacarpal is the second metacarpal, and so on in the ulnar direction.

Proximal refers to a location closer to the body; **distal** is farther from the body (Figure 8). For example, the wrist is distal to the elbow and is proximal to the fingers. The application of this terminology allows precise and accurate documentation of your examination of the patient and conveys your meaning clearly to other physicians who are either reviewing the records or being consulted in the care of the patient.

Bony Anatomy

Each of the digits of the hand is supported by a single metacarpal. The thumb consists of two phalanges (proximal and distal), and each of the other digits consists of three phalanges (proximal, middle, and distal). Accordingly, the thumb only has one interphalangeal joint while the other digits have a proximal and a distal interphalangeal (PIP, DIP) joint. The junction of

the metacarpals with the phalanges is called the metacarpophalangeal (MCP) joint (Figures 7, 9A, 10, 11). At the head of the first (thumb) metacarpal are two sesamoid bones (Figure 9B). Sesamoid bones are round bones that form within tendons or ligaments and protect them from excessive wear; they are called "sesamoid" because of their resemblance to sesame seeds.

The metacarpals articulate proximally with the carpal bones. The eight carpal bones form a complex, three-dimensional structure that articulates proximally with the distal radius and ulna, allowing movement of the wrist in four directions: flexion, extension, and radial and ulnar deviation. Because of their overlapping position, it is difficult to visualize the carpal bones radiographically (Figures 12, 13). The carpal bones are held together by a strong and complex arrangement of supporting ligaments. Tears of these ligaments can lead to alteration of the carpal bone position, which can result in wrist pain, arthritis, and wrist collapse.

The hand bones are endochondral in origin—they form from ossification of cartilage elements. The process of ossification occurs throughout childhood, and radiographs of children reflect this bony immaturity as open epiphyses (Figure 14).

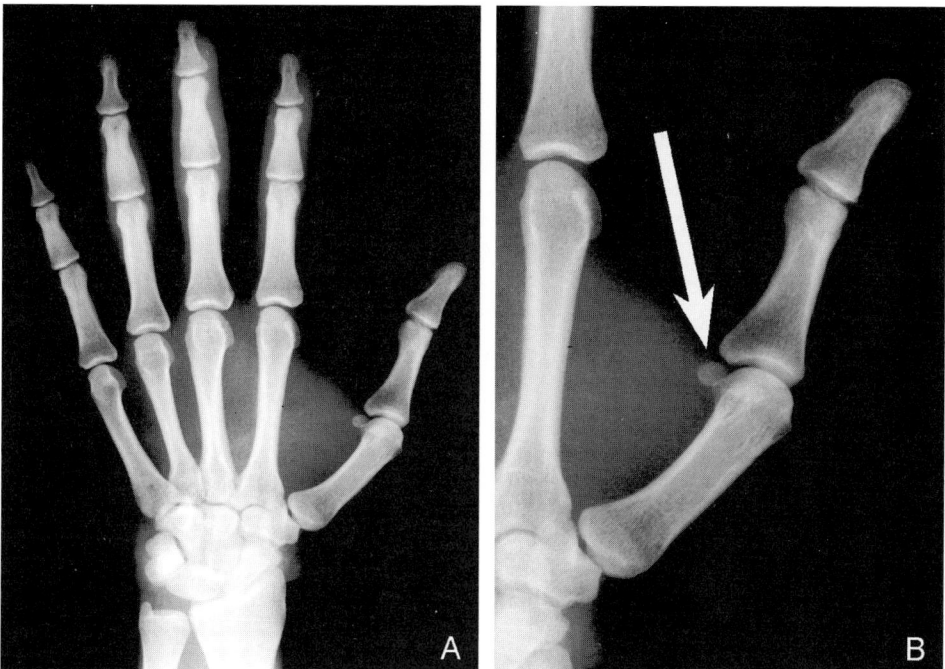

FIGURE 9. **A,** Normal x-ray of the bony anatomy of the hand (compare to Figure 7). **B,** Close-up of thumb, with arrow pointing to sesamoid bone at the metacarpal head.

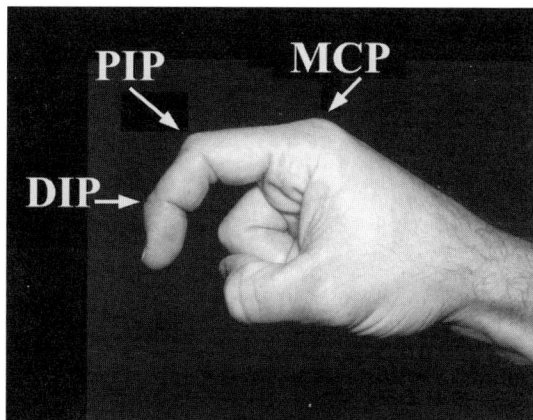

FIGURE 10. Surface anatomy of the lateral aspect of the hand showing the distal interphalangeal (DIP), proximal interphalangeal (PIP), and metacarpophalangeal (MCP) joints.

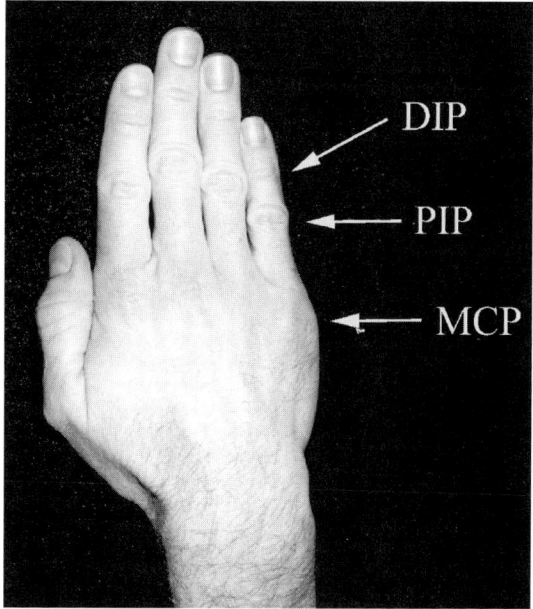

FIGURE 11. Surface anatomy of the dorsal aspect of the hand showing the DIP, PIP, and MCP joints.

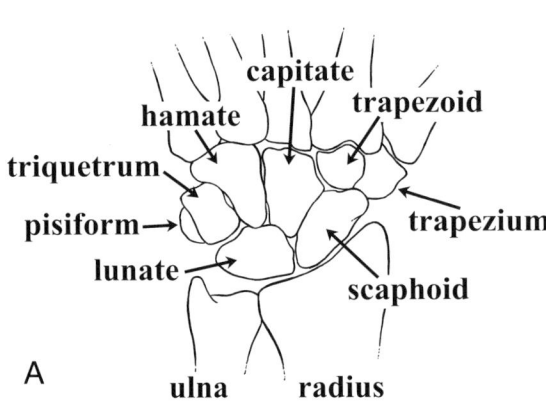

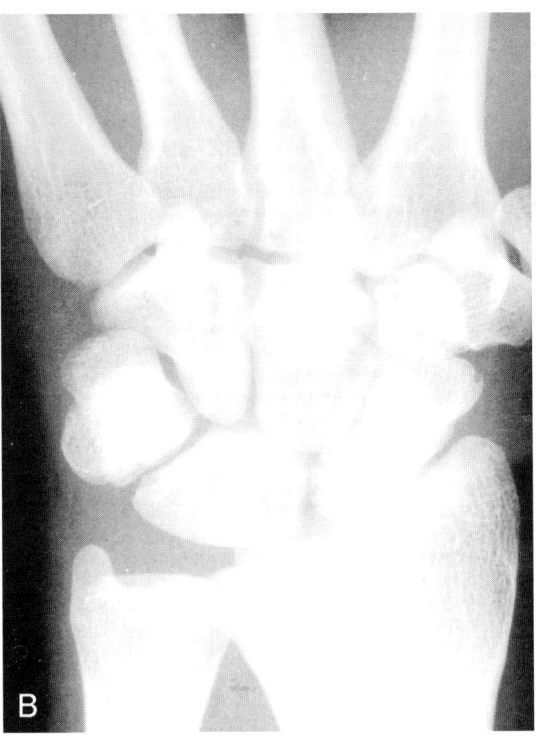

FIGURE 12. **A,** The carpal bones. **B,** X-ray of the carpal bones. Due to their overlapping and complex anatomy, interpretation of carpal x-rays can be difficult. Check for equal joint spaces between the bones and no obvious derangement of the normal anatomic position.

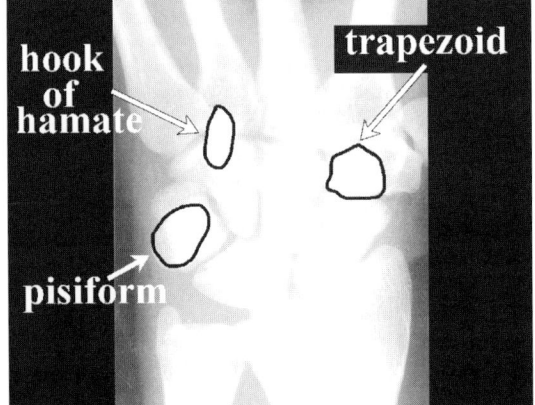

FIGURE 13. The overlapping areas of the carpal bones are outlined. The pisiform lies volar and is palpable at the ulnar aspect of the distal wrist crease. The trapezium anchors the thumb, and the trapezoid anchors the second metacarpal: they overlap radiographically because the thumb is positioned volar as well as lateral to the trapezoid. The hook of the hamate also extends volarly (compare to Figure 12B).

Vascular Anatomy

The hand has a dual blood supply, with vascular inflow provided by the radial and ulnar arteries (Figure 15). Venous outflow is provided through a rich network of veins along the dorsum of the hand, although vena comitantes also travel on the volar side with the radial and ulnar arteries. The ulnar artery usually is the dominant blood supply to the hand. In approximately 80% of the population, there is sufficient collateral flow between the radial and ulnar arteries that the entire hand can be adequately perfused by either artery alone (Figure 16). Anastomoses between these vessels occurs in the palm between the superficial arch (the termination of the ulnar artery) and deep arch (the termination of the radial artery).

In the 20% of the population that does not have adequate communication between these two arteries, the loss of either could result in finger ischemia and tissue loss unless corrective action is taken (Figure 17). A common clinical situation is one in which the radial artery has

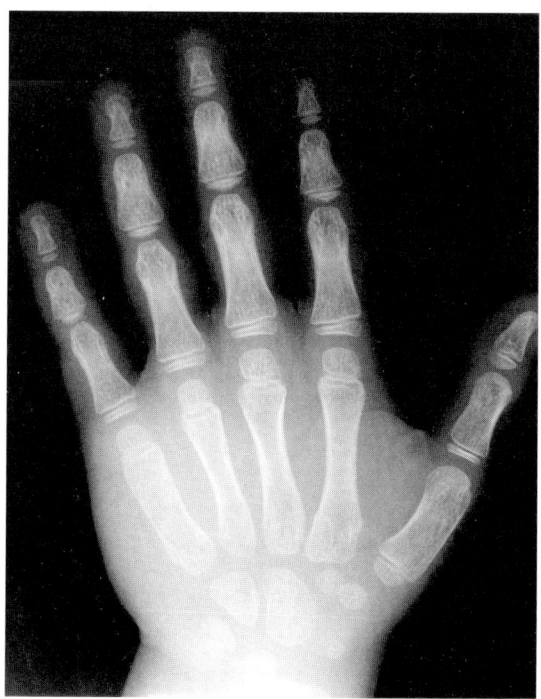

FIGURE 14. A radiograph of a 6-year-old child demonstrating open epiphyses (growth centers) and variable ossification, particularly of the carpal bones. Fracture identification can be difficult in the setting of an open growth plate; therefore, a contralateral view of the uninjured hand usually is obtained for comparison.

been injured after arterial puncture or cannulation, causing thrombosis. If there is not an adequate circulation to the radial aspect of the hand from the ulnar artery, ischemia of the thumb and/or index finger may occur. The easiest way to assess the adequacy of the communication between these arteries is with the Allen's test (see Chapter 2).

The ulnar artery forms the superficial arch and the radial artery forms the deep arch within the palm (Figures 15, 18). The common digital arteries arise from these arches to provide blood supply to the fingers via the digital arteries. The digital arteries of the fingers lie along the volar lateral aspect of each of the digits and are intimately associated with the digital nerves. The artery and nerve together are termed the **neurovascular bundle** (Figure 19). Knowledge of the location of the neurovascular bundle in the digits is helpful in the application of local anesthesia (see Chapter 3). Since there is a dual blood supply to each of the digits, survival is possible as long as one of the digital arteries remains patent. For this reason, usually only one artery is repaired during digital replantation.

In contrast to the other fingers, the neurovas-

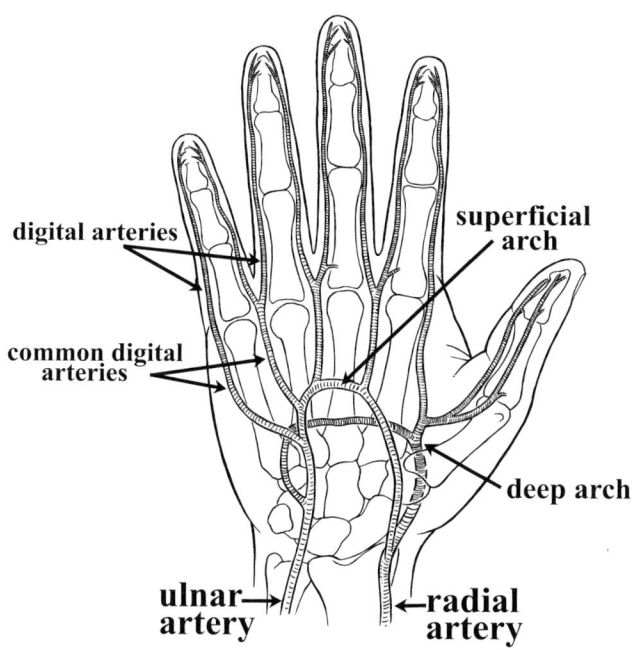

FIGURE 15. The arterial anatomy of the hand. There are two major arteries to the hand: ulnar and radial. In most people the ulnar artery is the dominant blood supply. The ulnar artery continues on to form the superficial arch, from which the common digital arteries arise. The radial artery terminates in the deep arch and principally supplies the radial aspect of the index finger and the thumb. The common digital arteries bifurcate at the level of the MCP joints to form the proper digital arteries. These travel with the digital nerves along the ulnar and radial aspects of each finger (see Figure 19).

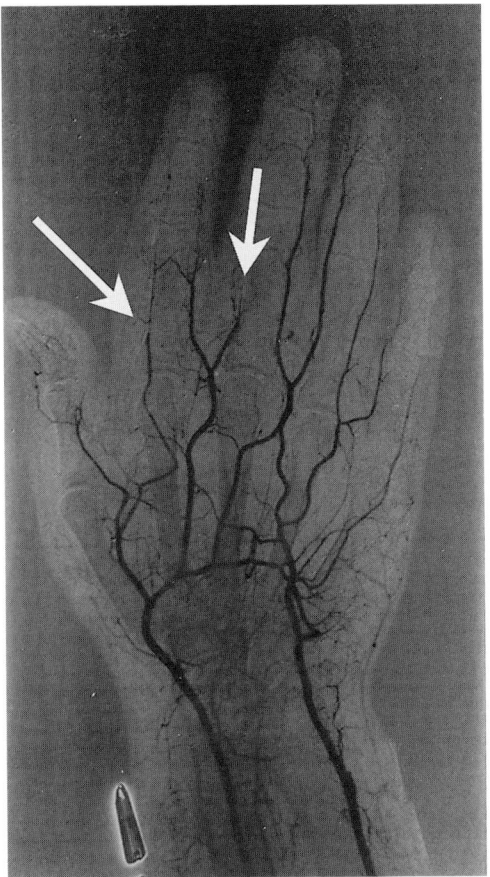

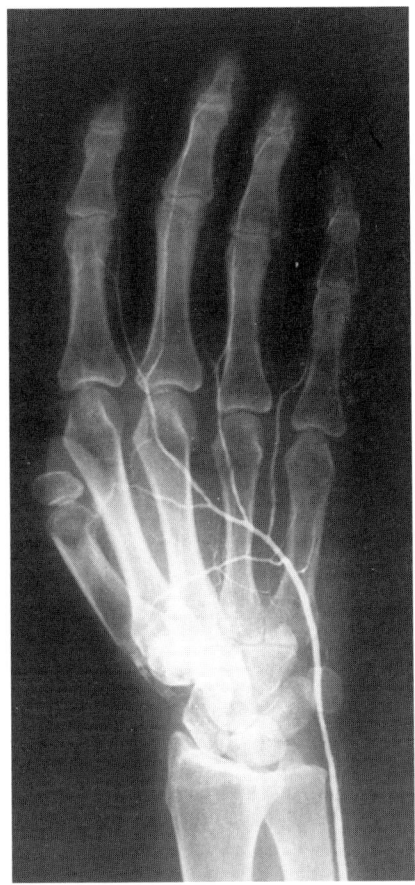

FIGURE 16. Arteriogram demonstrating patency of both the radial and ulnar arteries. This is not a normal arteriogram: the patient has a vasospastic disease (scleroderma) and presents with chronic ischemia of the fingers. Note the destruction of the proper digital arteries of the index and long fingers in particular (*arrows*).

FIGURE 17. Abnormal arteriogram. This patient has severe vasospastic disease, with complete occlusion of the radial artery and diffuse disease of the common and proper digital arteries. Insufficient collateral flow from the ulnar artery system to the radial side of the hand resulted in loss of the radial artery, critical thumb ischemia, and thumb loss.

cular bundles of the thumb are more centrally located and superficial (Figure 20). The thumb neurovascular bundles can be easily palpated at the central volar aspect of the thumb (over the flexor tendon) at the MCP joint. This is important to recognize when applying local anesthesia (digital block) to the thumb and when evaluating thumb lacerations for nerve or artery involvement.

Nerves

There are three major nerves that supply the upper extremity distal to the elbow: the radial, median, and ulnar nerves (Figures 21, 22). Each of these is a mixed nerve, providing sensory information to the brain as well as motor innervation to the musculature of the forearm and hand. Therefore, the function of these nerves can be

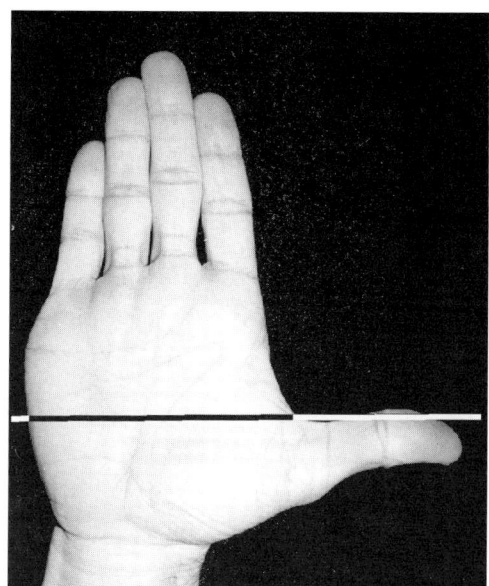

FIGURE 18. The anatomic level of the superficial palmar arch usually can be approximated by drawing a line across the hand perpendicular to the volar aspect of the thumb (fully abducted).

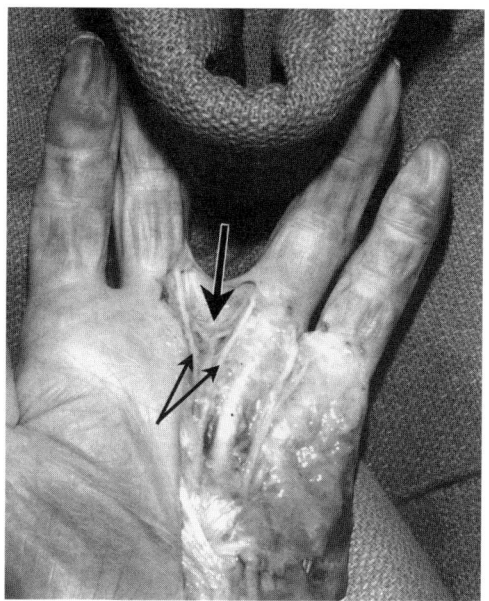

FIGURE 19. In this cadaver dissection, note the bifurcation of the common digital artery into the two proper digital arteries (*large arrow*) and the associated digital nerves to the ulnar aspect of the long finger and the radial aspect of the ring finger (*small arrows*). After the bifurcation of the common digital artery, there is a close association of the digital artery and nerve along the lateral aspect of the finger. This association is termed the neurovascular bundle.

evaluated by testing sensation as well as motor function (see Chapter 2).

SENSORY DISTRIBUTION

The radial nerve provides sensation primarily to the radial dorsal aspect of the hand. The ulnar nerve provides sensation to the ulnar aspect of the hand (specifically the ulnar one and a half digits) on both the volar and dorsal sides. The median nerve innervates the volar radial aspect of the hand, as well as the dorsal aspect of the index and long fingers distally (Figure 22).

MUSCLES AND TENDONS

A great deal of hand and finger motion is provided by muscles proximal to the hand, located in the forearm. As a matter of fact, the digits themselves have no muscles at all. An understanding of the innervation of the musculature that provides specific movement of the digits and hand enables the examiner to evaluate not only

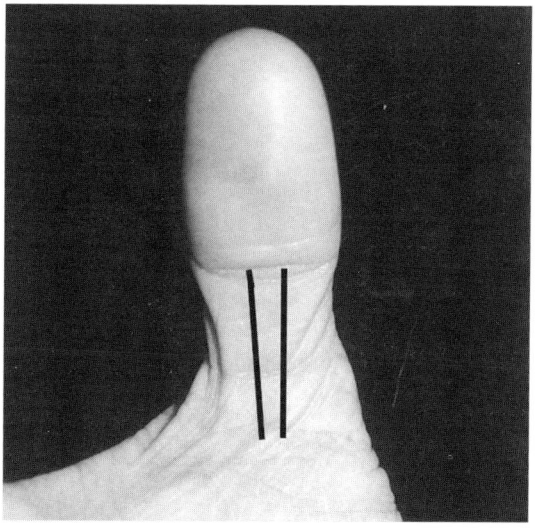

FIGURE 20. The neurovascular bundles of the thumb (*black lines*) lie more volar and medial than the neurovascular bundles of the other digits.

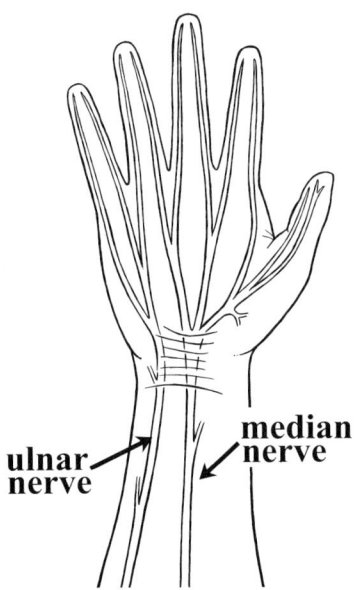

FIGURE 21. The ulnar and median nerves in the forearm, hand, and fingers. The median nerve enters the hand through the carpal tunnel; the ulnar nerve travels in a similar space at the wrist called Guyon's canal.

the muscle, but also the muscle's innervation. It is impossible to describe the function of the motor nerves without considering the muscles that they innervate. Therefore, for the purposes of this summary the muscles are grouped and discussed based on the nerves that motor them. Notice how each nerve provides a generalized function: extension (radial nerve), flexion (median nerve), and hand coordination (ulnar nerve).

Radial Nerve

The radial nerve travels along the dorsal-radial aspect of the arm (Figure 23). Along with its main motor branch, the posterior interosseous nerve, the radial nerve provides extension of the wrist, extension of the MCP joints, and extension of the thumb (Table 1). The dorsal muscles of the forearm, therefore, function as extensors. The tendons of these muscles pass underneath the extensor retinaculum, just proximal to the wrist. The extensor retinaculum is a strong, fibrous pulley that is

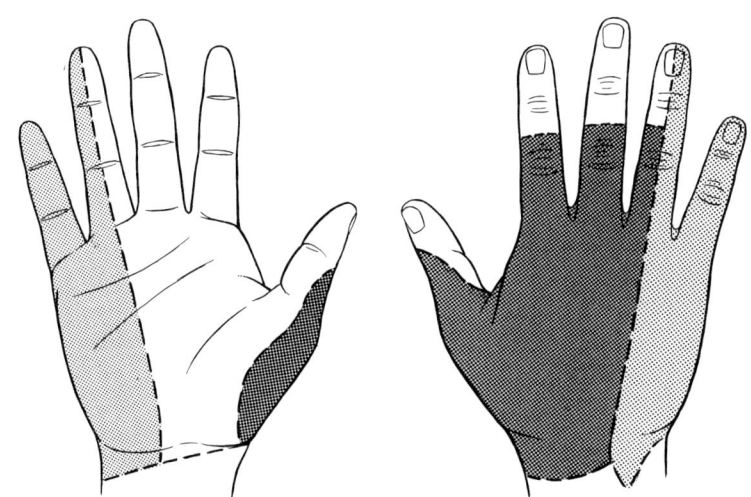

FIGURE 22. Cutaneous innervation from the median, ulnar, and radial nerves. The ulnar nerve (*light shading*) supplies the ulnar one and a half digits both volarly and dorsally. The volar sensation is provided by the digital nerves of the neurovascular bundles. Dorsal sensation is provided by the dorsal sensory branches (see Figure 46). The median nerve (*white area*) provides the volar sensation to the radial aspect of the hand via the proper digital nerves and supplies the dorsal distal index and long fingers and the radial half of the ring finger distally. The radial nerve (*dark shading*) provides sensory information for the radial dorsal aspect of the hand. Knowledge of these territories is useful when assessing nerve function.

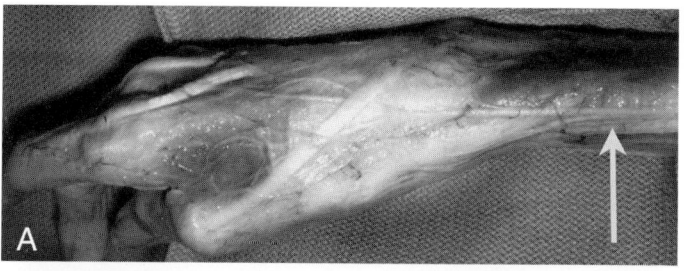

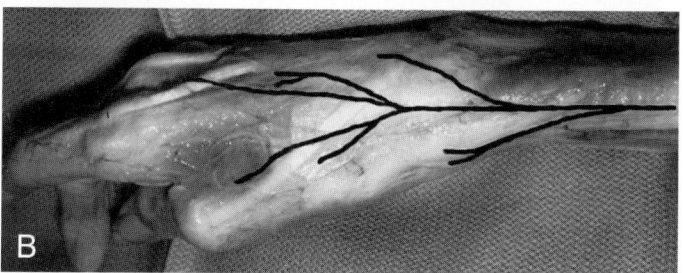

FIGURE 23. A, Cadaver dissection showing the distal trunk of the radial nerve proximal to the wrist (*arrow*). At this level, the radial nerve divides into multiple branches to provide cutaneous sensation to the radial dorsal aspect of the hand. See Figure 22 to correlate these branches with the cutaneous distribution of radial innervation. **B,** The larger radial nerve branches are outlined to more clearly demonstrate their location.

densely adherent to the distal radius and ulna, preventing bowstringing of the tendons during extension (Figures 24, 25).

The tendons are isolated into six separate compartments underneath the retinaculum. The anatomic snuff box is bordered by the first and third compartment tendons (Figure 26).

The first extensor compartment lies most radially and contains the abductor pollicis longus and the extensor pollicis brevis (EPB). The abductor pollicis longus inserts at the base of the first metacarpal and functions to radially deviate the thumb, and the EPB inserts at the base of the proximal phalanx of the thumb and functions to extend the proximal thumb (Figure 27). The third extensor compartment contains the extensor pollicis longus tendon,

TABLE 1. Dorsal Forearm and Hand: Radial Nerve

Extensor Compartment	Muscle	Action
First	Abductor pollicis longus*	Extend and abduct thumb (metacarpal)
	Extensor pollicis brevis*	Extend thumb (proximal phalanx)
Second	Extensor carpi radialis brevis	Extend wrist
	Extensor carpi radialis longus	Extend and radially deviate wrist
Third	Extensor pollicis longus*	Extend thumb (distal phalanx)
Fourth	Extensor digitorum communis*	Extend MCPs
	Extensor indicis proprius*	Extend MCP (index finger)
Fifth	Extensor digiti quinti*	Extend MCP (small finger)
Sixth	Extensor carpi ulnaris*	Extend wrist and deviate ulnarly

*Innervation: posterior interosseous nerve (the major motor branch of the radial nerve)
MCP = metacarpophalangeal

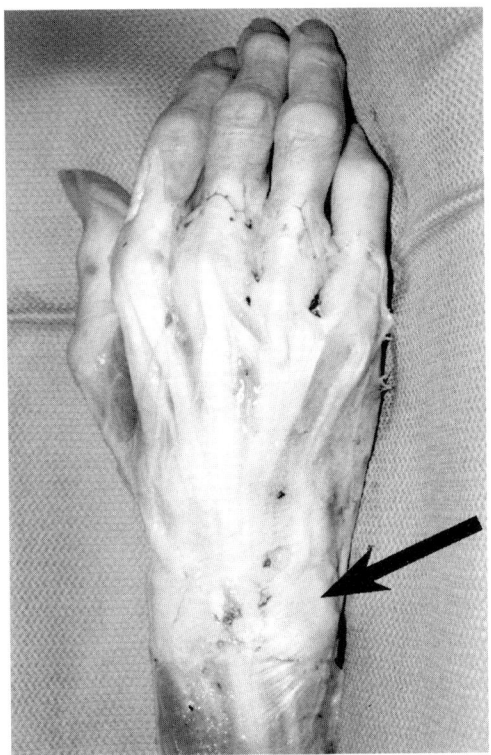

FIGURE 24. The extensor retinaculum (*arrow*) is a thick, fibrous structure that functions as a pulley to maintain the extensor tendons in position at the wrist and prevent bowstringing.

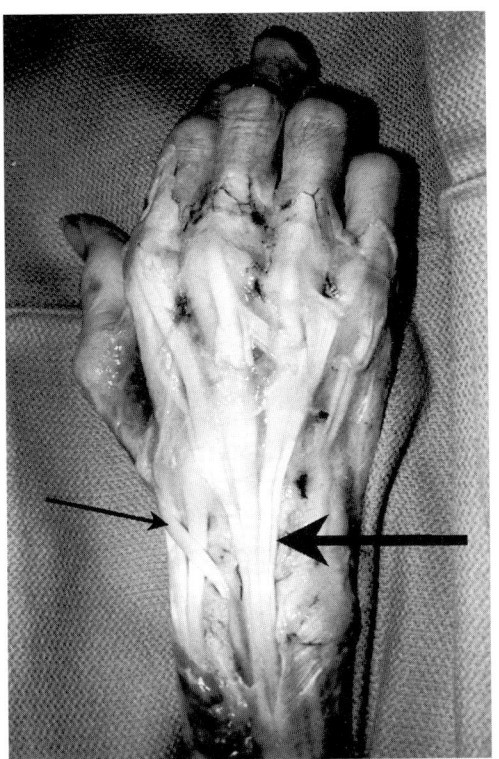

FIGURE 25. Same specimen as in Figure 24 after removal of the extensor retinaculum demonstrates the in-situ position of the extensor tendons at the wrist. Also visible are the position of the extensor pollicis longus (*small arrow*) and the contents of the fourth extensor compartment—the EDC and EIP (*large arrow*).

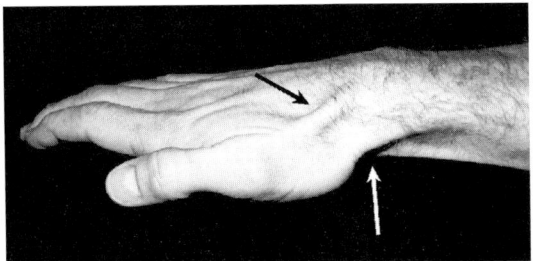

FIGURE 26. The anatomic snuff box, found at the radial border of the hand, is formed volarly by the tendons of the abductor pollicis longus and EPB (*white arrow*). The dorsal aspect of the snuff box is defined by the tendon of the extensor pollicis longus (*black arrow*) (see Figures 25 and 28). The primary wrist extensor tendons—ECRL and ECRB—as well as the radial artery and usually one or two branches of the superficial radial nerve (see Figure 23) lie within the snuff box.

which inserts at the base of the distal phalanx of the thumb and functions to strongly extend it (Figure 28).

Between the first and third extensor compartments (at the level of the wrist) are the extensor carpi radialis longus (ECRL) and the extensor carpi radialis brevis (ECRB). These are the primary wrist extensors, and they lie within the second extensor compartment. They insert at the base of the second and third metacarpals (Figure 29).

The fourth extensor compartment contains the extensor digitorum communis (EDC) and the extensor indicis proprius (EIP). The EDC functions to extend the fingers, particularly at the MCP joints (Figure 30). The EIP has the

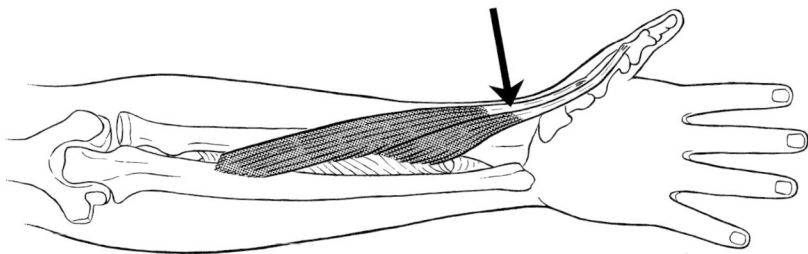

FIGURE 27. The first extensor compartment contains the abductor pollicis longus (*arrow*) and the extensor pollicis brevis. These tendons form the radial border of the anatomic snuff box, which is easily palpable with active thumb extension (see Figure 26).

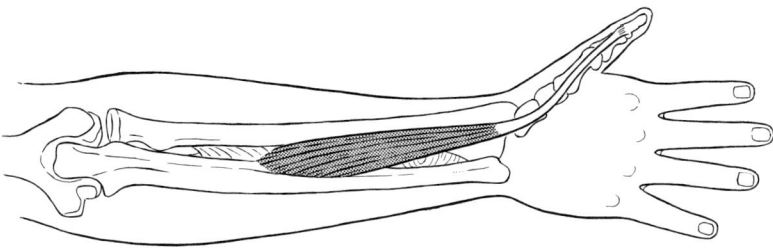

FIGURE 28. The dorsal (top) aspect of the anatomic snuff box is formed by the extensor pollicis longus tendon which lies within the third extensor compartment.

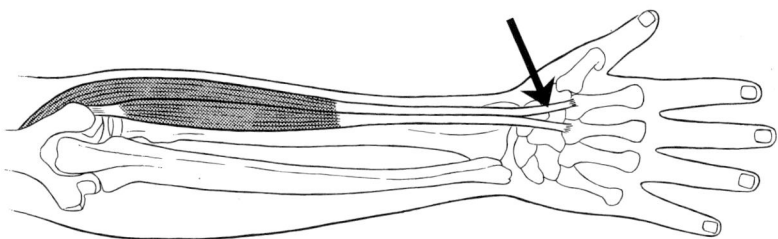

FIGURE 29. The ECRL (*arrow*) and the ECRB are the primary wrist extensors. The ECRL attaches at the base of the second metacarpal, and the ECRB attaches at the base of the third metacarpal. These tendons occupy the second extensor compartment at the base of the anatomic snuff box.

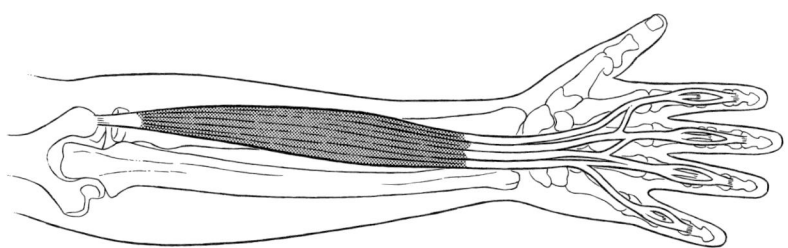

FIGURE 30. The EDC (*shaded area*) functions to extend the fingers, particularly at the MCP joints (see Figure 25).

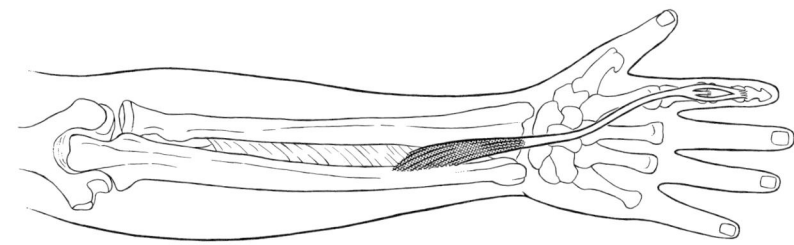

FIGURE 31. The extensor indicis proprius (EIP; *shaded area*) lies within the fourth extensor compartment with the EDC. The two tendons have the same function, but the EIP affects only the index finger and allows more independent extension of that digit. At the level of the MCP joint, the EIP tendon usually lies ulnar to the EDC tendon.

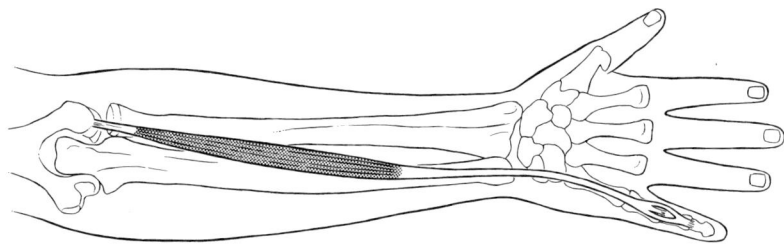

FIGURE 32. The extensor digiti quinti tendon (*shaded area*) lies within the fifth extensor compartment and is analogous to the EIP in that it extends only the MCP of the small finger.

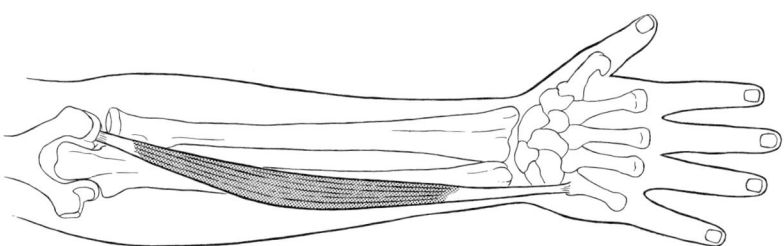

FIGURE 33. The extensor carpi ulnaris lies within the sixth and most ulnar extensor compartment. It functions to extend and ulnarly deviate the wrist.

same function as the EDC, but extends only the index finger (Figure 31). The index finger, therefore, has two tendons for extension.

The fifth extensor compartment contains the extensor digiti quinti, which is analogous to the EIP in that it extends only the MCP of the small finger (Figure 32). The extensor carpi ulnaris lies within the sixth extensor compartment. It attaches to the base of the fifth metacarpal and functions to extend and ulnarly deviate the wrist (Figure 33).

All of the muscles within the extensor compartments are innervated by the posterior interosseous nerve, which is the terminal motor branch of the radial nerve. The exception to this are the ECRL and the ECRB, which are innervated by the radial nerve prior to the takeoff of the posterior interosseous nerve.

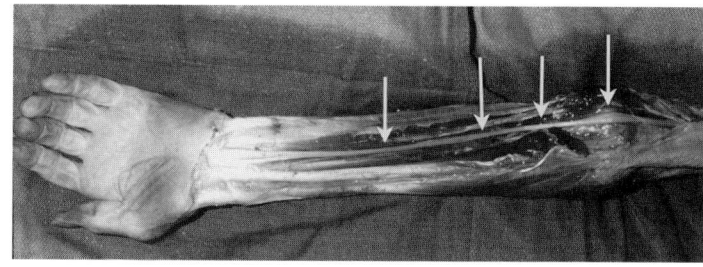

FIGURE 34. Cadaver dissection of the deep tissues of the forearm, demonstrating the location of the median nerve from the antecubital fossa (*most proximal arrow*) to the wrist, where it enters the carpal tunnel (see Figure 21).

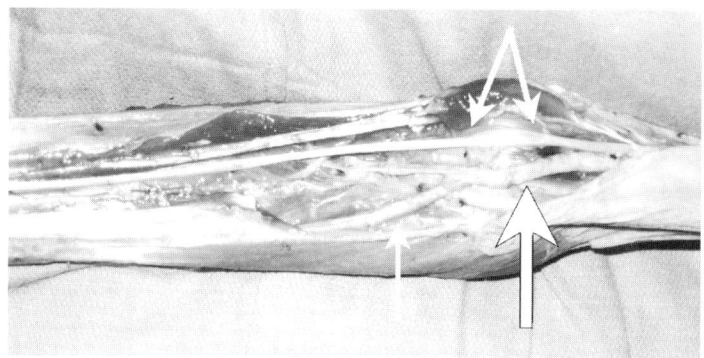

FIGURE 35. The relationship of the median nerve (*double arrow*) at the antecubital fossa to the brachial artery (*large arrow*). Immediately distal to the elbow, the brachial artery bifurcates into the radial (*small arrow*) and ulnar arteries.

Median Nerve

The median nerve travels along the volar-central aspect of the forearm (Figures 34, 35). Its function can be summarized as providing pronation, flexion of the wrist and fingers, and thumb opposition (Table 2). This generalization is not as "pure" as that for the radial nerve, because the ulnar nerve also supplies some flexion function, as we shall see in the following section. Nevertheless, as a generalization this is a useful way to summarize the function of this nerve.

The median nerve innervates the pronator teres, which originates above the elbow at the humerus and also inserts at the proximal ulna. Since the pronator teres crosses the elbow joint, it serves two functions: flexing the elbow and pronating the forearm (Figure 36).

The flexor carpi radialis inserts at the base of the second metacarpal and functions to flex the wrist, as well as deviate it radially. The palmaris longus is present in approximately 80% of the population and is a weak flexor of the wrist. The

TABLE 2. Volar Forearm and Hand: Median Nerve

Muscle	Action
Pronator teres	Pronate forearm, flex elbow
Flexor digitorum super-ficialis	Flex proximal interphalangeal joint
Flexor carpi radialis	Flex wrist, radially deviate
Palmaris longus	Weakly flex wrist
Flexor pollicis longus*	Flex thumb interphalangeal joint
Pronator quadratus*	Pronation
Flexor digitorum profundus (index, long fingers)*	Flex distal interphalangeal (index and long fingers)
Abductor pollicis brevis,[†] opponens pollicis, and[†] flexor pollicis brevis[†]	Thumb abduction and pronation: opposition
Lumbricals (index, long fingers)	Coordinate movement of fingers; extend interphalangeal joints, flex metacarpophalangeal joints

* Anterior interosseous branch
[†] Thumb intrinsic muscles—thenar mass

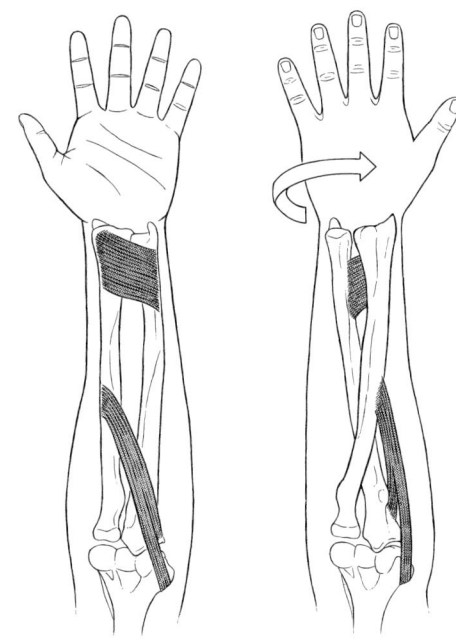

FIGURE 36. Function of the pronator teres and pronator quadratus. *Left,* the pronator quadratus and pronator teres are both completely relaxed. *Right,* with contraction, the radius is pronated, drawing the thumb toward the body (direction of arrow). The pronator teres' function as an elbow flexor (not shown) can be exploited to differentiate between the actions of the pronator quadratus and the pronator teres: by flexing the elbow completely and then asking the patient to pronate, all pronation is accomplished by the pronator quadratus alone, because the pronator teres is placed at a mechanical disadvantage with full elbow flexion.

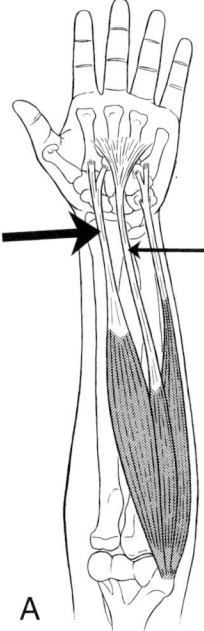

A

FIGURE 37. **A,** The major flexors of the wrist—the flexor carpi radialis (*large arrow*) and the palmaris longus (*small arrow*)—are both innervated by the median nerve. The palmaris longus is absent in approximately 20% of the population. **B,** Demonstration of the relative positions of the flexor carpi radialis and the palmaris longus in a normal subject.

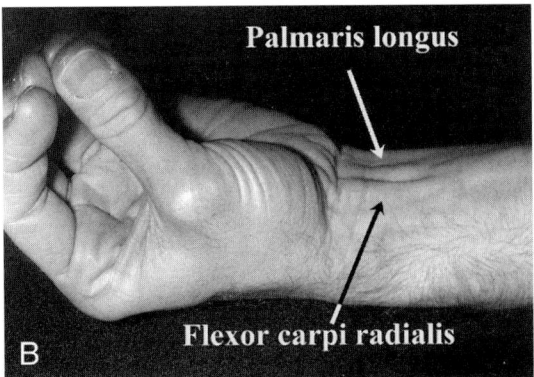

Palmaris longus

Flexor carpi radialis

B

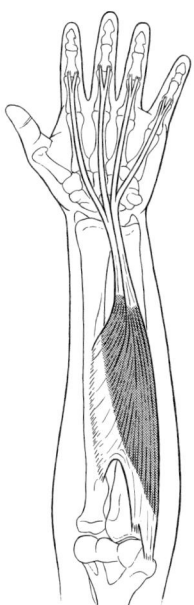

FIGURE 38. The FDS travels through the carpal tunnel and inserts at the base of each middle phalanx, functioning to flex the PIP joint of each finger.

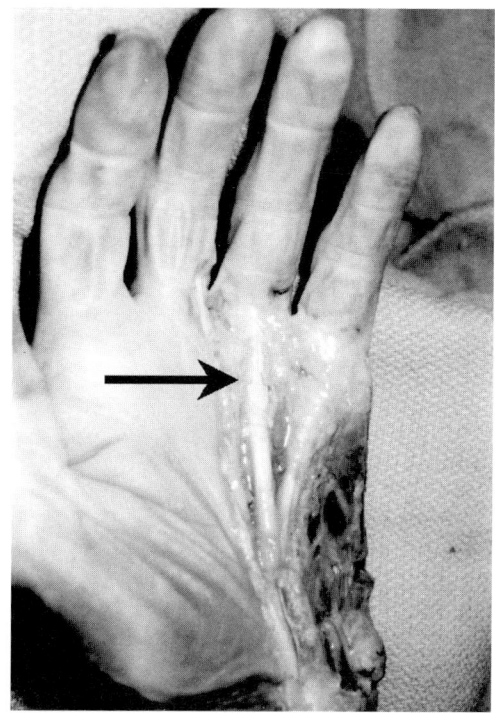

FIGURE 39. Cadaver dissection demonstrating the location of the flexor tendons within the palm of the ulnar two digits. At this level, the FDS is superficial to the profundus tendon; therefore, the FDS is visible. Note the divided A-1 pulley (*arrow*), preserved in the fifth finger for comparison. This pulley is a fibrous structure that marks the beginning of the fibro-osseous tunnel, previously referred to as "no man's land" because of poor tendon healing and a predilection for adhesion formation after tendon repair in this zone. Patients who present with "trigger finger" usually have a localized nodule in the FDS, which becomes entrapped or blocked by the A-1 pulley. The pulley can be divided easily in an outpatient procedure to restore full flexion and extension without triggering.

flexor carpi radialis lies radial to the palmaris longus at the volar wrist (Figure 37).

The flexor digitorum superficialis (FDS) inserts at the bases of the middle phalanges of the four fingers and flexes the PIP joints (Figure 38). Within the palm, the FDS of each finger travels volar (or "superficial," from the palmar aspect) to the flexor digitorum profundus (FDP) of that finger. At the base of each finger, the FDS tendon splits into two slips, which then insert at the base of the middle phalanx. This splitting allows the underlying FDP tendon to travel between the slips to reach the distal phalanx (Figures 39–42).

The anterior interosseous nerve is a separate motor branch of the median nerve that provides innervation to three muscles: the flexor pollicis longus, the pronator quadratus, and the FDP to the index and long fingers. The FDP tendons insert at the bases of the distal phalanges and flex the DIP joints; the flexor pollicis longus inserts at the base of the distal phalanx of the thumb and flexes the interphalangeal joint of the thumb (Figure 43). The pronator quadratus, a broad,

flat muscle that lies between the radius and ulna (volar to the interosseous membrane), functions to pronate the forearm (see Figure 36).

Like the FDS, the FDP and flexor pollicis longus enter the hand through the carpal tunnel, traveling with the median nerve. The carpal tunnel is an anatomic structure that is formed on three sides by the bones of the carpus, with the volar "roof" formed by dense fibers of the transverse carpal ligament. Swelling of the contents of the carpal tunnel or chronic irritation of the

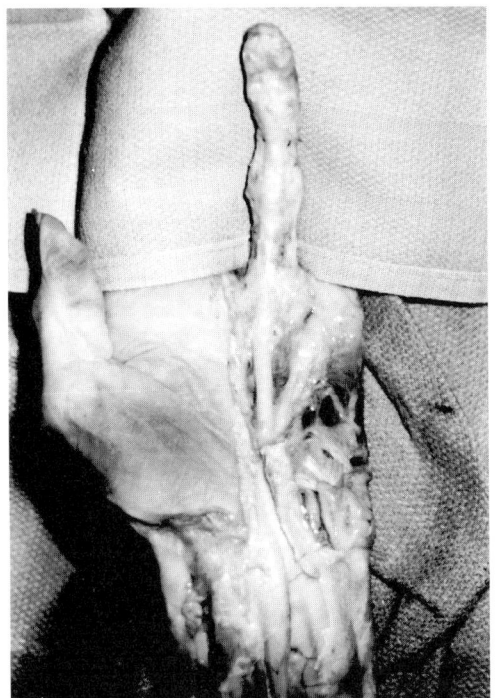

FIGURE 40. Further dissection in which the volar and dorsal skin has been removed from the ring finger. The retaining pulleys and fibro-osseous tunnel of the flexor tendons have been left intact.

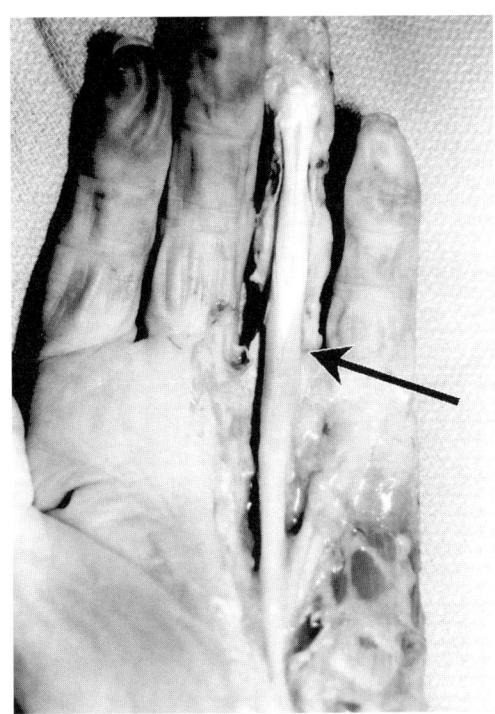

FIGURE 41. The FDS and FDP in-situ, after removal of the pulleys and synovial tissue of the fibro-osseous tunnel. Note the level (*arrow*) at which the FDS splits into two slips, allowing the FDP to pass through. These slips wrap around the FDP and attach to the base of the middle phalanx. Proximal to the split, only the FDS is visible; however, distal to the split, the FDP tendon is visible as well.

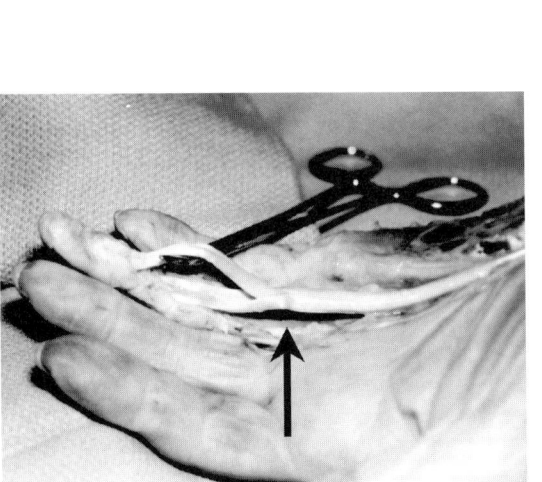

FIGURE 42. Lateral view of the FDS tendon splitting (*arrow*) and curving around the FDP to attach to the middle phalanx. The hemostat clamp is elevating the FDP tendon as it travels to insert at the base of the distal phalanx.

median nerve at this level can lead to "carpal tunnel syndrome"—a compression neuropathy of the median nerve.

The terminal motor branch of the median nerve emerges in the palm and innervates the muscles of the thenar eminence: the abductor pollicis brevis, the opponens pollicis, and the flexor pollicis brevis (Figure 44). These muscles together are responsible for thumb opposition (see Figure 4).

Ulnar Nerve

The ulnar nerve primarily provides motor innervation to the "intrinsic" muscles of the hand (Table 3). These muscles work as a group to coordinate the function of the fingers, allowing

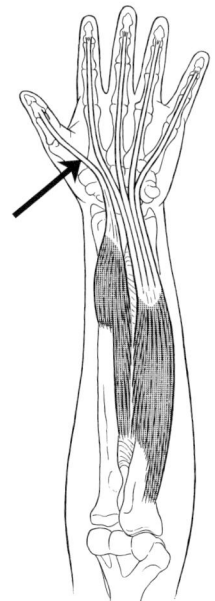

FIGURE 43. The FDP tendons—the only flexors of the DIP joints—insert at the bases of the distal phalanges and function to flex the fingers. The flexor pollicis longus (*arrow*) is analogous to the FDP, in that it flexes the distal phalanx of the thumb.

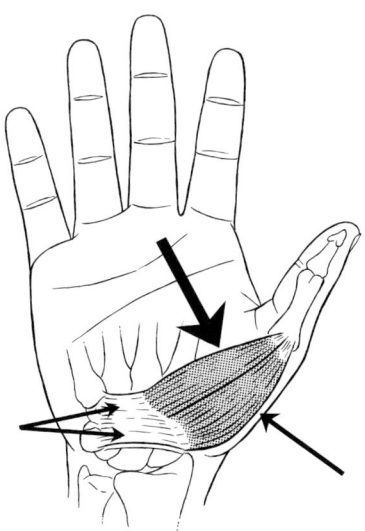

FIGURE 44. The muscles of the thenar eminence are responsible for thumb opposition. The opponens pollicis muscle (not shown) lies deep to the flexor pollicis brevis (*large arrow*) and the abductor pollicis brevis (*small arrow*). These muscles originate from the thick, fibrous tissue of the transverse carpal ligament—the roof of the carpal tunnel (*double arrows*).

TABLE 3.   Volar Forearm and Hand: Ulnar Nerve

Muscle	Action
Flexor carpi ulnaris	Flex wrist, ulnarly deviate
Flexor digitorum profundus (ring and 5th)	Flex distal interphalangeal joint (ring and 5th)
Abductor digiti quinti*†	(analogous to dorsal interosseous)
Flexor digiti quinti*†	(analogous to dorsal interosseous)
Opponens digiti quinti*†	Flexes and supinates 5th metacarpal
Volar interossei*	Adduct fingers, weak flexion metacarpophalangeal
Dorsal interossei*	Abduct fingers, weak flexion metacarpophalangeal
Lumbricals (ring and 5th)*	Coordinate movement of fingers; extend interphalangeal joints, flex metacarpophalangeal joints
Adductor pollicis*	Adduct thumb toward index finger
Lumbricals (ring, small)*	Coordinate movement of fingers; extend interphalangeal joints, flex metacarpophalangeal joints

* Hand intrinsic muscles
† Hypothenar mass

delicate and fine movement and precise positioning. Acute loss of ulnar nerve innervation may produce a more subtle loss of finger function than similar damage to either the median or radial nerves. However, this injury ultimately produces a devastating loss of hand function.

The ulnar nerve travels along the volar-ulnar aspect of the forearm, from the cubital tunnel at the elbow (just posterior to the medial epicondyle) to Guyon's canal at the wrist (Figures 45–47; also see Figure 21). It innervates the flexor carpi ulnaris, which inserts on the pisiform, and functions to flex and ulnarly deviate the wrist (Figure 48). The only other muscle innervated in the forearm by the ulnar nerve is the FDP to the ring and small fingers, which flexes the distal interphalangeal joints of these digits (see Figures 41–43).

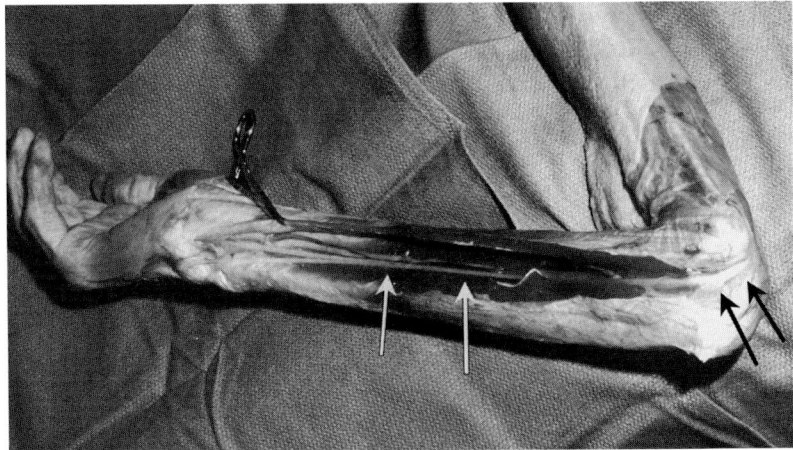

FIGURE 45. In this cadaver dissection the ulnar nerve is demonstrated within the cubital tunnel (*black arrows*). It lies immediately posterior to the medial epicondyle, and at this location it is relatively vulnerable to painful trauma ("funny bone"). The ulnar nerve then travels along the ulnar border of the forearm (*white arrows*).

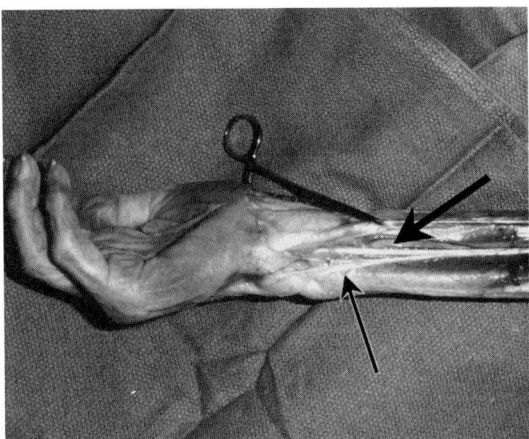

FIGURE 46. The main trunk of the ulnar nerve (*large arrow*) enters Guyon's canal at the level of the wrist. The dorsal sensory branches of the ulnar nerve (*small arrow*) travel distally to provide sensation to the dorsal ulnar aspect of the hand (see Figure 22). The clamp is retracting the flexor carpi ulnaris radially, allowing visualization of the ulnar nerve at this location.

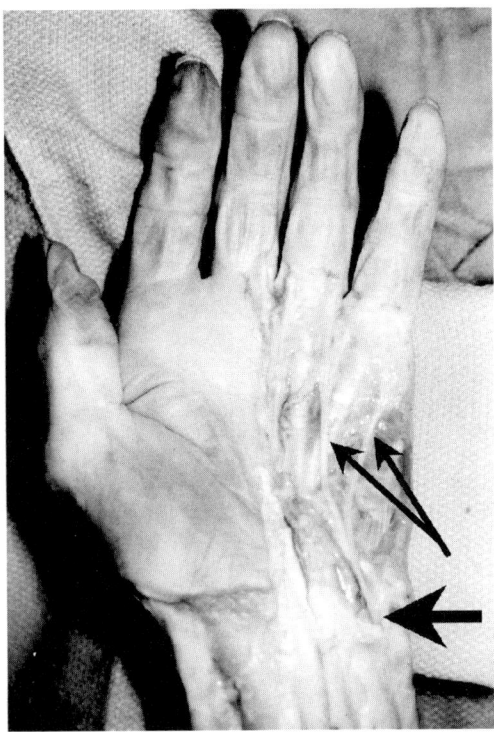

FIGURE 47. The ulnar nerve (*single arrow*) courses from the carpus through the mid-palm. It divides into sensory branches to the fifth finger and the ulnar aspect of the ring finger (*double arrows*). Note the flexor tendons' position deep to the nerves. The motor branches of the ulnar nerve (not shown) supply the intrinsic muscles of the hand.

The median nerve provides all of the finger flexion at the PIP joints (via the FDS) as well as flexion at the DIP of the index and long fingers. The ulnar nerve innervates the FDP to the ring and the fifth fingers. By innervating the flexor carpi ulnaris and the ulnar FDP, the ulnar nerve overlaps the median nerve flexion function on the ulnar side of the hand. *These two overlap areas represent the only ulnar nerve–innervated muscles proximal to the hand.*

The intrinsic muscles of the hand include the interosseous muscles, the lumbricals, the hypothenar group (abductor digiti quinti, flexor digiti quinti, and opponens digiti quinti), and the median nerve–innervated thenar muscles (abductor pollicis brevis, opponens pollicis, flexor pollicis brevis). The **interosseous muscles** are divided into two types: dorsal and volar. As their name implies, they are located between the metacarpals and function to adduct (volar

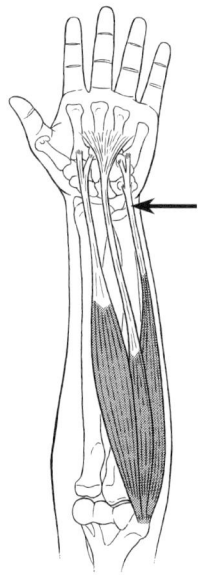

FIGURE 48. The flexor carpi ulnaris (*arrow*) functions to flex the wrist and ulnarly deviate it.

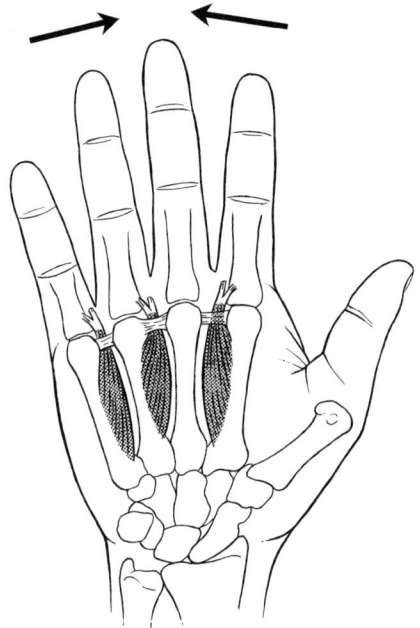

FIGURE 49. The volar interossei function to adduct (*direction of arrows*) the fingers. There are no volar interossei attached to the long finger because it is the axis.

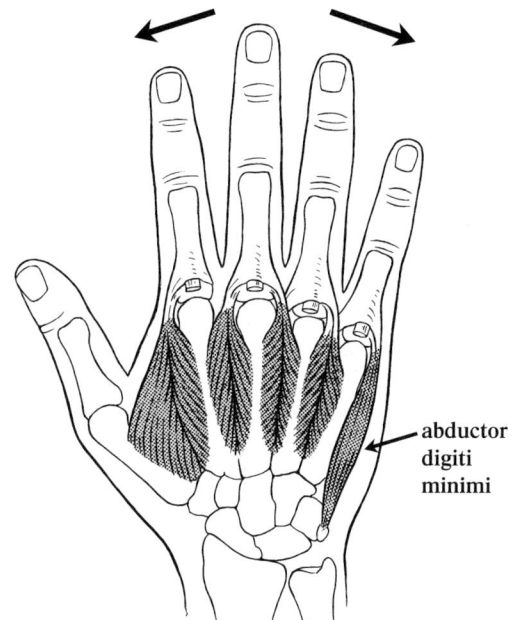

abductor digiti minimi

FIGURE 50. The dorsal interossei function to abduct (*direction of arrows*) the fingers away from the axis of the hand (the long finger ray). Therefore, the long finger has two dorsal interossei. The ring finger and the index finger each have one to draw them away from the axis. The adductor digiti minimi muscle abducts the fifth finger.

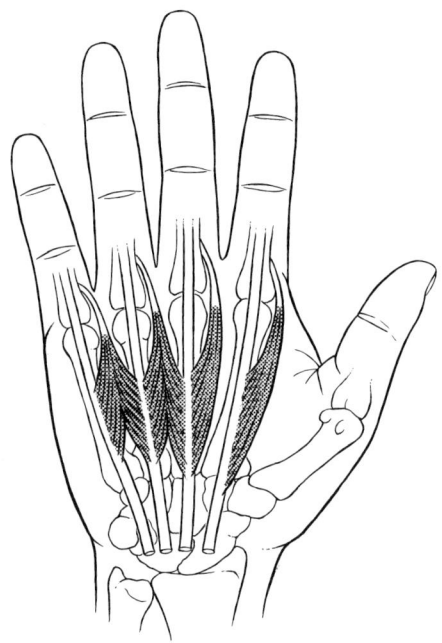

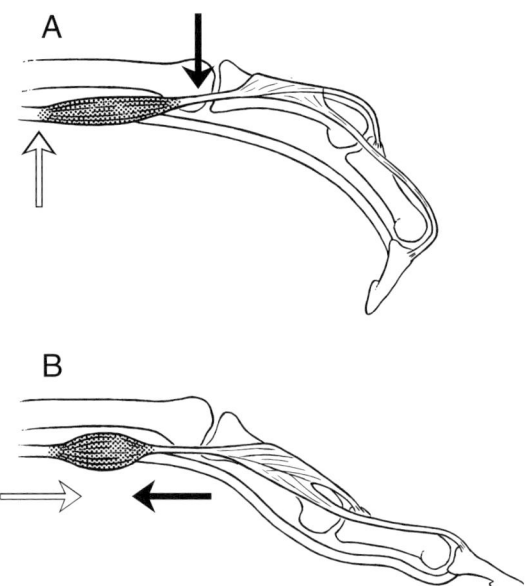

FIGURE 51. The lumbrical muscles (*shaded*) originate from the FDP tendons and insert on the extensor mechanisms of the fingers (see Figures 52 and 54–56).

FIGURE 52. Lumbrical muscle function. **A,** The lumbrical muscle at rest, originating from the FDP tendon (*white arrow*) and inserting on the lateral band of the extensor mechanism (*black arrow*). **B,** During finger extension the lumbrical muscle contracts, which pulls the FDP tendon distally (*white arrow*) while simultaneously extending the finger via the extensor mechanism (*black arrow*). By relaxing the FDP tendon via lumbrical muscle contraction, the finger can extend without having to overcome antagonistic pull from the FDP.

interosseous; Figure 49) or abduct (dorsal interossei; Figure 50) the digits. In addition, the interossei weakly flex the MCP joints. Remember that adduction of the fingers draws them toward the long finger. Therefore, there are only three volar interossei muscles: one each at the index, ring, and small fingers. There are four dorsal interossei, which serve to pull the fingers away from the long finger: two on the long finger (movement in either the radial or ulnar direction would be abduction), one for the index finger, and one for the ring. The fifth finger is abducted by a muscle analogous to the interossei (the abductor digiti quinti), but since it is not *between* bones, it would be a misnomer to label it as an interosseous muscle.

The **lumbricals** have no bony insertion: they originate on the FDP tendon in the palm and insert on the extensor tendon of the finger. When contracted, the lumbricals extend the finger (at the interphalangeal joints) and simultaneously pull the FDP tendon distally—relaxing it and

thus allowing the finger to extend more easily (Figures 51, 52).

The abductor digiti quinti and flexor digiti quinti function as interosseous muscles, except that since they lie on the ulnar border of the hand, they are not between bones. Nevertheless, they serve the same function of finger abduction and weak flexion of the proximal phalanx. The opponens digiti quinti functions to flex and mildly rotate the fifth metacarpal into the palm.

The final muscle innervated by the ulnar nerve is the adductor pollicis, an important muscle which adducts the thumb into the hand and provides "key pinch" (Figure 53).

The interosseous and lumbrical muscles combine with the extrinsic extensor tendons to form the **extensor mechanism** for the fingers.

The anatomy of the extensor mechanism is complex and intricate (Figures 54–56). To generalize, it is important to recognize that the intrinsic muscles function to extend the PIP and DIP joints of the digits and flex the metacarpophalangeal joints (Figure 57). The "extrinsic extensors" (extensor digitorum communis, extensor indicis proprius, extensor digiti quinti) function to extend the metacarpophalangeal joints and also contribute fibers that assist with PIP and DIP extension.

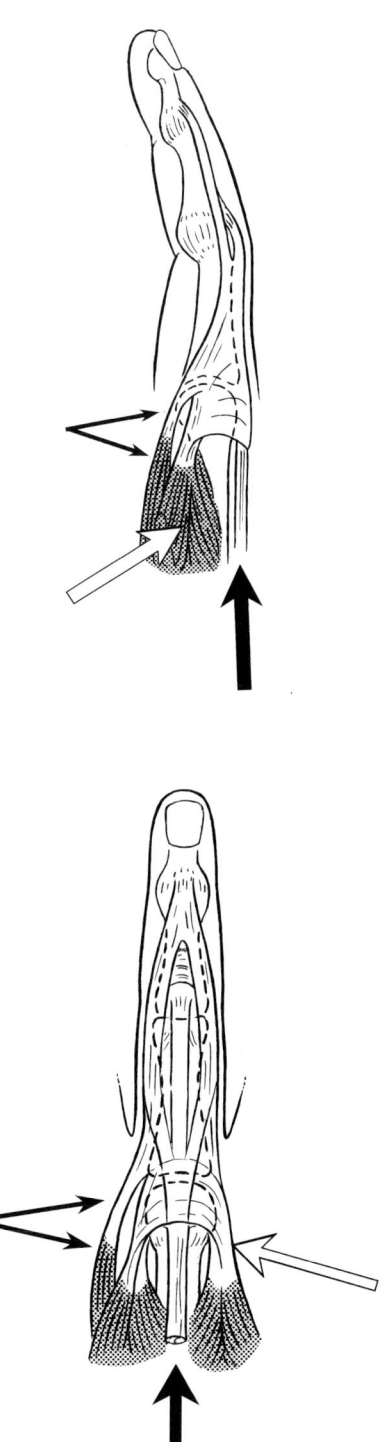

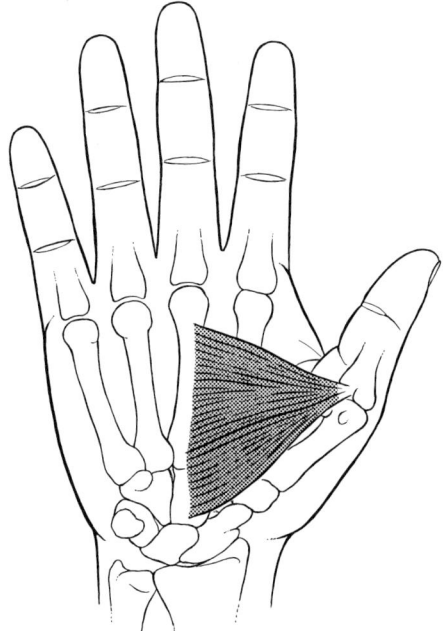

FIGURE 53. The adductor pollicis (*shaded*) inserts at the base of the proximal phalanx of the thumb and functions to strongly adduct the thumb into the palm.

FIGURE 54. The extensor mechanism of the finger receives contributions from the volar and dorsal interossei (*white arrows*), the lumbrical muscles (*double arrows*), and the long extensors (EDC, EIP, extensor digiti quinti; *black arrows*). These fibers coalesce to form a strong, fibrous sheet that functions to extend the finger. The interossei and lumbrical muscles form the lateral band of the extensor mechanism, and the extrinsic extensor forms the central tendon.

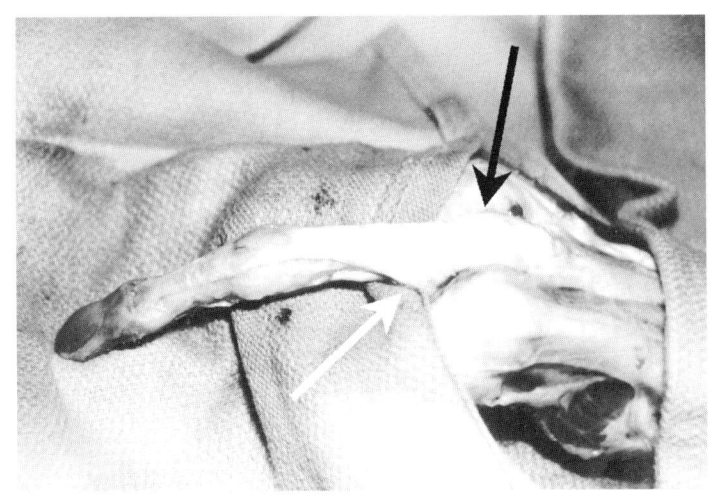

FIGURE 55. In this cadaver dissection of the extensor mechanism of the finger, note the contributions of the extrinsic extensors (EDC; *black arrow*) and the intrinsic contribution (lumbrical and interosseous muscles; *white arrow*). The extensor mechanism of the finger grossly appears to be a thin sheet of fibers, and delineation of specific structures is difficult.

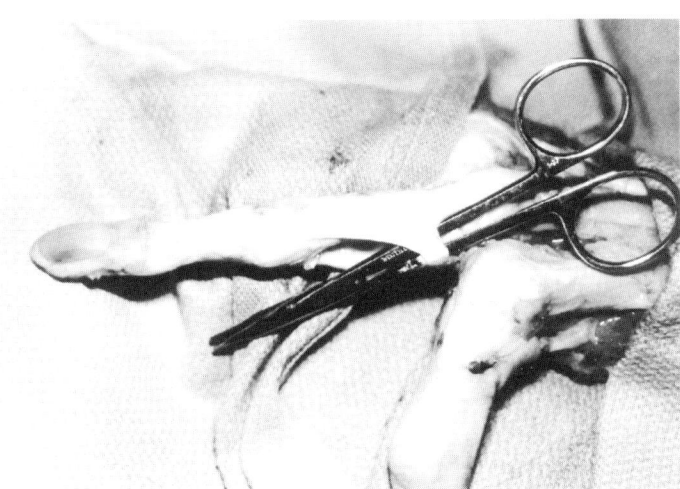

FIGURE 56. Here, the lateral band (the contribution from the intrinsic musculature) has been dissected free and is held out by the hemostat. Note that the tension applied to the lateral band functions to extend both the DIP and PIP joints (compare to Figure 55). The interosseous muscles weakly flex the MCP joints; assist in extending the interphalangeal joints by contributing to the lateral band of the extensor mechanism; and adduct or abduct the fingers.

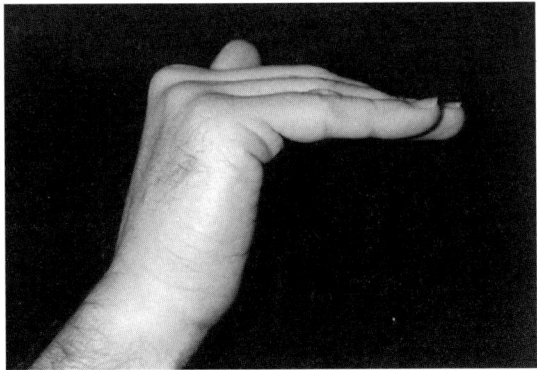

FIGURE 57. Position of maximum function of the intrinsic muscles of the hand: MCP flexion and PIP and DIP extension.

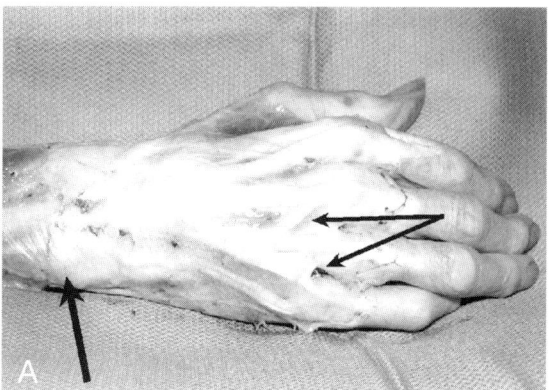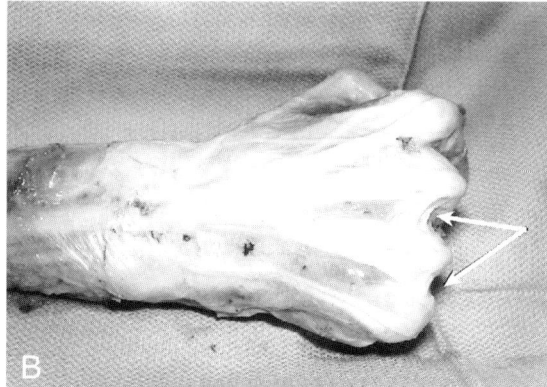

FIGURE 58. **A,** The juncturae tendinum (*double arrows*) are fibrous interconnections between the extensor tendons at the distal dorsal hand. They maintain coordinated extension at the MCP joints and can assist in extension of an adjacent finger if the primary extensor tendon has been cut. The *single arrow* points to the extensor retinaculum. **B,** With full fist flexion, the juncturae migrate distally to assist in stabilization of the MCP joints. The juncturae typically are palpable in the normal individual on full fist flexion.

Juncturae Tendinum

The juncturae tendinum are located between the extensor tendons at the distal aspect of the hand (Figure 58). They are relatively constant in location and function to connect the extensor tendons of the digits. The juncturae tendinum make individual finger extension difficult, as extension of one finger tends to pull the adjacent fingers into extension. Perhaps the earliest elective hand surgery was division of the juncturae in a musician to allow greater independent extension of the fingers.

Of importance to the clinician is that a complete transection of an extensor tendon might not be obvious if the juncturae from adjacent fingers are providing extension to the injured digit during examination.

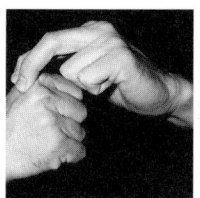

2 Examination of the Hand

History

The patient's medical history is a critical component in the evaluation of a hand problem or injury. It is important to note the patient's age and gender, as well as the presence of other medical problems. In addition, the physician should inquire specifically about issues that are germane to hand problems: is the patient a diabetic, a smoker, arthritic? Have there been previous injuries or problems with the hand? Hand dominance (is the patient right-handed or left-handed?) also is important to document. When evaluating patients in your office (i.e., non-trauma cases), attempt to define exacerbating and relieving factors of the pain or complaints. When evaluating injuries, ask the patient to describe exactly how the injury occurred, characterize the pain or problem, and determine how long it has been troubling. This type of information can clarify the etiology of the problem and furnish clues as to possible solutions.

Knowledge of the patient's occupation and hobbies can give a sense of how the hands are used. For example, a construction worker uses his or her hands in a different way than a touch typist and has different needs that must be considered when evaluating complaints of injury or chronic problems, particularly with regard to subsequent solutions. Information about extracurricular activities that are an important part of the patient's life (such as playing musical in-

struments) can give insight into the impact of the injury and the most appropriate treatment options.

Physical Examination

It is important to develop a consistent examination process that is thorough and complete for use on *every* patient examined. In the emergency department, it is easy for the clinician to be distracted by a large, gaping, and profusely bleeding laceration over the thumb and miss the fracture of the ring finger that also is present. By maintaining a consistent examination and going over the entire hand in a *systematic and organized* fashion, the examiner is much less likely to miss an injury or associated problem at the time of presentation.

VISUAL INSPECTION

Spend a moment looking at the patient's hand. Notice if the skin is calloused or soft, indicating whether the hands are used in manual labor or not. In a trauma situation, examine the wounds. Are they "sharp" (such as with simple lacerations), or are they stellate, "crush-type" injuries, which imply much deeper and more widespread tissue damage. Evaluate the color of

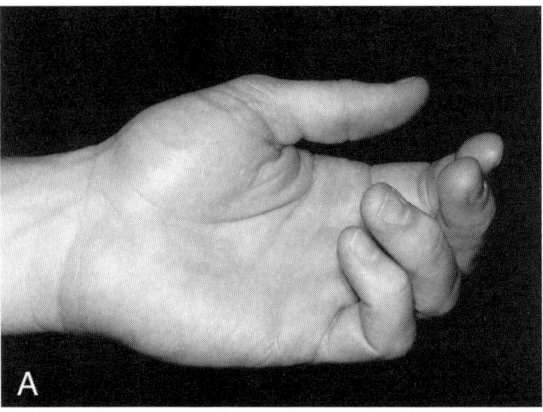 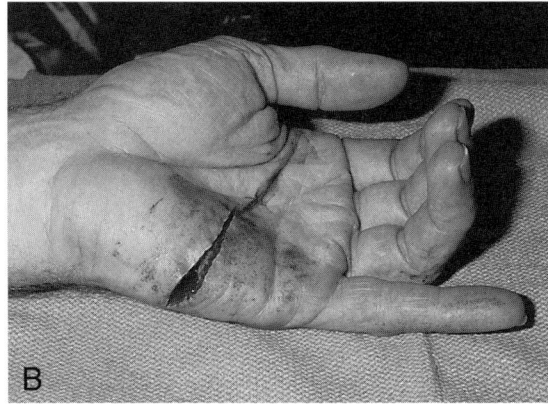

FIGURE 1. **A,** The normal cascade of fingers at rest. Notice that the fingers form a gentle cascade, with the index finger slightly flexed and a gradual increase in flexion of the ulnar digits. **B,** Abnormal finger cascade in hand at rest, with no resting flexion of the fifth finger. This individual suffered a laceration on the ulnar border of the hand that completely transected the flexor digitorum superficialis and flexor digitorum profundus of the fifth finger.

the hand to gather clues about vascular status, force of injury, and potential occult damage to the underlying tissue. For example, a very pale digit may be ischemic, while a dark purple color and congestion may indicate venous obstruction. Diffuse ecchymosis may provide evidence of a severe crush injury.

Examine the resting finger and hand position: at rest, the fingers fall into a normal "cascade" (Figure 1A). Division of the flexor tendons results in an abnormal posture at rest

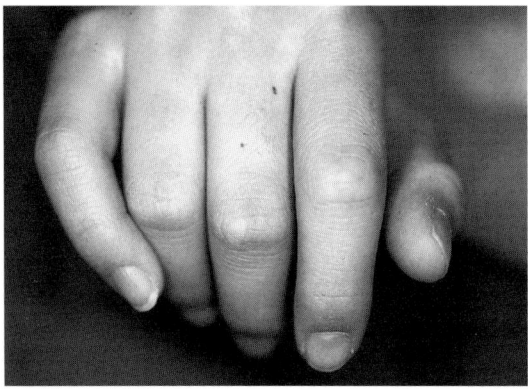

FIGURE 2. Angular deviation of the fifth digit. This patient suffered a fracture of the proximal phalanx of the fifth finger which resulted in a rotational deformity of the finger.

(Figure 1B). The loss of a normal cascade can be an important clue to underlying tendon injury. However, it is important to remember that a patient can have a transected flexor digitorum superficialis with an intact flexor digitorum profundus and maintain a normal cascade, due to the inherent tone of the intact profundus tendon. Fractures of the phalanges may result in finger rotation or produce an angular deviation (Figure 2). Any rotational or angular deformities of the fingers is strongly suspicious for underlying bony injury.

Examine the musculature of the hand, particularly at the first web space (Figure 3A) and the thenar eminence. Is there evidence of muscle atrophy? The elderly have a certain degree of muscle atrophy as a natural result of aging, but atrophy also can be evidence of an underlying neural problem such as longstanding nerve compression (i.e., carpal tunnel syndrome or cubital tunnel syndrome). In carpal tunnel syndrome, which affects the median nerve, late symptoms might include wasting of the muscles of the thenar eminence (which are innervated by the median nerve). Injuries or entrapment of the ulnar nerve can result in atrophy of the hand intrinsic muscles, which usually is most visible at the dorsal first web space (Figure 3B).

Look at the hand and forearm as a whole.

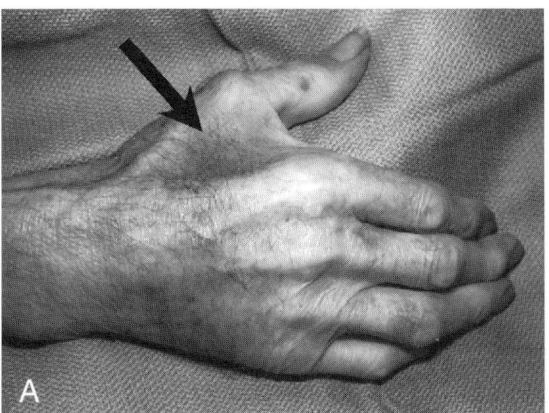
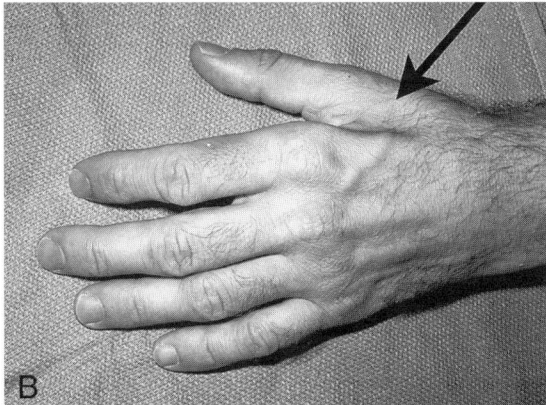

FIGURE 3. **A,** Muscle atrophy of the first dorsal web space (*arrow*) can be evidence of nerve injury, such as results from longstanding nerve compression. Muscle atrophy is relatively common within the elderly population; therefore, it is important to compare both hands to note any asymmetry. In this patient, the atrophy was due to aging and not to an underlying neural injury. **B,** Wasting of the first web space (due to wasting of the first dorsal interosseous muscle) in a patient with longstanding ulnar nerve damage resulting from cubital tunnel syndrome.

Gently move the fingers, wrist, and forearm through their normal ranges of motion. Do these movements cause pain? Check for any areas of focal tenderness over the bony structures, which can be indications of underlying bony injury.

Have a low threshold for obtaining radiographs if there is any question of bony injury. When inspecting radiographs, be sure to apply a systematic and methodical approach to each film, taking time to check the entire hand to avoid missing an occult bony injury. One approach is to "start at the top," checking the phalanges, then the metacarpals, and so on. What exactly should you look for when evaluating radiographs? Check the "edges" of the bone, making sure the cortical surfaces are smooth (Figures 4–7). Any sharp defects are indicative of fracture. Confirm that the joint spaces appear roughly equal in size. Note that while it is important to completely examine the entire film to avoid missing an occult injury, it is equally important to focus on the areas where the patient complains of tenderness.

If you are uncomfortable reading hand films, are unsure about a specific area in particular, and don't have a radiologist to confirm your diagnosis, a handy trick is to obtain radiographs of the patient's contralateral hand (assuming it is uninjured) for comparison. This method is of particular value when evaluating children's hands (Figure 8), because children's epiphyseal plates have not closed and their bony ossification is variable. In fact, it is a good idea to obtain contralateral views in *all* children under the age of 12. Most radiology departments charge significantly less for comparison views.

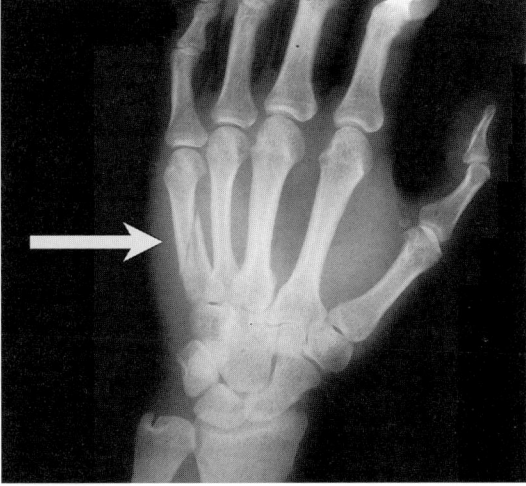

FIGURE 4. Spiral fracture of the fifth metacarpal. The obliquely oriented fracture is clearly visible at the midshaft of the fifth metacarpal (*arrow*).

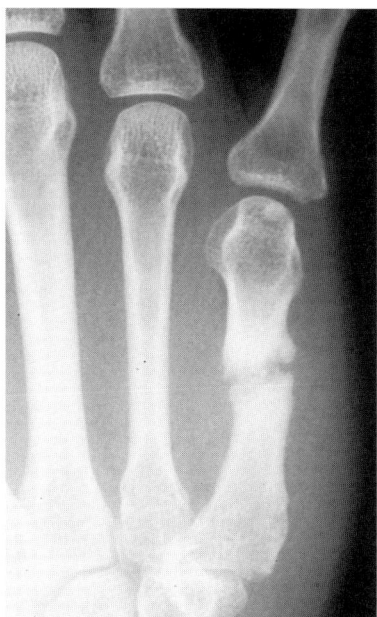

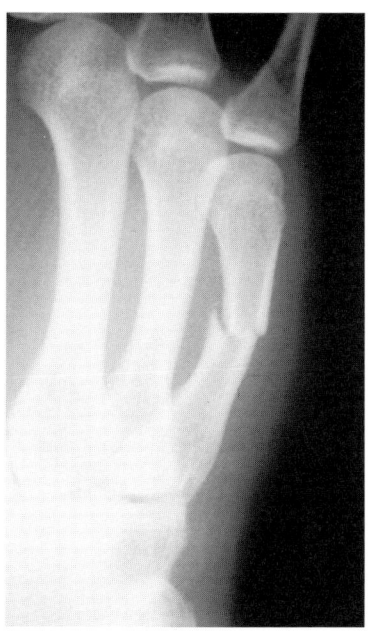

FIGURE 5. Chronic nonunion of fifth metacarpal. This patient hurt the hand about 6 weeks earlier, but did not seek medical attention. Note the "fuzzy" edges to the bone ends (compared to the acute fracture in Figure 6), which are indicative of partial and incomplete healing and are evidence of the nonacute nature of the problem.

FIGURE 6. Transverse fracture of the fifth metacarpal. Note the irregularity of the cortical bone at the area of the fracture, indicative of bony disruption.

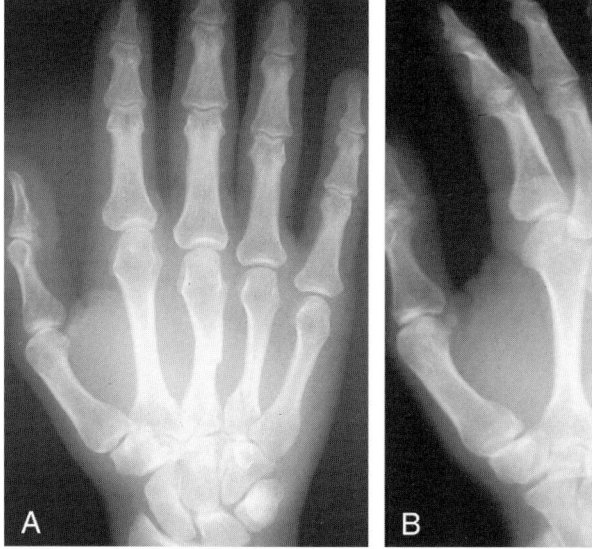

FIGURE 7. Transverse fracture of the third metacarpal. **A,** The cortical defect and stepoff of the third metacarpal are not immediately apparent on the anteroposterior view. **B,** In contrast, the bony defect with stepoff and displacement is obvious on the oblique view. This example emphasizes the importance of obtaining multiple views when evaluating hand injuries. A fracture can be invisible on one view, but obvious from a different perspective. Note that the joint spaces between the carpal bones are approximately equal in size—a normal finding.

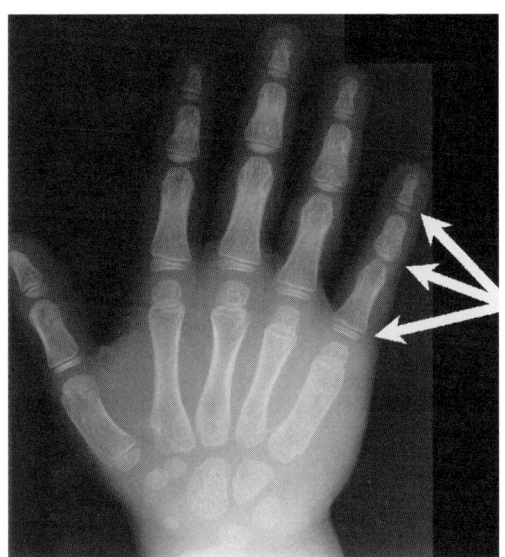

FIGURE 8. Radiograph of a 6-year-old demonstrating open growth plates of the phalanges (*arrows*) and metacarpals, as well as incomplete ossification of the carpal bones. Because it sometimes is difficult to discern a fracture from an open growth plate, it often is advisable to obtain radiographs of the contralateral (uninjured) hand for comparison.

A special mention is in order for **scaphoid fractures.** The scaphoid is the most commonly fractured carpal bone (Figure 9). A common etiology is falling forward on an outstretched hand. If a scaphoid fracture is unrecognized or untreated, it can progress to chronic nonunion, which can lead to chronic wrist pain and disabling degenerative arthritis of the wrist. Recognition of these risks is critical because, quite commonly, scaphoid fractures cannot be radiographically detected in the acute setting—not even by the most talented radiologist. The presumptive diagnosis (in this setting) is made based on a high degree of suspicion, which in turn is founded on the history combined with the symptom of tenderness within the anatomic snuff box.

If the examiner feels that there is a possibility of a scaphoid fracture, treatment consists of placement in a thumb spica splint, with referral to a hand specialist for follow up 1 week later. At the follow-up visit, the radiographs can be repeated (tomograms are helpful, as well) and the snuff

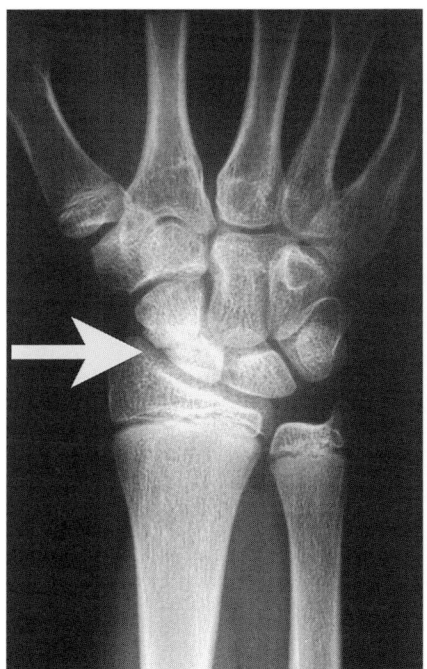 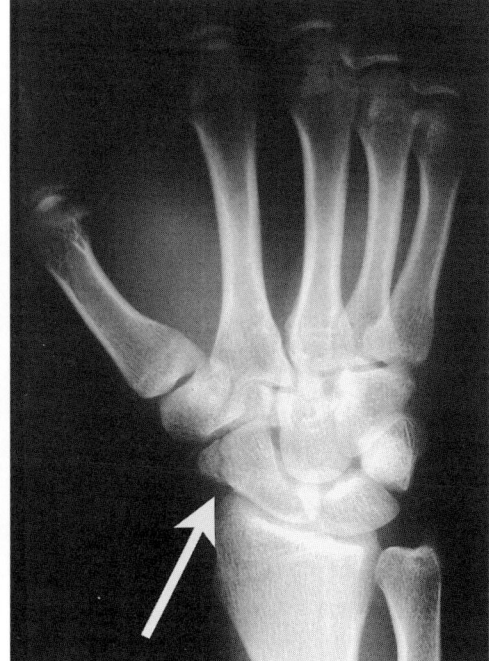

FIGURE 9. Scaphoid fractures (*arrows*).

box re-examined to definitively make the diagnosis. If a fracture is present, it is usually evident on radiograph within 1–2 weeks after injury. Due to the potentially devastating consequences of an untreated scaphoid fracture, in these cases it is better to err on the side of caution, and splint the hand if there is any doubt. Not all acute scaphoid fractures are invisible on radiograph, and not all scaphoid fractures progress to nonunion, wrist arthritis, and collapse. However, it is best to be cautious to avoid these potential complications.

VASCULAR EXAMINATION

There are many ways to assess the vascular status of the hand or digit. In addition to observance of skin color, the radial and ulnar arteries often can be palpated at the volar wrist. A Doppler probe can be used to analyze the blood flow not only in these arteries, but also as far distally as the volar pulp at the distal phalanx. A standard, pencil-type Doppler probe can detect the vascular signal when placed at the volar pulp of a healthy finger (Figure 10).

If after visual inspection and Doppler exam there still is some question as to the vascular status, pinprick of the affected part with a 22-gauge needle may be helpful. Both the color and the quality of the blood expressed can help determine if a vascular problem exists. A completely ischemic part will not bleed at all, whereas one with venous congestion will bleed

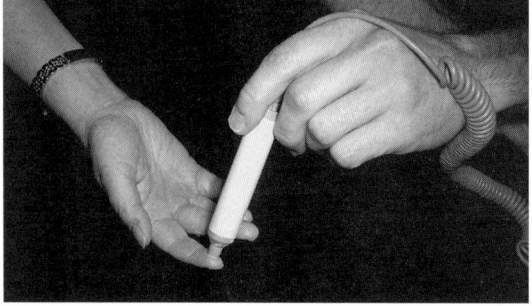

FIGURE 10. Examination of the vascular adequacy of the finger using a pencil-type Doppler probe. When placed on a distal volar fingertip pad, the arterial signal should be easily audible. Individual digital arteries can be selectively evaluated using this probe.

quite briskly with very dark (almost black) blood. Normal perfusion is indicated by moderately brisk bleeding of bright red blood.

A proximal vascular injury can be particularly challenging to diagnose, because the collateral circulation in the hand may obviate any distal ischemia. For example, consider a traumatic laceration involving the ulnar artery in the forearm. With adequate collateral flow in the hand (an "intact arch"), it could easily demonstrate no ischemic effects. Indeed, Doppler exam of the ulnar artery at the volar wrist (distal to the transection) could detect a good arterial signal (via distal anastomosis from the radial artery). To exclude or diagnose this type of injury, each artery should be "doppled" while the examiner occludes the other artery at the wrist with firm pressure, eliminating back flow and preventing a false negative exam.

Allen's test is used to confirm the adequacy of perfusion to the hand by either the radial or ulnar artery alone. It always should be performed prior to any planned manipulation of these vessels (such as radial artery line placement) to avoid the potentially devastating consequences of distal ischemia if the artery becomes injured or thrombosed. To perform this test, the examiner occludes both the radial and ulnar arteries at the volar wrist, and the patient is asked to tightly squeeze and open the fist several times (Figure 11A and B). The blood is forced out of the hand, and the palmar skin appears pale. The patient then holds the fingers extended, and the examiner removes the pressure from *either* the radial *or* ulnar artery while maintaining pressure on the other (Figure 11C). The palm is closely observed: a rapid blush of reperfusion in the distal palmar skin and all the digits confirms good crossover perfusion. The test is then repeated, releasing the contralateral artery after squeezing the blood from the hand, to confirm the findings. If the thumb and index finger do not show a good blush of reperfusion after release of the ulnar artery (while still occluding the radial artery), it is likely that inadequate crossover perfusion from the ulnar side of the hand exists, and any cannulation or manipulation of the radial artery should be avoided to prevent possible ischemic loss.

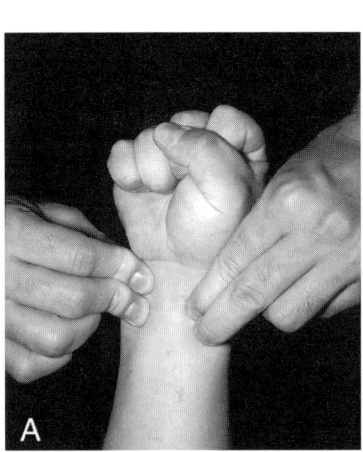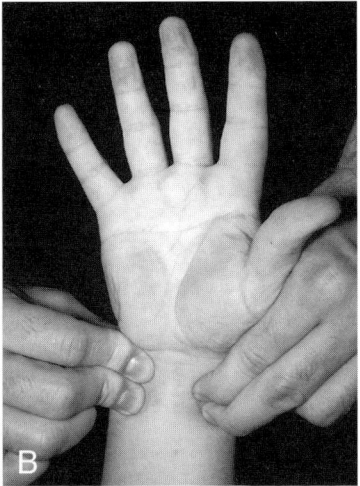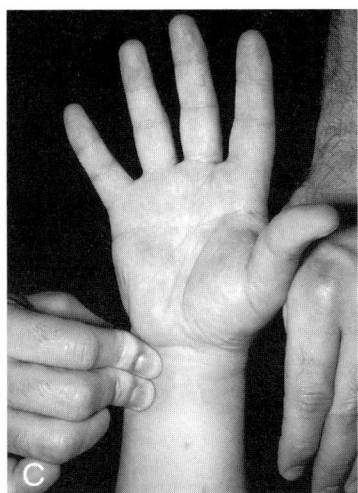

FIGURE 11. Allen's test assesses the collateral circulation in the hand. **A,** The examiner applies direct pressure over the radial and ulnar arteries at the wrist. Then the patient tightly squeezes and opens the fist several times to force the blood out. **B,** While pressure over the radial and ulnar arteries is maintained, the patient holds the fingers in extension. The palmar skin is visibly pale. **C,** The radial artery is released while occlusion is maintained over the ulnar artery. In this example, particular attention is paid to the ulnar aspect of the hand to insure that good perfusion occurs from the radial artery.

NERVE EXAMINATION

The major nerves to the hand provide sensory information as well as transmit motor impulses; therefore, nerve function can be analyzed with both sensory and motor tests. This dual function can be exploited to help distinguish a tendon injury from a nerve injury when a patient is unable to perform a particular action, such as thumb extension. Testing for sensation is relatively straightforward. While the borders between regions covered by the nerves are not precisely consistent from individual to individual, certain areas are purely innervated by only the ulnar nerve, median nerve, or radial nerve. The volar small finger is the best place to assess ulnar nerve sensation; the volar index finger is the best place to test for median nerve sensation; the dorsal first web space is the best place to assess for radial sensory innervation (Figure 12).

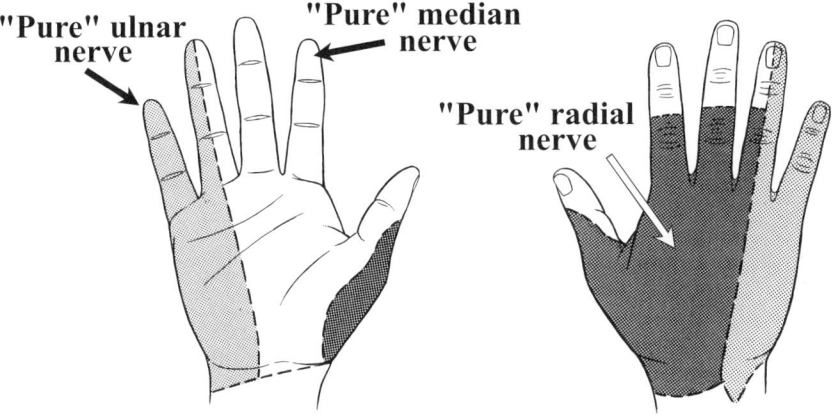

FIGURE 12. "Pure" areas of innervation. Borders may differ slightly among individuals.

Sensory Tests

The ability of the digital nerves to provide sensation to the fingers must be assessed in patients who have sustained lacerations or other injury to the hand or fingers. The best way to evaluate this function is to test moving two-point discrimination. A calipers is the ideal tool, starting with the points approximately 5–6 millimeters apart. The points of the calipers are *lightly* brushed across the radial or ulnar aspect of the finger being examined (testing either the radial or ulnar digital nerve). The examiner alternates between brushing one and both points of the calipers across the side of the fingertip (Figure 13). The patient (with eyes closed) is asked to discern whether one or two points is felt moving across the finger. The ability to distinguish one versus two points at 5–6 millimeters apart is considered normal in most people. If the patient cannot distinguish one from two, the distance between the caliper points is increased until he or she can make the determination. Failure of the two-point discrimination test when the calipers are greater than 10 millimeters apart is considered abnormal and raises suspicion of nerve injury. Individuals with a complete nerve transection have a dense anesthesia on that aspect of their digit.

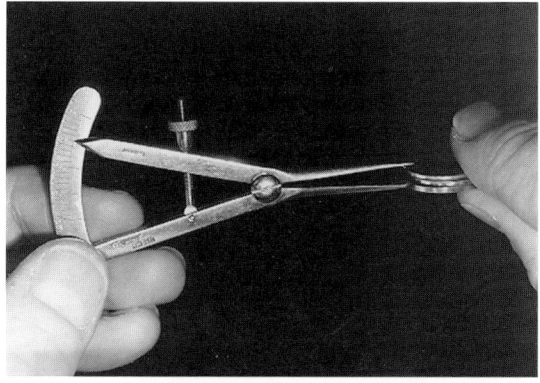

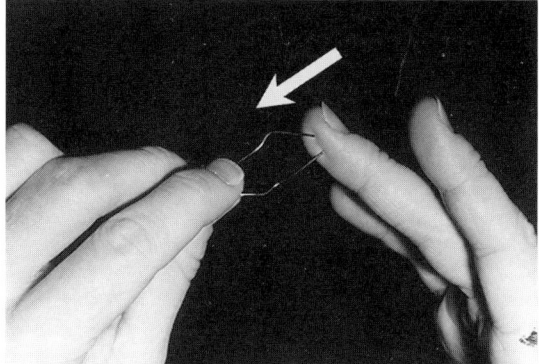

FIGURE 14. When calipers are not available for measuring two-point discrimination, a paper clip and a ruler can be used in the same fashion. For convenience, three stacked pennies are exactly 5 millimeters thick, and this distance is a good starting point in assessing digital nerve function.

There are many other methods of assessing sensation in the digits, including static two-point discrimination, monofilament testing, and light touch. The moving two-point method is preferable because it is easy to perform and to reproduce.

If a calipers is not available in the emergency department, an easily constructed alternative can be assembled by unfolding a paper clip and placing the two tips exactly three pennies apart (Figure 14), which is exactly 5 millimeters apart. If the patient cannot discern one versus two points, the tips of the paper clip can be adjusted further apart and the test repeated. Once the smallest distance that the patient can distinguish as two points is established, the distance between the tips of the paper clip can be measured with a standard pocket ruler.

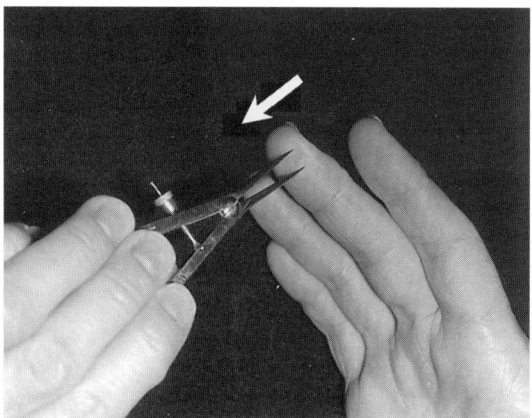

FIGURE 13. Evaluating digital nerve function by testing moving two-point discrimination. Calipers are lightly brushed on either the ulnar or radial aspect of the digit, alternating between one and two points. Normally, the two distinct points of the caliper tips can be distinguished at 5–6 millimeters apart.

Motor Tests

When examining a patient, remember that there are three possible reasons why a motion (such as finger flexion) is not executed:

1. The tendon or muscle is cut
   or
2. The nerve to that muscle is cut or damaged
   or
3. The patient doesn't want to move the part, either due to pain or secondary gain.

The art of medicine is in trying to distinguish which of these is the case. It may be helpful to refer to Tables 1–3 in Chapter 1 to review the actions of the muscles and the groups of muscles innervated by the radial, median, and ulnar nerves.

Sometimes (particularly in the acute injury setting) the patient may be in too much pain to perform the movement that you request. If this is the case, try this: place the patient's finger or hand in the position of maximal function of the muscle you are testing, and ask that it be held in that position. If the patient is able to do this, then the tested musculotendinous unit and its nerve are intact. For example, when testing the flexor pollicis longus, completely flex the thumb interphalangeal joint for the patient. Then ask the patient to simply maintain that position after you release the thumb. This usually is less painful for the acutely injured patient to execute than moving the finger actively (Figure 15).

Proximal Injuries

When evaluating proximal injuries (for example, a stab wound to the forearm), assessment of nerve injury or transection can be accomplished by testing the distal sensation in a "pure" area (see Figure 12). In addition, the knowledge of specific motor functions provided by each nerve can help verify that the major nerve is intact.

Ulnar Nerve. Examination of the interosseous muscles is one way to evaluate ulnar

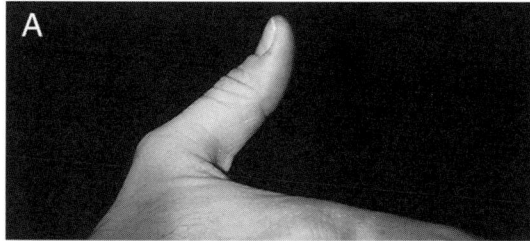
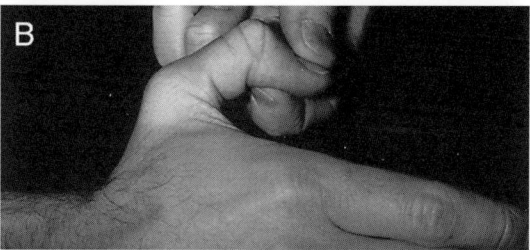
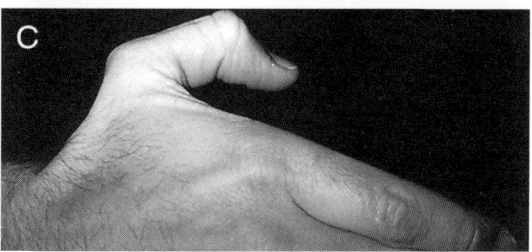

FIGURE 15. Testing often is confounded by the patient's pain as a result of their injuries. **A,** If a patient is unable to move a certain motor unit—for example, to flex the interphalangeal (IP) joint of the thumb as a test of the flexor pollicis longus—it may be unclear to the examiner whether the reason is tendon or nerve injury, or pain. **B,** A useful trick is to place the finger or hand in the position of maximum function. Here, the examiner flexes the thumb IP joint for the patient. **C,** The patient is instructed merely to hold the finger in that position. In most circumstances, this is less painful than actively moving the finger, and the ability to hold the digit in the position of maximum function gives evidence that the musculotendinous unit and its innervation are intact.

nerve motor function. The patient points the index finger straight out and resists ulnar deviation to test the first dorsal interosseous muscle (Figure 16A). In addition, the ability to abduct and adduct the fingers and to cross the fingers indicates that the ulnar nerve is intact (Figure 16B).

Median Nerve. The distal motor branches of the median nerve innervate the thenar emi-

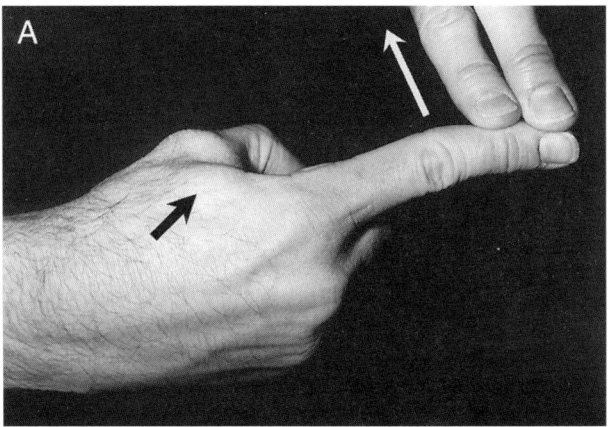

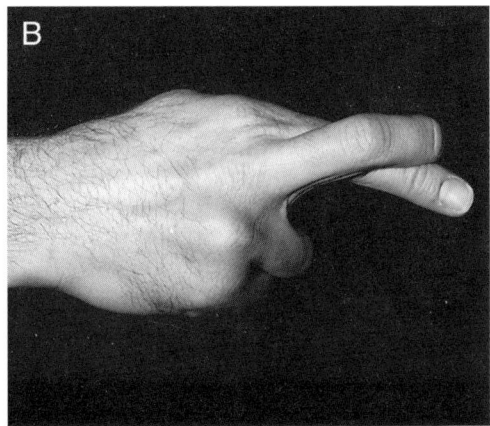

FIGURE 16. **A,** Test of the first dorsal interosseous muscle to assess adequacy of ulnar nerve. The patient is instructed to point the finger straight ahead and, by exerting upward force (*white arrow*), resist downward pressure by the examiner. The first dorsal interosseous muscle (*black arrow*) can be palpated as it contracts. Compare to Figure 3B, which demonstrates first dorsal interosseous atrophy due to ulnar nerve injury. **B,** Quick test of ulnar nerve function: crossing the fingers. This motion uses both the volar and dorsal interossei, and the ability to perform this maneuver confirms proximal ulnar nerve function.

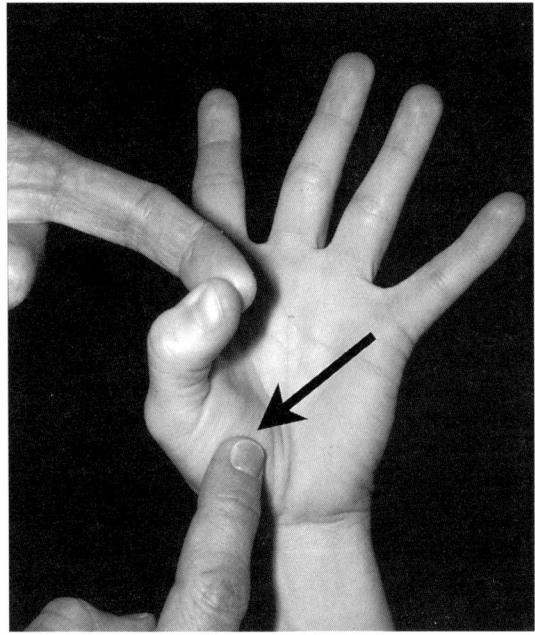

FIGURE 17. The muscles of the thenar eminence produce thumb opposition and are innervated by the median nerve. A quick assessment of median nerve function can be performed by having the patient forcefully oppose the thumb; the examiner can palpate the muscles of the thenar eminence (*arrow*) to confirm good muscular contraction.

nence, which is responsible for thumb opposition. These muscles provide the ability to abduct the thumb forcefully away from the palm and to pronate it towards the fifth finger (Figure 17). While the patient is performing this maneuver, palpate the thenar eminence to confirm contraction of these muscles. The proximal median nerve also can be assessed by testing the flexor pollicis longus (Figure 18A) or the flexor digitorum profundus (Figure 18B).

Radial Nerve. The radial nerve, solely responsible for wrist and metacarpophalangeal (MCP) extension, can be quickly and easily assessed by testing these functions. The inability to extend either the wrist or the MCP joints should raise suspicion of a radial nerve injury. Remember that the intrinsic muscles of the hand (specifically the interosseous and lumbrical muscles) can provide extension of the fingers at the interphalangeal joints and are innervated by the ulnar nerve. A patient could have a complete radial nerve transection and still be able to extend his or her fingers.

Each of these tests of the motor nerves is suggested only as a quick way to assess motor

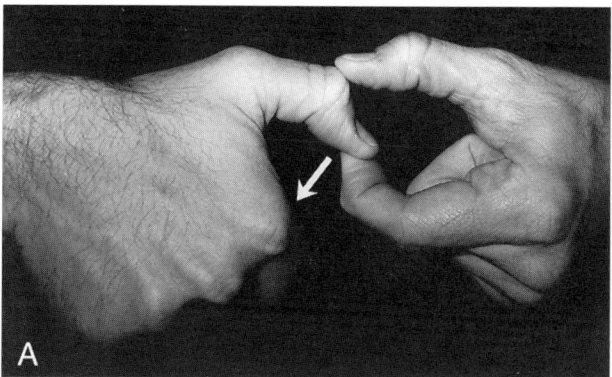
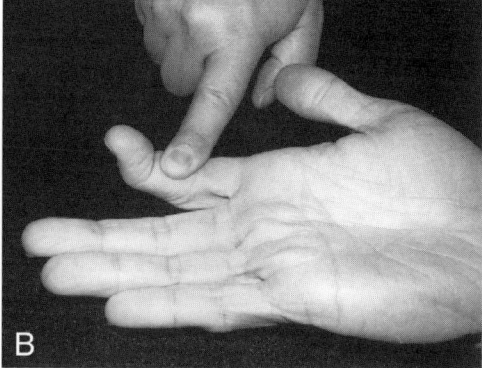

FIGURE 18. **A,** Rapid assessment of proximal median nerve function by testing the flexor pollicis longus. The patient flexes the thumb interphalangeal joint and exerts force (*arrow*) against resistance. **B,** Another test focuses on the flexor digitorum profundus (FDP). The patient flexes the finger while the examiner holds the middle phalanx still. By immobilizing the middle phalanx, flexion from the flexor digitorum superficialis is blocked, and the function of the FDP is isolated.

nerve function in a proximal injury. The physician's ability to assess these specific motor functions is dependent on the individual patient and the type of injury. For example, a patient with a crush injury to the fingers would be completely unwilling and most likely unable to attempt crossing the fingers to assess ulnar nerve function. Examiner flexibility is important: be prepared to test other muscles innervated by the nerve in question (if possible) to assess proximal nerve status.

MUSCULOTENDINOUS UNIT EXAMINATION

Each muscle of the arm and hand can be individually tested, providing insight into the function and integrity of not only the muscle, but also its tendon and innervation. The following section is a discussion of the specific testing maneuvers for each muscle.

Dorsal Forearm and Hand (Radial Nerve)

The extensor carpi radialis longus and brevis function as the primary wrist extensors. They insert at the base of the second and third metacarpals. To test their function, the patient forcefully extends the wrist with fingers slightly flexed while the examiner's hand rests lightly over the index and long metacarpals (Figure 19). Remember that other muscles can act to extend the wrist, such as the extensor carpi ulnaris. However, if the extensor carpi ulnaris is the only muscle participating in wrist extension, the hand ulnarly deviates. During this test, the fingers and thumb are lightly curled to eliminate possible weak participation by the extensor digitorum communis (EDC), extensor indicis proprius, and extensor digiti quinti.

The abductor pollicis longus (APL) forms the volar border of the anatomic snuff box (Figure 20A). The APL tendon can be easily palpated while the patient forcefully abducts the thumb metacarpal (Figure 20B and C). The extensor pollicis brevis (with the APL) forms the inferior border of the anatomic snuff box. This muscle is tested by the patient extending the MCP joint of the thumb (extending the proximal phalanx; Figure 21). Remember that the APL inserts at the base of the metacarpal, while the extensor pollicis brevis inserts on the proximal phalanx of the thumb and serves to extend it. The extensor pollicis longus tendon forms the dorsal aspect of the anatomic snuff

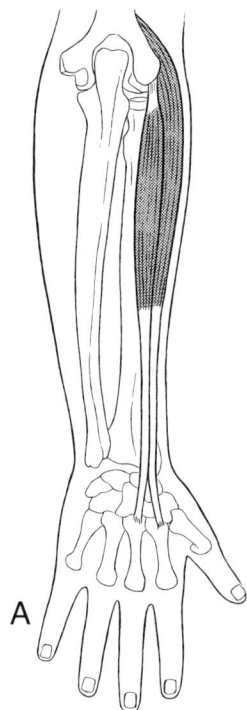

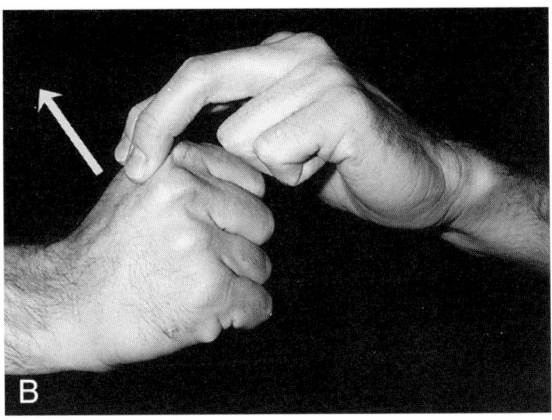

FIGURE 19. **A,** Testing of the extensor carpi radialis longus and brevis. **B,** The patient forcefully extends the wrist against resistance, keeping the fingers and thumb lightly curled to eliminate participation by other muscles.

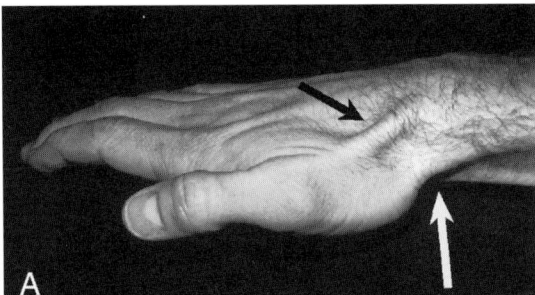

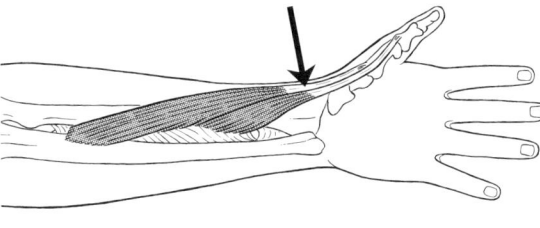

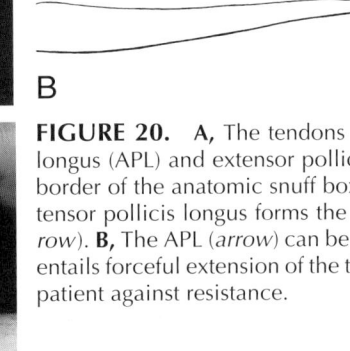

FIGURE 20. **A,** The tendons of the abductor pollicis longus (APL) and extensor pollicis brevis form the volar border of the anatomic snuff box (*white arrow*). The extensor pollicis longus forms the dorsal border (*black arrow*). **B,** The APL (*arrow*) can be easily tested. **C,** The test entails forceful extension of the thumb metacarpal by the patient against resistance.

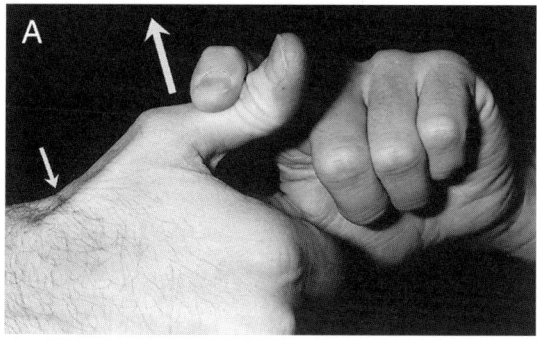

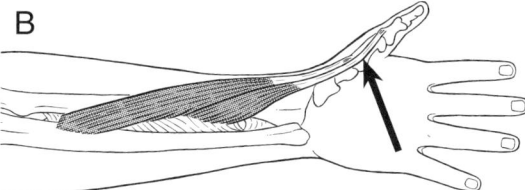

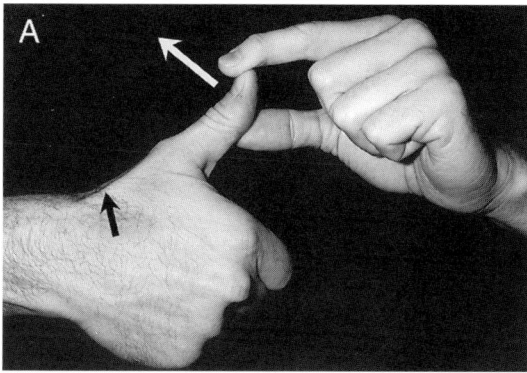

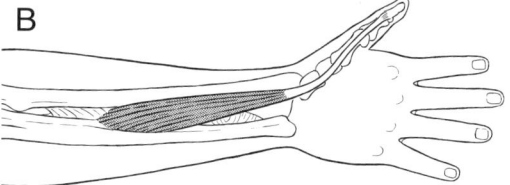

FIGURE 21. **A,** The extensor pollicis brevis is tested by the patient forcefully extending (*large arrow*) the thumb proximal phalanx against resistance. Remember that this tendon (*small arrow*) is located *volar* to the extensor pollicis longus. **B,** Extensor pollicis brevis (*arrow*).

FIGURE 22. **A,** The extensor pollicis longus is tested by the patient extending the interphalangeal joint of the thumb (*black arrow*) against resistance (*white arrow*). **B,** Extensor pollicis longus.

box (see Figure 20A) and is tested by the patient forcefully extending the thumb interphalangeal joint against resistance (Figure 22). The tendon can be palpated during this maneuver.

The extensor digitorum communis (EDC) travels across the dorsal aspect of the hand to all of the fingers. Its function is evaluated by the patient extending the MCP joints against resistance (Figure 23). When evaluating the EDC for possible injury (such as in a dorsal hand laceration), have a high degree of suspicion for **occult EDC transections.** These injuries can be easily missed due to the pull from the adjacent junctura tendinae: even if the EDC to the long finger is completely transected, the patient may be able to extend the finger due to the action of the junctura from the index and ring fingers. In addition, MCP extension also is accomplished via the extensor indicis proprius and extensor digiti quinti in the index and small fingers, respectively. An-

other reason to have a high index of suspicion for tendon injury in dorsal hand wounds is because the soft tissue of the dorsum is very thin, making the extensor tendons more susceptible to injury.

If the MCP is being extended by an adjacent junctura, it usually is a weaker extension than in the uninjured digits, and the patient typically complains of pain while attempting the manuever. If there is any question as to the status of the tendons in this circumstance, the best thing to do is to completely anesthetize the injured area with local infiltration of lidocaine (after completing the examination for possible nerve injury). Then the wound can be thoroughly explored, rinsed out with saline, and repaired with sutures. A common error in this situation is **inadequate exploration,** particularly if the laceration is not large enough to facilitate full exposure of the tendon. Be sure to observe the excursion of the tendon while the patient completely flexes and extends the fingers. It is not uncommon for a

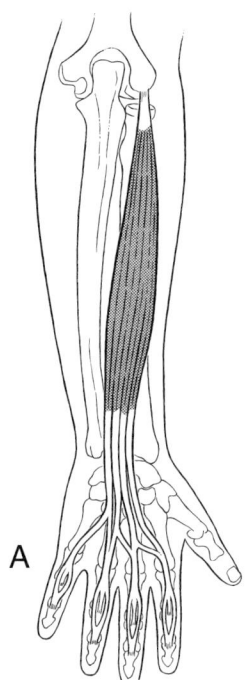

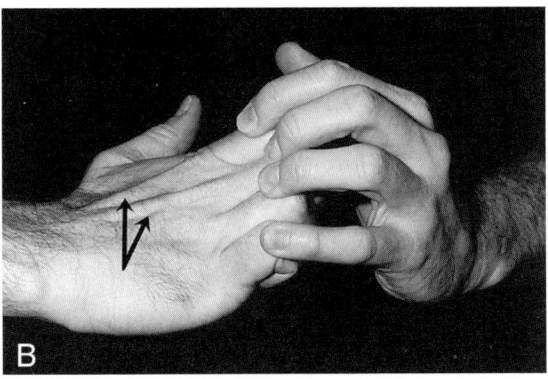

FIGURE 23. **A,** The extensor digitorum communis (EDC). **B,** The EDC is tested by the patient forcefully extending the metacarpophalangeal joints against resistance. Note the EDC tendons during this attempted extension (*arrows*).

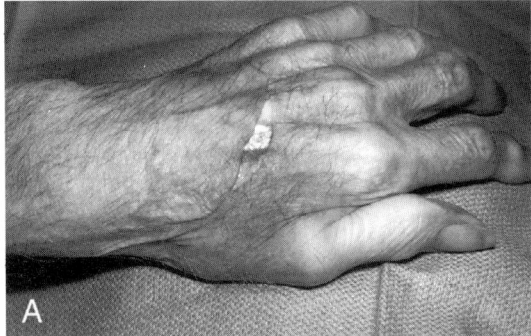

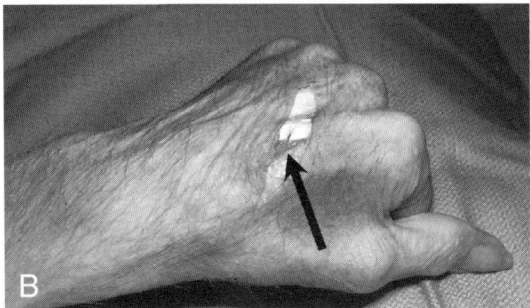

FIGURE 24. A hand that suffered a laceration on the dorsal aspect overlying the extensor tendons. **A,** Simple inspection of the underlying tendon with the hand at rest reveals no injury to the tendon. **B,** However, when the fingers are flexed the tendon glides forward, and the partial laceration becomes evident (*arrow*).

tendon at the base of a wound to appear completely normal until full finger flexion brings into view a lacerated end. This situation results from laceration occuring with the fingers flexed, a typical hand position in altercations. When examined in the emergency department, the fingers and wrist rest in extension, and the injured tendon glides proximal to the skin laceration (Figure 24).

The extensor indicis proprius can be selectively tested by the patient forcefully extending the index MCP while keeping the remainder of the fingers flexed (Figure 25). By flexing the other fingers, the EDC cannot participate in index finger MCP extension. Similarly, the extensor digiti quinti can be selectively tested by the patient forcefully extending the MCP of the small finger while keeping the other fingers flexed into a fist (Figure 26).

The extensor carpi ulnaris functions as both a wrist extensor and an ulnar deviator. It is isolated by the patient forcefully extending and ulnarly deviating the wrist. The examiner can palpate the tendon just distal to the ulna on the dorsal-ulnar aspect of the hand during this maneuver (Figure 27).

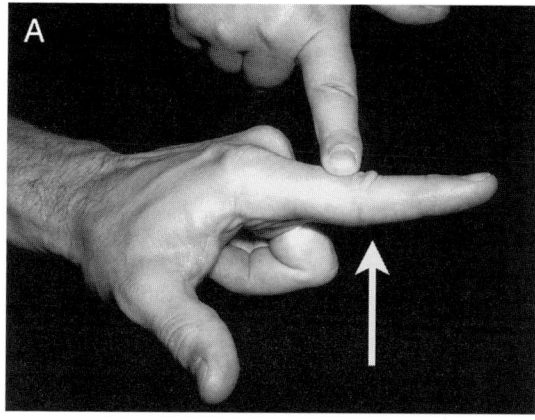

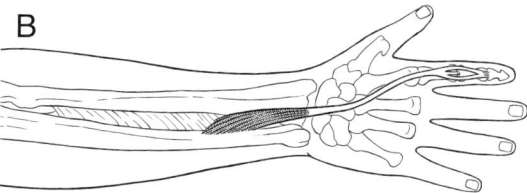

FIGURE 25. **A,** The extensor indicis proprius can be selectively tested by having the patient forcefully extend the index MCP. The remainder of the fingers are maintained in flexed position to prevent the EDC from participating. **B,** Extensor indicis proprius.

Volar Forearm and Hand (Median Nerve)

The pronator teres functions to both pronate the forearm and flex the elbow. It is tested by the patient extending the elbow and forcefully pronating the forearm (Figure 28). This maneuver places the muscle in maximal stretch and gives it a mechanical advantage over the pronator quadratus, which also functions to pronate the arm. Unfortunately, pronation still can be achieved by the pronator quadratus in this position; it is difficult to completely isolate the pronator teres in function tests.

The flexor digitorum superficialis deserves special consideration in examination of the hand. An intact ability to flex the fingers does not rule out injuries to the superficialis, because this action also can be performed by the flexor digitorum profundus. Isolation of the flexor digitorum superficialis (which flexes the middle phalanx) is achieved by the examiner holding the adjacent fingers in full exten-

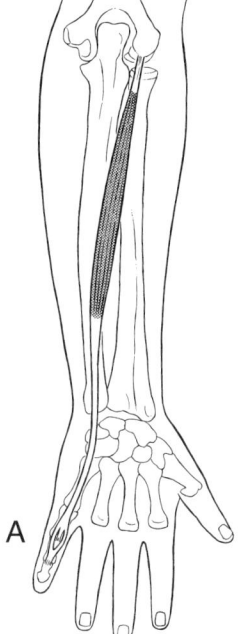

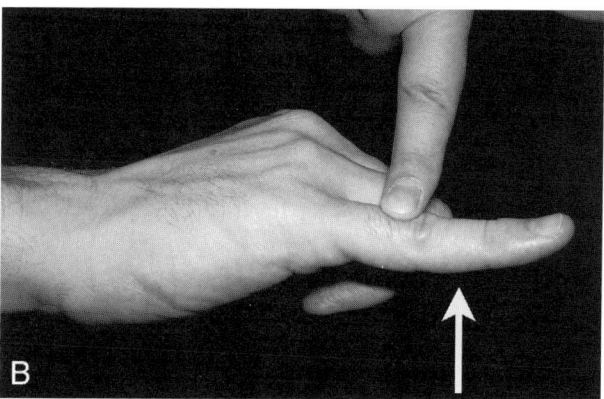

FIGURE 26. **A,** Extensor digiti quinti. **B,** These tendons are selectively tested by extending the fifth metacarpophalangeal joint while flexing the other fingers to eliminate participation by the extensor digitorum communis.

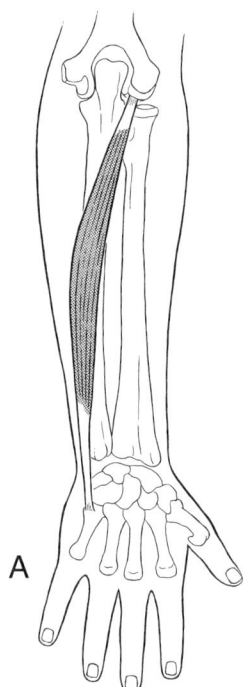

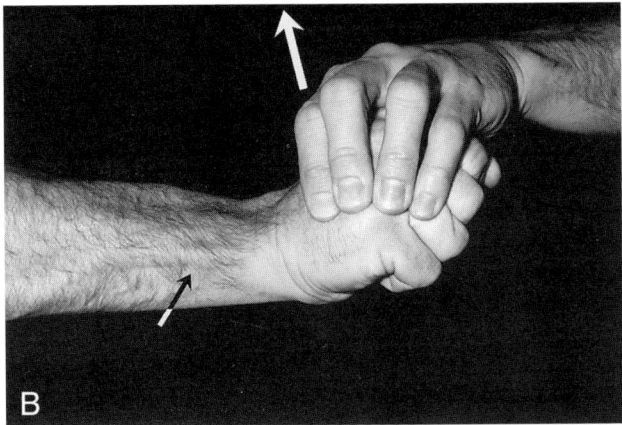

FIGURE 27. **A,** The extensor carpi ulnaris functions as a wrist extensor and an ulnar deviator. **B,** It can be tested by the patient forcefully extending (*large arrow*) and ulnarly deviating the wrist. The physician should palpate the tendon (*small arrow*) while the patient performs this maneuver.

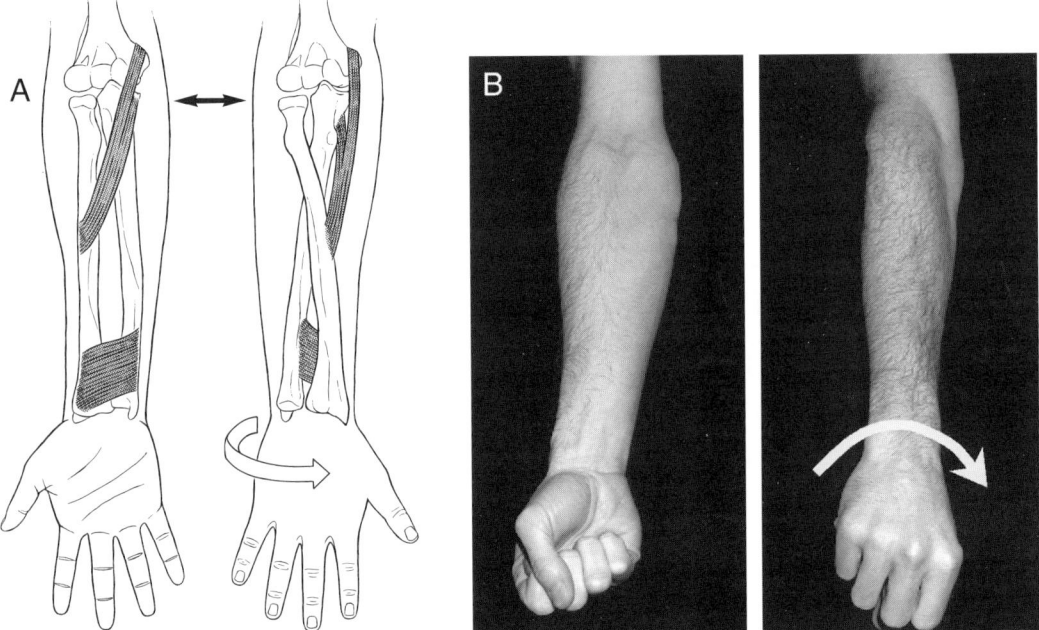

FIGURE 28. **A,** The pronator teres (*double arrow*) crosses the elbow and functions to pronate the forearm and flex the elbow. **B,** This muscle is tested by placing it on maximum stretch by fully extending the elbow and supinating the forearm (*left*). The patient is then asked to pronate the forearm (*right*).

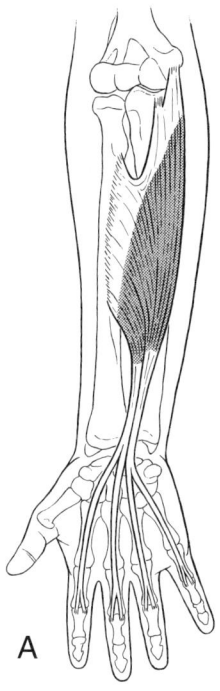

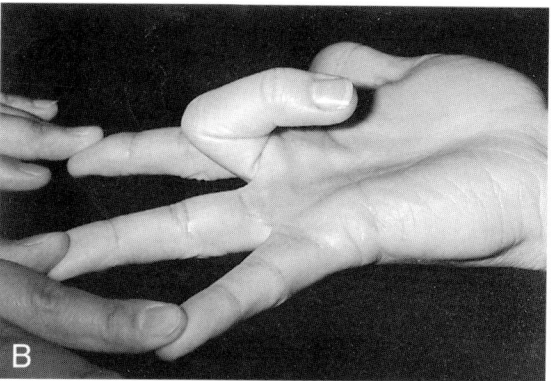

FIGURE 29. **A,** Flexor digitorum superficialis (FDS). **B,** This muscle is tested by holding the adjacent digits in extension while the patient flexes the middle finger. With the adjacent digits in extension, the only musculotendinous unit able to function is the FDS.

sion while the patient flexes the finger in question (Figure 29). This maneuver prevents the flexor digitorum profundus from flexing the finger and isolates the superficialis tendon for evaluation. The profundus tendon is blocked because it has a common muscle belly: the flexor digitorum profundus of one finger cannot function independently of the other fingers. Conversely, each flexor digitorum superficialis has its own muscle belly and flexes independently.

The flexor carpi radialis is one of the primary flexors of the wrist. This tendon can be palpated immediately radial to the palmaris longus tendon (if present) with the wrist in forceful flexion and the fingers cupped (Figure 30). The palmaris longus tendon (which can act as a weak wrist flexor) can be palpated with the same manueuver. Remember that up to 20% of the population does not have a palmaris longus.

The flexor pollicis longus can be evaluated by the patient flexing the thumb interphalangeal joint against resistance (Figure 31). The flexor digitorum profundus of each digit is tested by the patient flexing the distal interphalangeal joint with the middle phalanx held in extension by the examiner (Figure 32).

The pronator quadratus is easier to test than the pronator teres. The pronator quadratus is isolated by the patient flexing the elbow and then forcefully pronating the arm. Elbow flexion eliminates participation from the pronator teres by placing it at a mechanical disadvantage (Figure 33).

The thenar musculature (abductor pollicis brevis, opponens pollicis, and flexor pollicis brevis) can be tested by the patient forcefully abducting the thumb from the plane of the palm and pronating it across to oppose the ring or small finger (Figure 34).

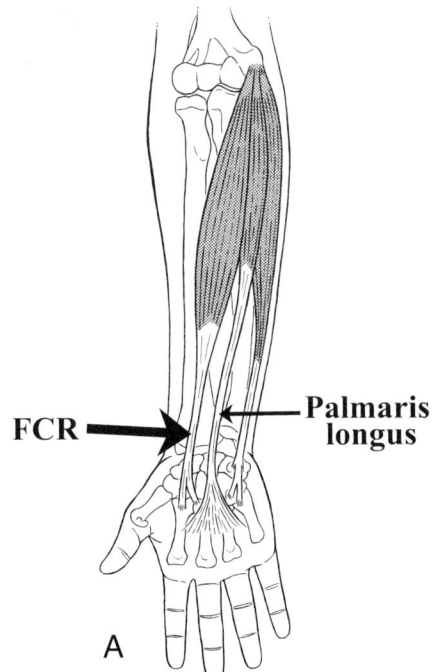

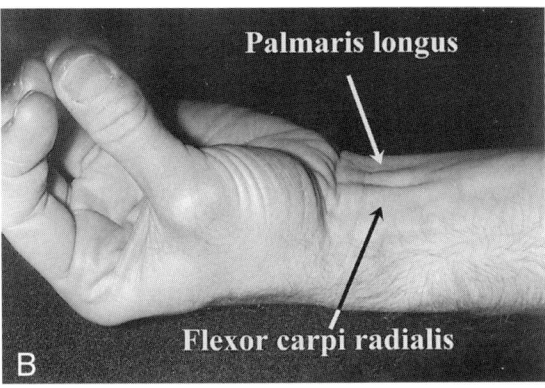

FCR → **Palmaris longus**

FIGURE 30. **A,** Flexor carpi radialis (FCR) and palmaris longus. **B,** These tendons can be easily palpated by having the patient slightly flex the wrist with the fingers held together.

A

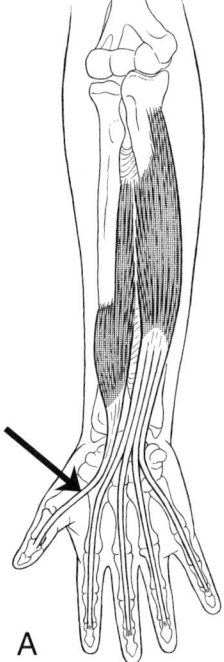

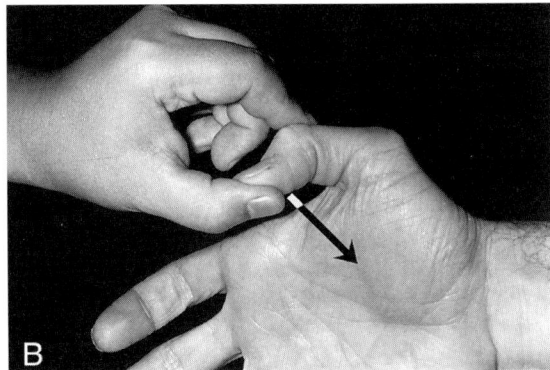

FIGURE 31. **A,** The function of the flexor pollicis longus (*arrow*) is to flex the interphalangeal joint of the thumb. **B,** This function can be tested by the patient performing this motion (*arrow*) against resistance.

A

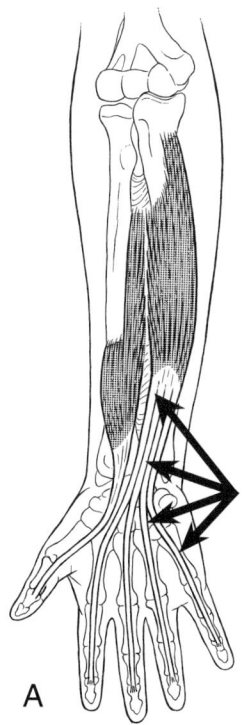

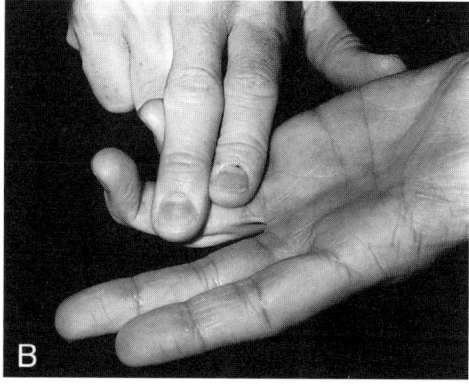

FIGURE 32. **A,** Flexor digitorum profundi (*arrows*). **B,** These tendons can be tested by the patient flexing the distal phalanx while the examiner blocks the middle phalanx from flexing.

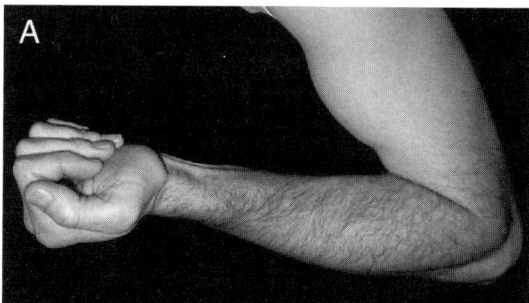

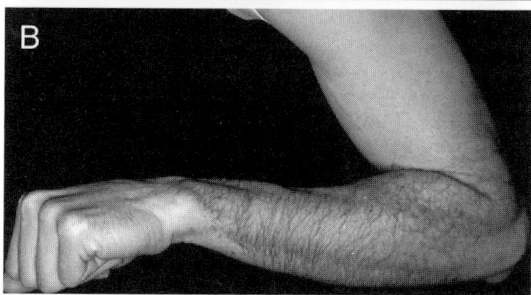

FIGURE 33. Testing of the pronator quadratus. **A,** The patient completely flexes the elbow and supinates the forearm. **B,** Then the patient forcefully pronates the arm. While in this position, most pronation is accomplished by the pronator quadratus rather than the pronator teres (see Figure 28).

Volar Forearm and Hand (Ulnar Nerve)

The flexor carpi ulnaris functions as a wrist flexor and ulnar deviator. It can be easily palpated at the volar wrist when the patient flexes and ulnarly deviates the wrist (Figure 35).

The volar interossei muscles function to adduct the fingers. They are tested by the patient forcefully adducting the fingers (Figure 36). The examiner places his or her own fingers between the patient's to gauge the strength of the adduction.

The patient forcefully abducts the fingers in testing the dorsal interossei (Figure 37). Remember that the dorsal and volar interosseous muscles can be tested as a unit by having the patient cross the fingers (see Figure 22).

The adductor pollicis is a strong muscle that functions to draw the thumb toward the index finger. It is tested by the patient forcefully bringing the thumb adjacent to the index finger (Figure 38).

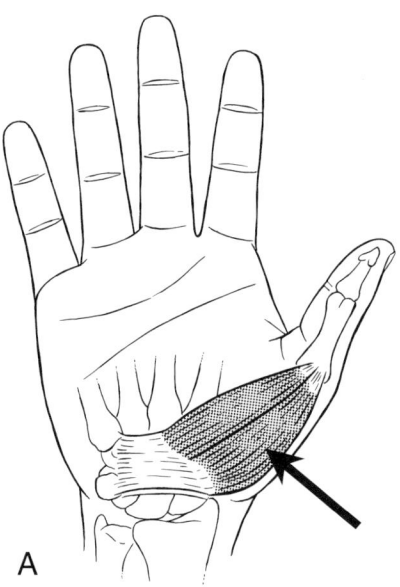

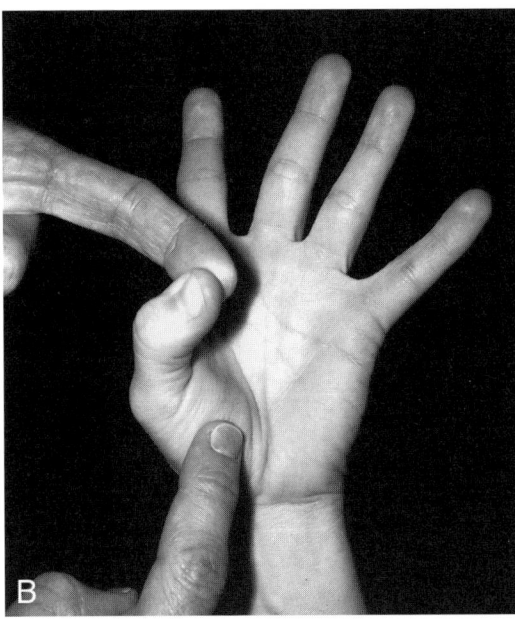

FIGURE 34. **A,** Thenar musculature (*arrow*). **B,** Testing is conducted by the patient forcefully opposing the thumb, abducting and pronating it. During this action the physician can palpate the thenar eminence to feel the muscles contracting.

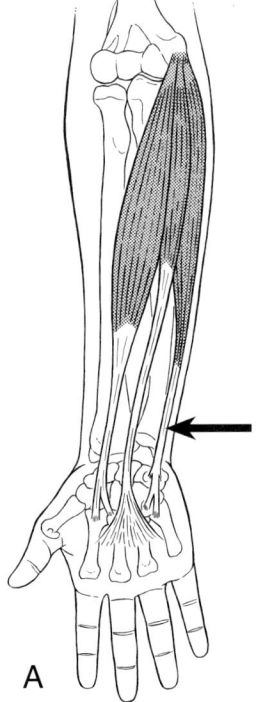

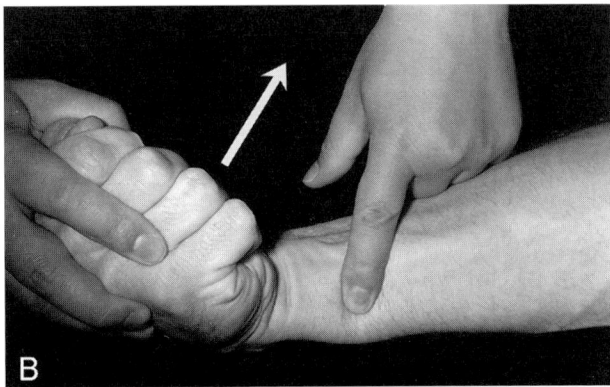

FIGURE 35. **A,** Flexor carpi ulnaris (*arrow*). **B,** The patient forcefully flexes and ulnarly deviates the wrist against resistance to test this unit. Palpate the tendon during this motion to confirm flexion by the flexor carpi ulnaris and not (for example) by the flexor carpi radialis.

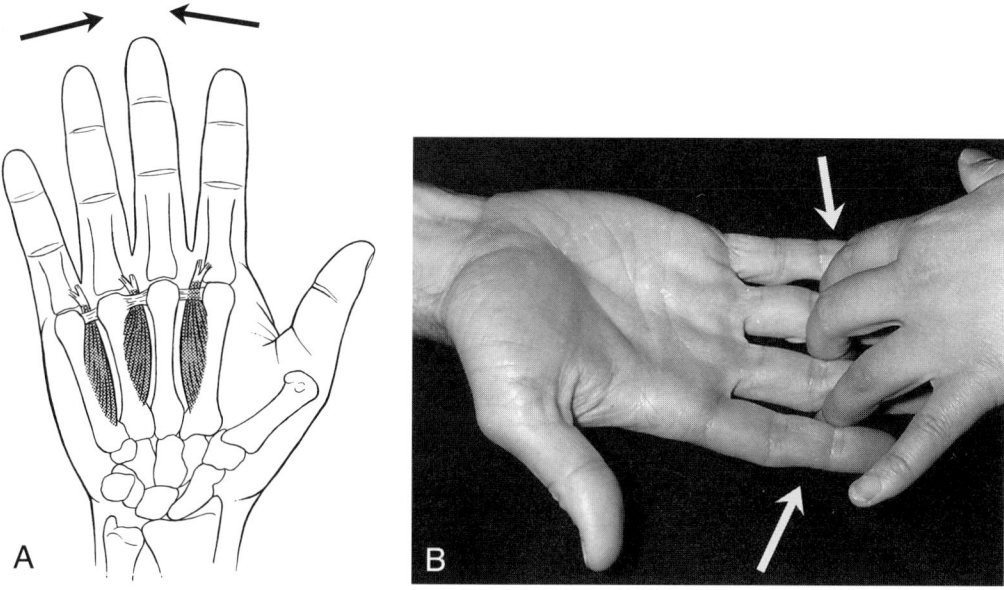

FIGURE 36. **A,** Volar interossei (*shaded areas*). These muscles are tested by the patient forcefully adducting (*arrows*) the fingers. **B,** The physician gauges the strength of these muscles by placing his or her own fingers between the patient's during this maneuver.

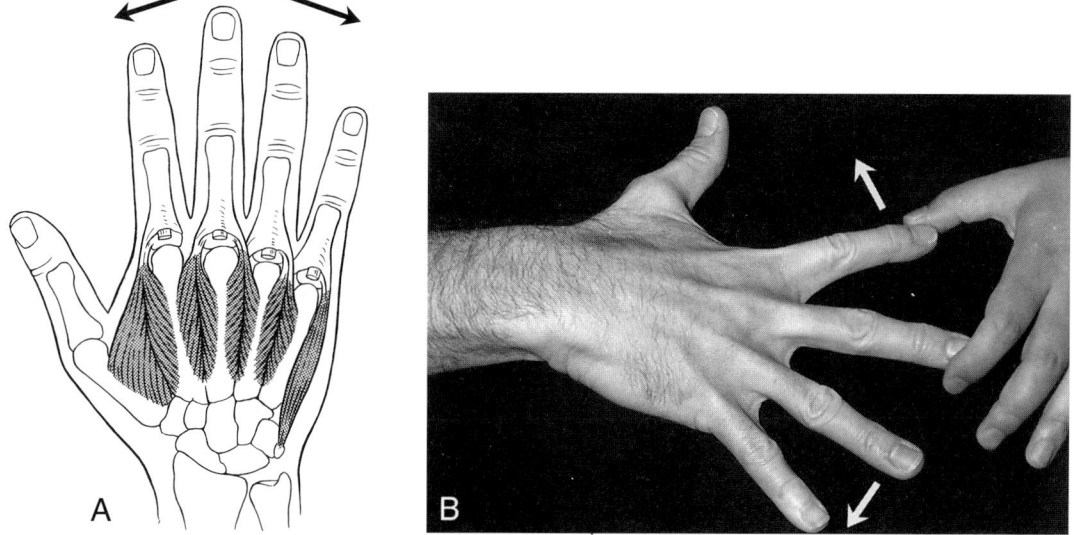

FIGURE 37. **A,** Dorsal interossei (*shaded areas*). **B,** The dorsal interossei, which function to abduct the fingers (*arrows*), can be tested by the patient forcefully abducting the fingers against resistance.

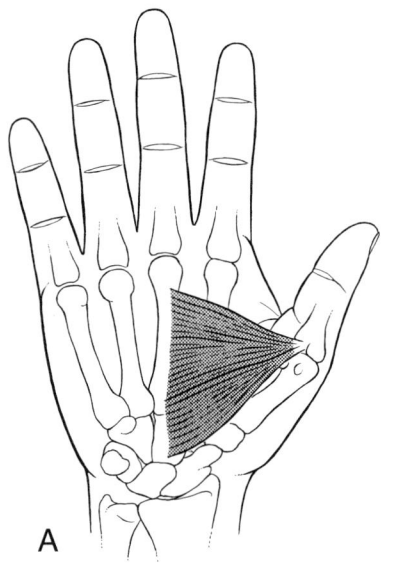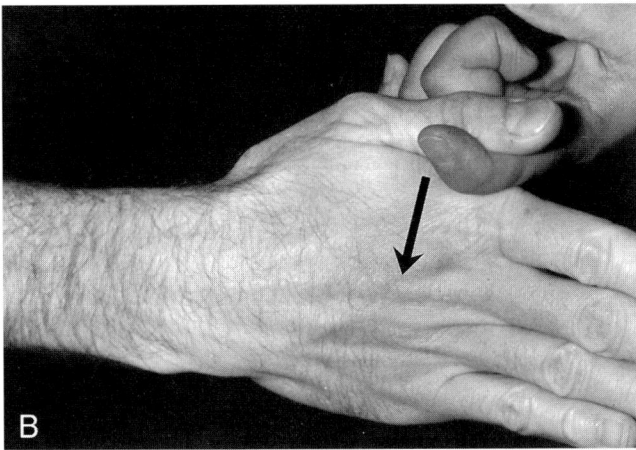

FIGURE 38. **A,** Adductor pollicis (*shaded area*). **B,** Test this muscle by having the patient tightly squeeze the thumb toward the hand against resistance.

Case Examples

The following case studies illustrate various hand injuries, describe approaches to their evaluation, and outline appropriate treatments.

CASE NO. 1

History

A 25-year-old woman presents to the emergency department after sustaining a crush-type injury to her hand. By her report, she was driving an automobile and her free (left) hand was located outside the window when she was side-swiped by another vehicle. The injury occurred approximately 1 hour prior to presentation. She is right-hand dominant and currently is not employed outside the home. She is a nonsmoker and denies any other medical problems. Her only medications are birth control pills. The patient's main complaint upon presentation is of diffuse and generalized pain throughout the hand. She denies any focal areas of tenderness.

Physical Examination

Observation. The hand and fingers are edematous, and there are several superficial abrasions over the dorsal and palmar aspects of the hand (Figure 39). There are no deep lacerations through the skin. The patient's hand is diffusely tender to palpation. The fingers and thumb are in a normal position at rest, with no angular or rotational deformities.

Nerve. The patient's moving two-point discrimination is 5 millimeters for all digits.

Vascular. Doppler signal indicates perfusion at the distal volar fingertips of all digits. Allen's test confirms good crossover vascularity with patent ulnar and radial arteries.

Musculotendinous. The patient has full active range of motion of all digits and wrist, although limited somewhat by pain.

Bone. The patient's entire hand is diffusely tender, particularly on the dorsal aspect. There are no focal areas of tenderness. Radiographs of the hand and fingers demonstrate no acute fractures or dislocations.

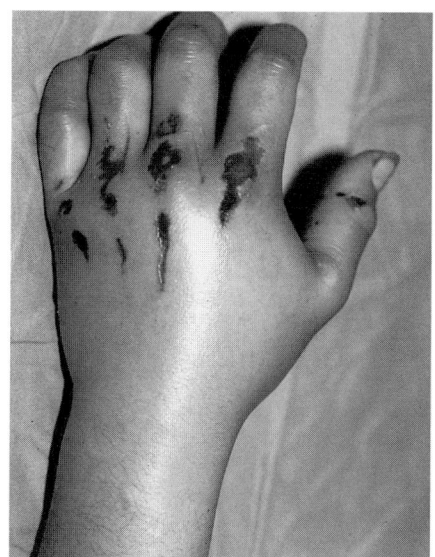 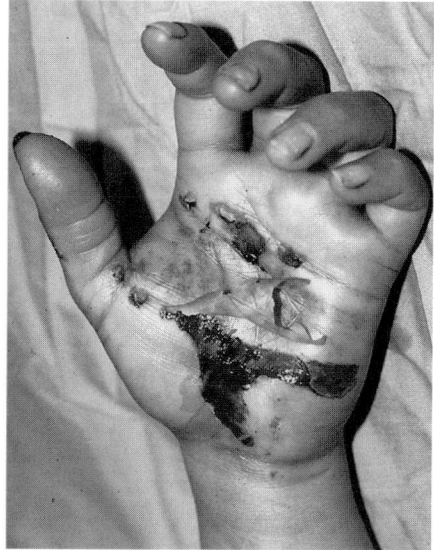

FIGURE 39. Case No. 1: crush-type injury with scraping.

Diagnosis

This patient's injury comprises hand contusion and superficial abrasions.

Treatment

Application of antibiotic ointment to the abrasions, splinting for comfort, analgesics, and antibiotics.

CASE NO. 2

History

A 44-year-old woman presents to the emergency department after her right hand was caught in a conveyer belt at work. The patient is right-hand dominant and is a nonsmoker. She denies any other medical problems and is currently on no medications. Hobbies include needlepoint and sewing.

Physical Examination

Observation. There is a large, avulsion-type injury along the entire dorsal aspect of the hand, as well as a second laceration over the dorsal proximal wrist (Figure 40). Examination reveals several lacerated tendons visible at the base of the

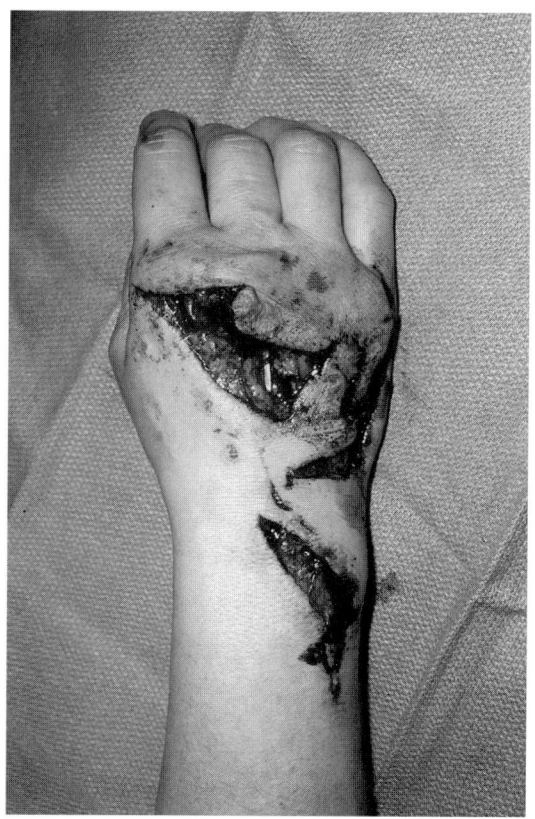

FIGURE 40. Case No. 2: avulsion and laceration injury.

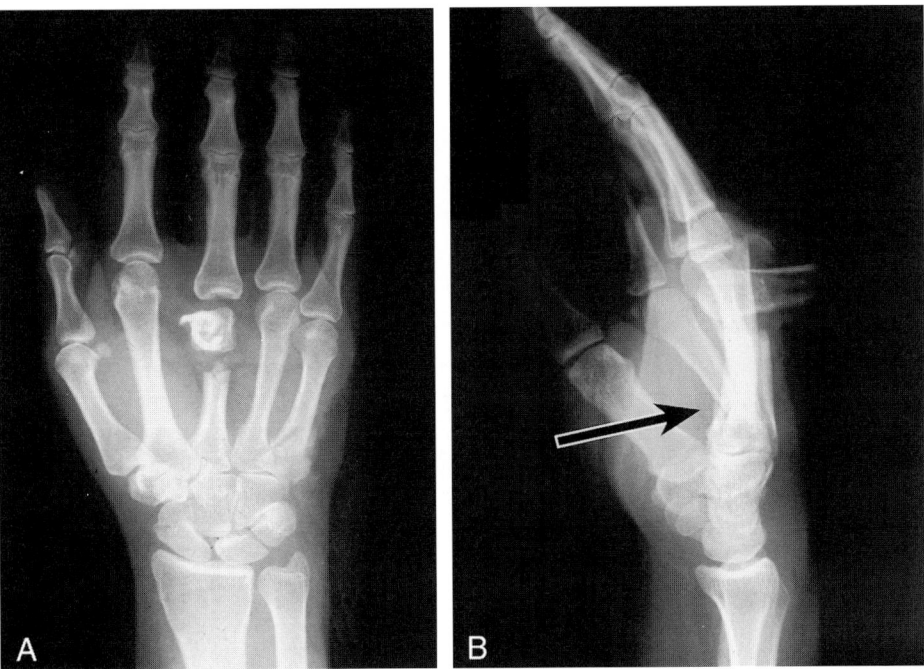

FIGURE 41. Case No. 2 radiographs. **A,** Anteroposterior view. **B,** Lateral view. Note the fracture of the fifth metacarpal (*arrow*), which is difficult to appreciate on the anteroposterior view.

wound and a large, bony fragment protruding dorsally. The wound has some particulate debris in it, but is not badly contaminated. Examination of the finger position shows the long finger to be somewhat shortened, but there are no angular or rotational deformities. The hand appears pink, with no evidence of vascular insufficency.

Nerve. Moving two-point discrimination reveals good sensation (5 millimeters) at the distal fingers and thumb.

Vascular. Good capillary refill, with an audible Doppler signal at the distal fingers. Allen's test reveals intact radial and ulnar arterial inflow.

Musculotendinous. The patient can slightly flex her fingers, but a severe amount of pain limits her efforts. She cannot extend the MCP joints of the long, ring, and fifth fingers, but can extend the index finger. She has limited and weak flexion of the thumb interphalangeal joint.

Bone. The patient complains of exquisite tenderness throughout the dorsal aspect of her hand. Radiographs (Figure 41) demonstrate fractures of the second, third, fourth, and fifth metacarpals, as well as a chip fracture of the thumb volar distal phalanx consistent with an avulsion injury to the flexor pollicis longus.

Diagnosis

Severe avulsion and laceration injury to the dorsal aspect of the dominant hand, with transection of multiple extensor tendons (EDC), multiple metacarpal fractures, and avulsion fracture of the flexor pollicis longus.

Plan

Referral to hand surgery specialist for operative debridement, repair of tendons, and reduction of fractures.

Discussion

This patient's case illustrates an important principle in the evaluation of radiographs. Perusal of the anteroposterior view of her hand (Figure 41A) shows an obvious fracture of the third metacarpal and a fracture of the thumb distal phalanx. The fracture of the fifth metacarpal may not be appreciated until the lateral view is seen (Figure 41B). The lateral view also provides a better view of the intra-articular fracture of the index metacarpal. *Always obtain multiple views when evaluating hand injuries for fractures to avoid missing injuries that are not visible on every view.*

CASE NO. 3

History

A 35-year-old woman presents to the office complaining of persistent pain in her right index finger. She is a smoker (one pack per day) with no other medical problems. When questioned, she complains of pain and swelling of 3-day duration, since an accident she sustained while riding her horse. The patient relates that while holding the reins, the horse suddenly pulled his head backward, wrenching her hand. She has had an ace wrap over the finger and hand since that time, and has been placing heating pads over the painful digit. She also has been taking over-the-counter nonsteroidal anti-inflammatory drugs. The patient states that the pain is worse at night, particularly when the hand is in a dependent position for an extended period of time.

Physical Examination

Observation. The right index finger is edematous, especially over the proximal phalanx, and appears to have a slight rotational deformity. There are no external wounds or lacerations (Figure 42).

Nerve. Sensory exam is normal, with moving two-point discrimination of 5 millimeters in all fingers.

Vascular. Digits are pink, rather than pale or dusky blue, indicating good capillary refill.

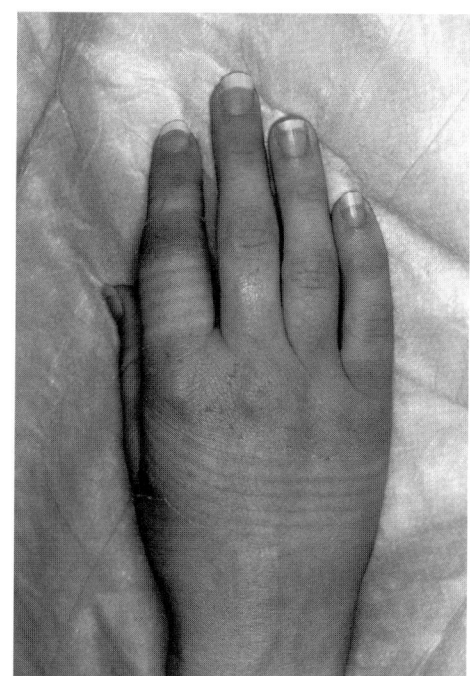

FIGURE 42. Case No. 3: proximal phalanx fracture of the index finger.

There is a strong Doppler signal at the distal pulp of all the fingers. Allen's test confirms patent radial and ulnar arteries, with good crossover perfusion.

Musculotendinous. The patient has active range of motion of all digits, although full extension and flexion of the index finger is difficult to obtain secondary to pain.

Bone. The proximal phalanx is exquisitely tender, and range of motion is limited at the MCP and proximal interphalangeal joints secondary to pain. Radiographs (Figure 43) reveal a comminuted fracture of the proximal phalanx.

Diagnosis and Plan

Proximal phalanx fracture; refer to a hand surgeon for open reduction and internal fixation of the fracture.

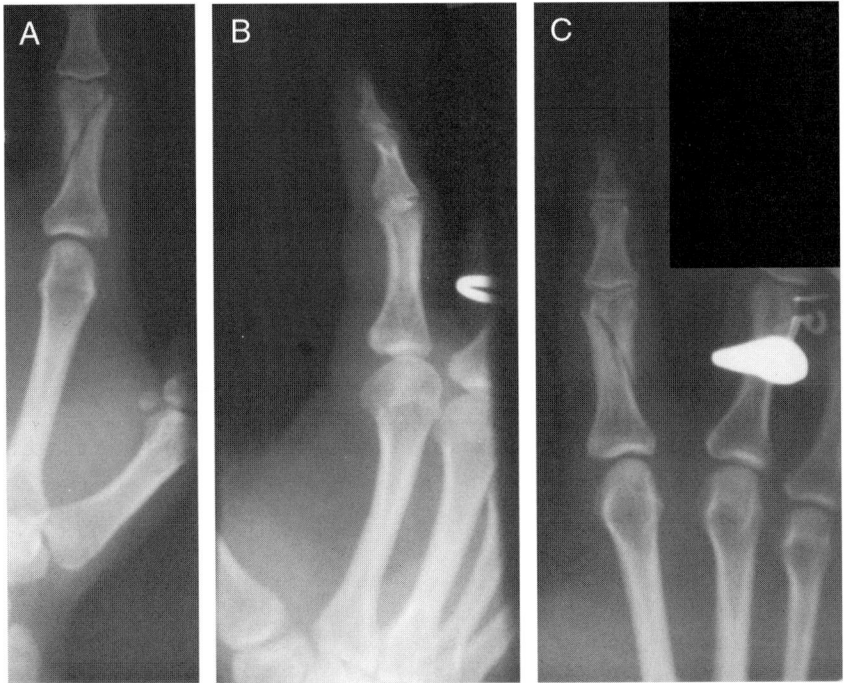

FIGURE 43. Case No. 3 radiographs. **A,** Anteroposterior view. **B,** Oblique view. **C,** Posteroanterior view.

CASE NO. 4

History

A 19-year-old man was involved in an altercation and sustained a stab wound to his right volar forearm along the ulnar aspect. The patient complains of pain over the laceration, but has no other initial complaints. He admits to smoking two packs of cigarettes per day, but is currently on no medications and does not have any other medical problems. He is right-hand dominant, and is currently an unemployed construction worker.

Physical Examination

Observation. The hand at rest shows the fingers in normal positions, with a normal cascade (Figure 44). The patient has an ulnar volar wound which is not actively bleeding at the time of examination. The hand color appears normal; all digits are pink and viable. The wound is a sharp laceration-type, with no crush or avulsion component. It does not appear to be dirty or grossly contaminated.

Nerve. The patient has normal two-point discrimination of the thumb, index, and long finger, but cannot discern two points at 10 millimeters apart on the ulnar aspects of his ring and fifth fingers. Motor examination of the median nerve is normal, with good thumb opposition and strong flexion of the flexor digitorum profundus (FDP) at the distal phalanx of the index finger.

Vascular. All fingers have brisk capillary refill with an audible Doppler signal at the distal pulp. The Doppler signal also is strong at the wrist at both the ulnar and radial arteries. However, the hand becomes pale and the Doppler signals at the digits and the ulnar artery are lost when the radial artery is compressed at the wrist.

Musculotendinous. The patient can extend the fingers and can actively bring them into full flexion into the palm, making a fist. Specific testing of the FDP of each finger demonstrates normal flexion of the distal pha-

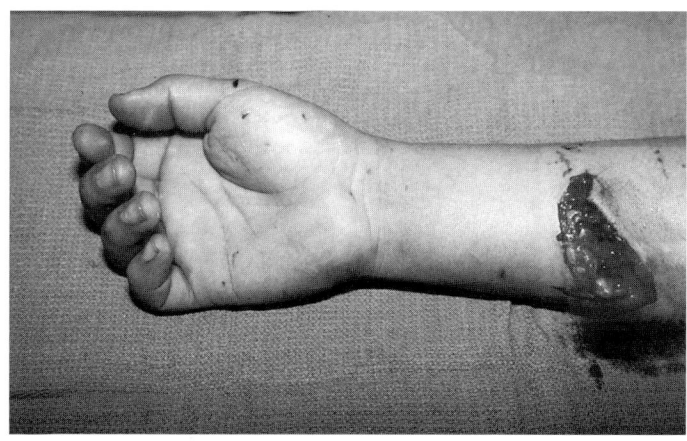

FIGURE 44. Case No. 4: sharp laceration-type injury at ulnar aspect of volar forearm.

langes. However, the patient is unable to flex his ring finger with the long and fifth fingers held in extension. Similarly, he is unable to flex the fifth finger with the ring finger held in extension. He can actively oppose his thumb to his fifth finger, but cannot cross his fingers and adduct or abduct them. He is able to actively flex his wrist, with radial and ulnar deviation.

Bone.   The patient has no bony tenderness of the radius or ulna, and passive range of motion of the fingers causes minimal discomfort. Radiographs of the forearm show absence of foreign body and no bony injury.

Diagnosis

Ulnar artery transection (forearm), ulnar nerve transection (forearm), transection of the flexor digitorum superficialis (FDS) to the ring and fifth fingers.

Discussion

Several injuries in this patient may have gone unnoticed if a thorough examination had not been performed. The fingers at rest demonstrated a normal cascade, and the patient was able to flex his fingers completely into the palm. To the casual observer these signs might have implied that no tendinous injury was sustained. However, specific testing of the FDS revealed that there was no FDS function to the ring and fifth fingers, consistent with transection. In fact, the normal cascade of these fingers was maintained by the resting tension of the FDP tendon. *Loss of the resting cascade occurs with transection of **both** flexor tendons of a specific digit; if only one tendon is injured, there may be no alteration in this posture.* Similarly, the patient was able to flex the fingers completely, due to the action of each digit's FDP.

Evidence of ulnar nerve injury was provided by the lack of sensation in the ulnar nerve distribution, as well as by the paralysis of the ulnar-innervated intrinsic muscles. Since the median nerve was noted to be completely intact (normal distal sensation, good motor funtion), the loss of FDS function could be diagnosed as a direct injury to the musculotendinous unit, rather than to its innervation. This ulnar nerve injury occurred *distal* to FDP innervation of the ring and fifth fingers, and therefore their functions were not affected by the nerve transection.

On initial observation, the hand was well vascularized, and there was no sign of vascular insufficiency. However, by specifically occluding the radial artery the hand was demonstrated to be ischemic, indicating that it was being perfused solely by the radial artery. The Doppler signal at the ulnar artery could have given the examiner the impression that the ulnar artery was intact at the proximal wound. In fact, this signal arose from the radial artery's distal collateral flow.

Another clue to the presence of occult arterial injury was the diagnosis of proximal nerve injury. This diagnosis was made because the patient was anesthetic in the ulnar one and one-half digits of the hand and had lost use of the ulnar nerve–innervated muscles. Since the arteries and nerves of the arm, hand, and fingers travel closely together, always have a very **high degree of suspicion** of a concomitant arterial injury when there is evidence of a nerve injury. It is not uncommon for arterial injuries to cease active bleeding due to intense vasoconstriction, one of the body's defense mechanisms to prevent massive hemorrhage. Lack of active bleeding can falsely lead an examiner to dismiss the diagnosis of arterial injury.

Note that if a major artery (such as radial or ulnar) is only partially transected, vasoconstriction will not completely occlude the lumen, and dramatic bleeding will continue. This is one of the potentially lethal injuries to the upper extremity.

CASE NO. 5

History

A 40-year-old man was injured while working at an animal processing plant. He suffered a deep laceration to the ulnar aspect of his right hand, proximal to the wrist. By report, the patient lost a great deal blood at the scene. He admits to smoking 1½ packs of cigarettes per day and has a history of untreated hypertension. Past medical history is significant for carpal tunnel release of the injured hand, approximately 5 years prior to injury. He is right-hand dominant, and his job requires heavy lifting and use of heavy machinery.

Physical Examination

Observation. There is a large, obliquely oriented laceration at the ulnar volar aspect of the distal forearm. There is no active bleeding at the time of examination. The ring and fifth fingers appear pale and have lost their normal resting cascade, demonstrating no intrinsic flexion.

There are no angular or rotational deformities of the digits (Figure 45).

Nerve. The patient has 5 millimeter moving two-point discrimination at the thumb and the index and long fingers, but is completely insensate at the ring and fifth fingers.

Vascular. Examination reveals typical capillary refill and Doppler signals at the distal thumb and the index and long fingers. There is no Doppler signal at the ring or fifth fingers. With occlusion of the radial artery, the entire hand becomes ischemic, with no Doppler signal noted distal to the compressed radial artery.

Musculotendinous. The patient can weakly flex his wrist, with some radial deviation. He is unable to strongly flex in an ulnar direction. He has no active flexion of the ring and fifth fingers, but has healthy FDS and FDP functions of the index and long fingers. He is unable to adduct and abduct his fingers. He has good opposition of the thumb to the fifth finger.

Bone. Aside from moderate tenderness around the wound, the patient denies pain and focal tenderness. The digits are moved through full range of motion without pain or discomfort. Radiograph of the hand demonstrates no foreign bodies nor underlying bony injuries.

Diagnosis

Deep laceration at right ulnar wrist; transection of the ulnar nerve, ulnar artery, flexor carpi ulnaris, and FDP and FDS to the ring and fifth fingers.

Plan

Emergent consultation with a hand surgeon for revascularization, microscopic repair of ulnar nerve, and tendon repair.

Discussion

This case differs from Case No. 4 in that this patient did not have adequate crossover perfusion of the hand and, therefore, transection of the ulnar artery resulted in distal ischemia of the

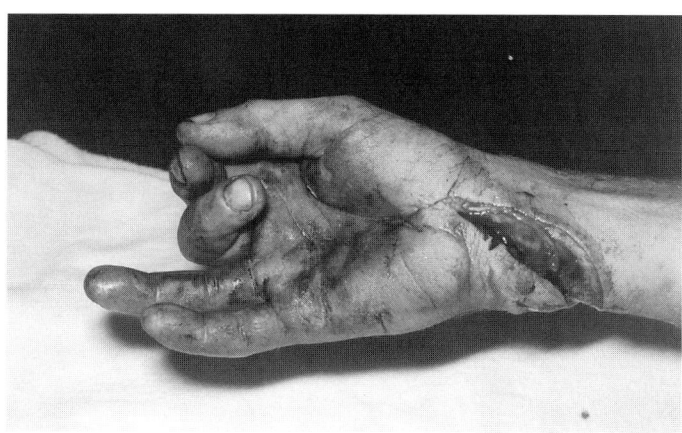

FIGURE 45. Case No. 5: deep laceration at ulnar wrist.

ulnar two digits. Distal ischemia of this type is a surgical emergency, and prompt intervention is indicated. Unlike the prior case, the normal cascade of the fingers at rest was lost, indicating transection of both the FDP and FDS to the affected fingers. Finally, the location of the laceration is highly suspicious for injury to the flexor carpi ulnaris, which lies immediately above and ulnar to the ulnar artery and nerve, which have been determined to be transected. Transection of the flexor carpi ulnaris was confirmed by physical examination.

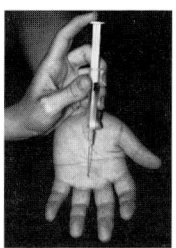

3 Anesthetic Techniques

This discussion on anesthetic techniques is provided to facilitate treatment of those injuries that can be addressed without further referral or consultation, within the emergency department or outpatient setting. A common error is to make the patient more comfortable by administering local anesthesia while waiting for the consulting physician to arrive. Obviously, the presence of a nerve block will confound the sensory and motor exams and make accurate diagnosis of any injuries extremely difficult, if not impossible. Pain can be successfully alleviated on a temporary basis by immobilization in a splint, elevation of the injured hand, and prudent administration of parenteral analgesics.

Lidocaine is the local anesthetic of choice in the hand. *Never* use lidocaine with epinephrine distal to the metacarpals; *always* take the time to draw up your own anesthetic solutions so that you know exactly what you are injecting. Some extremely devastating iatrogenic injuries (and correspondingly devastating malpractice awards) have arisen from erroneous infiltration of the wrong agent. The addition of epinephrine into the local anesthetic mix can cause a profound vasospasm, particularly at the level of the digits. In the face of an injury in which there may already be some compromise of arterial inflow, the addition of a vasoconstrictor may tip the balance toward critical ischemia of the finger or hand.

The maximum recommended lidocaine doses are 5 mg/kg without epinephrine and 7 mg/kg with epinephrine. The patient can tolerate another injection, if necessary, 45 minutes after infiltration. In a hypothetical patient weighing 70 kg, the lidocaine dose without epinephrine would be 5 mg × 70 kg = 350 mg, which is 35 ml of 1% lidocaine, or 70 ml of 0.5% lidocaine.

To maximize patient comfort, provide a block proximal to the area you will be working on if at all possible, rather than directly infiltrating the lidocaine within and around the wound. For example, a digital nerve block can render a finger completely insensate, allowing cleansing and repair of lacerations or other injuries. For larger palmar or dorsal hand injuries or multiple finger injuries, a wrist block can numb the entire hand, allowing exploration (if neccessary), irrigation of the wound, and closure. Sometimes a proximal block is not possible or practical, such as is often the case in otherwise uncomplicated forearm lacerations. In these situations, local infiltration of lidocaine may be the best option for providing local anesthesia.

Digital Block

When treating lacerations or other injuries of the finger, the digital block is the most expeditious way to provide local anesthesia. This technique is based on the knowledge that the neu-

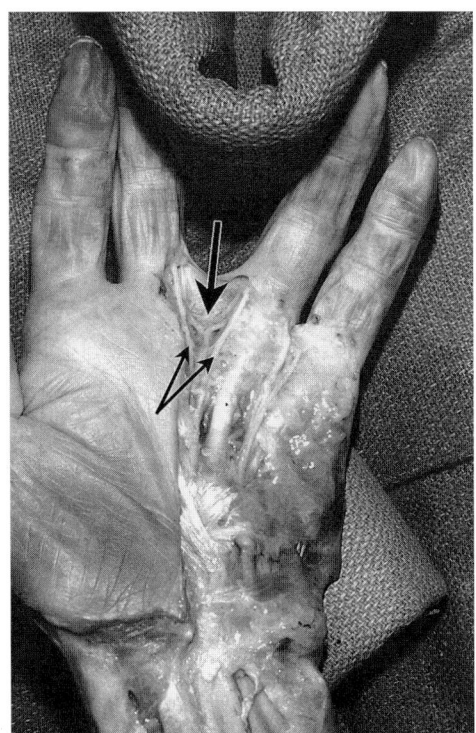

FIGURE 1. Dissection of the palm demonstrating the location of the neurovascular bundles. The digital arteries of the ulnar long and radial ring fingers (*large arrow*) are seen in close association with the digital nerves (*double arrow*) after their takeoff from the common digital artery.

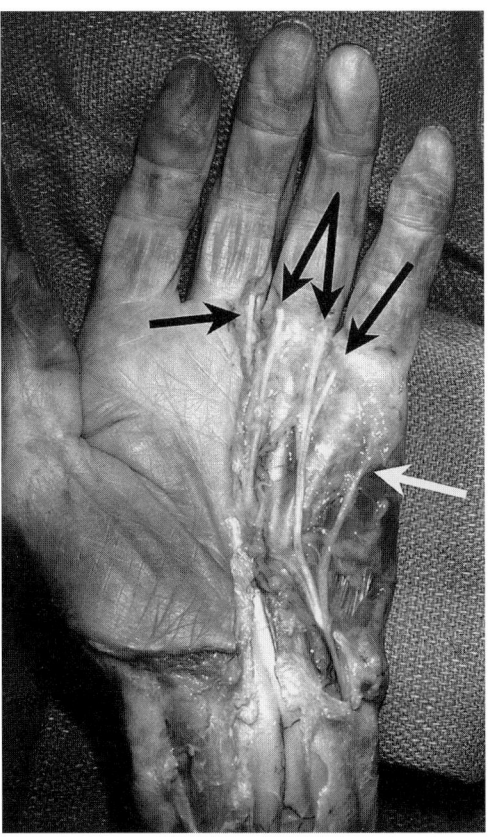

FIGURE 2. Location of the digital nerves to the long, ring, and fifth fingers. The nerves run along the lateral aspect of each finger (*black arrows*). Infiltration of 1% lidocaine adjacent to a digital nerve at the distal palm renders the distal aspect of that finger completely anesthetic. Clearly demonstrated here are the ulnar digital nerve to the long finger, the ulnar and radial digital nerves to the ring finger, and the radial digital nerve to the fifth finger. The ulnar digital nerve to the fifth finger (*white arrow*) has not been dissected free of the palmar fat at the distal palm.

rovascular bundles travel at the volar-lateral aspect of the fingers (Figures 1, 2). Infiltration of 2–3 ml of 1% lidocaine without epinephrine at the distal palm adjacent to each of these nerves provides an excellent level of local anesthesia (Figure 3A). To augment this, a dorsally based subcutaneous infusion just distal to the metacarpophalangeal joints ("ring block") acts on the dorsal innervation to render the finger completely anesthetic (Figure 3B). This dorsal infusion is particularly helpful when working at the dorsal proximal phalanx. Remember that the digital nerves send branches to innervate the dorsum of the finger *distal* to the proximal interphalangeal joint (PIP); for injuries proximal to this joint, a simple digital block alone does not provide adequate anesthesia.

When performing a digital block of the thumb, remember that the neurovascular bundles travel closer to the midline than in the other digits (Figure 4).

A digital block also can be performed via a dorsal approach, which may be less painful to the patient. A 25-gauge needle is inserted distal to and between the metacarpophalangeal (MCP) joints dorsally, and advanced volarly until it is close to the palmar skin (Figure 5). Approximately 2–3 ml of lidocaine then can be infiltrated to achieve the digital block.

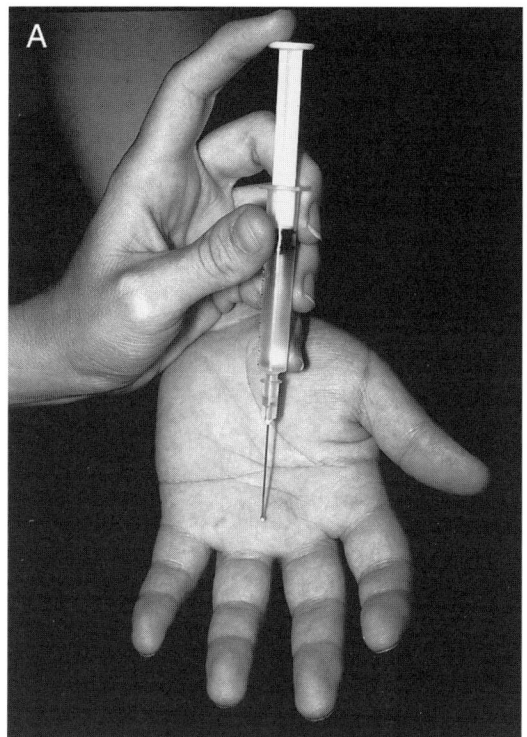

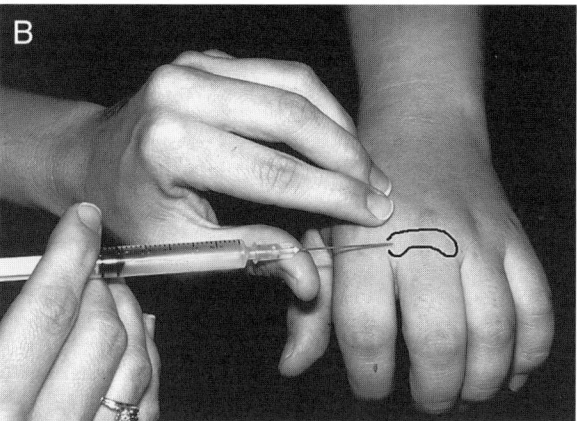

FIGURE 3. **A,** The digital block is performed by advancing the needle 5–6 ml beneath the skin and infiltrating 2–3 ml of lidocaine adjacent to the digital nerves of the affected finger. *Both* digital nerves to the finger must be blocked to completely anesthetize the entire digit. **B,** Dorsal finger "ring block." Digital nerves provide dorsal innervation *distal* to the PIP joint; dorsally based branches of either the ulnar or radial nerve provide dorsal innervation *proximal* to the PIP joint. A subcutaneous infiltration of lidocaine across the base of the finger (*outline*) blocks these branch fibers.

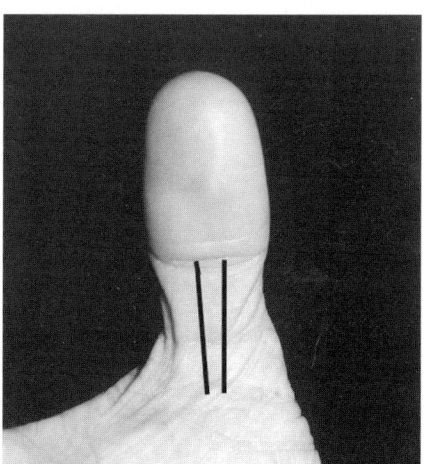

FIGURE 4. Approximate locations of the ulnar and radial digital nerves of the thumb.

FIGURE 5. Digital block—dorsal approach. The principles of lidocaine infiltration around the digital nerves are the same, but the injection is made just distal to the MCP joints on the dorsum of the hand. Remember that for a finger to be completely blocked, both its radial and ulnar nerves must be anesthetized.

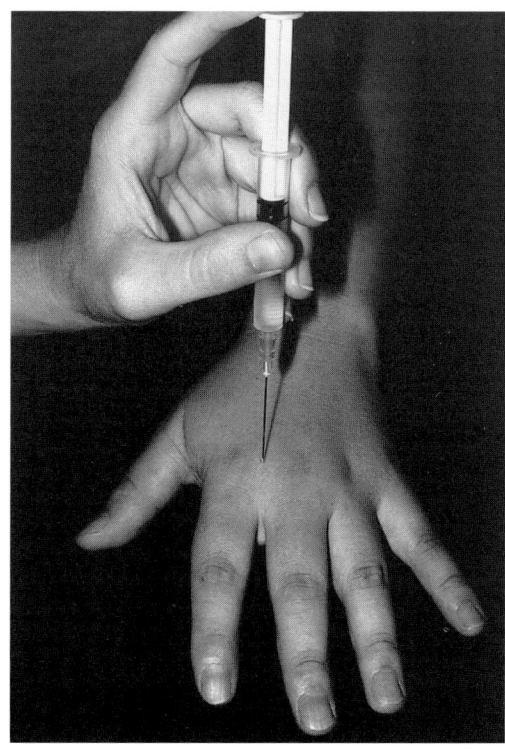

Wrist Block

The wrist block technique is an excellent method for obtaining dense anesthesia of the entire hand. The ulnar, median, and radial nerves are all blocked at the wrist level, providing anesthesia for repair of extensive injuries that involve multiple digits or the entire hand.

MEDIAN NERVE BLOCK

Using a 27- or 25-gauge needle, a small wheal is infiltrated subcutaneously just radial to the palmaris longus tendon. The needle for the nerve block should be at least 1½ inches long. Once the skin has been numbed, the needle is completely withdrawn and then advanced straight down and slightly distally, toward the median nerve and the flexor tendons that form the contents of the carpal tunnel (Figure 6A).

Prior to this maneuver, the patient is instructed to warn the physician if there is any feeling of "electrical shock" radiating to the fingers. The presence of this symptom warns the physician that the needle has pierced the median nerve. The objective is to place several milliliters of lidocaine *next* to the nerve, not *into* the nerve. Injection of lidocaine into a nerve can be extremely destructive and may cause permanent damage.

Once the needle has reached the approximate level of the nerve and tendons, the patient is asked to gently flex the fingers (Figure 6B). If the needle has penetrated one of the flexor tendons, the needle tip will move proximally as the fingers move. If this is the case, the needle

FIGURE 6. Wrist block—median nerve. **A,** The tendons of the flexor carpi radialis and palmaris longus (*marked lines*) border the injection site. Infiltrate a small skin wheal to numb the skin. Then advance a 25- or 27-gauge needle directly in, to the level of the carpal tunnel and the median nerve. Do not change direction once the tip has gone below the skin because the needle's bevel is razor sharp and can act as a cutting instrument. The objective is to place the lidocaine *around* the nerve, not into it. **B,** When the needle is correctly positioned, ask the patient to slowly flex the fingers. Proximal movement of the needle tip with finger flexion is an indication that it has entered a flexor tendon. A final indication that the needle is in the correct location is that the lidocaine is injected easily, without resistance. The patient should begin to experience paraesthesia and numbness of the median nerve distribution within 5 minutes.

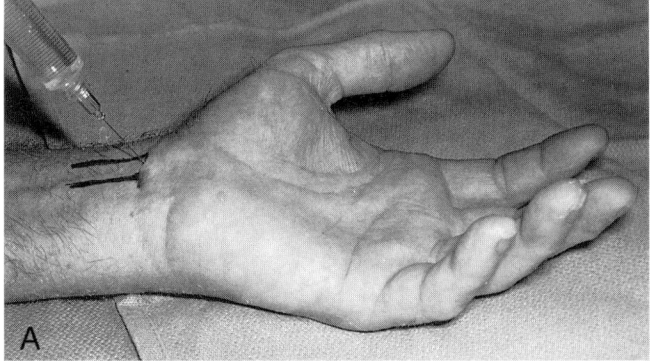

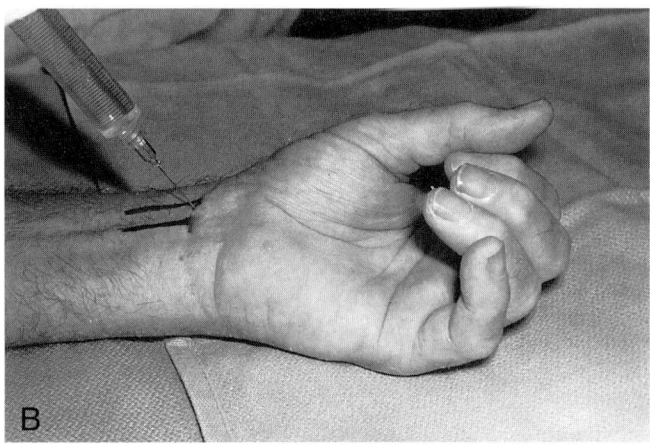

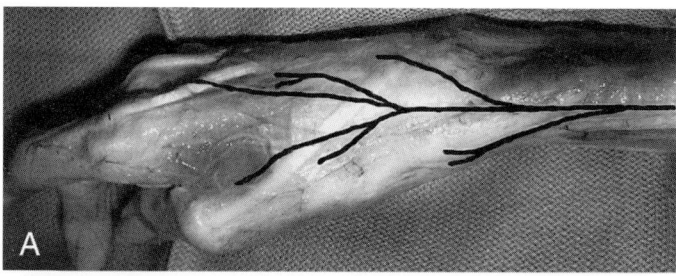

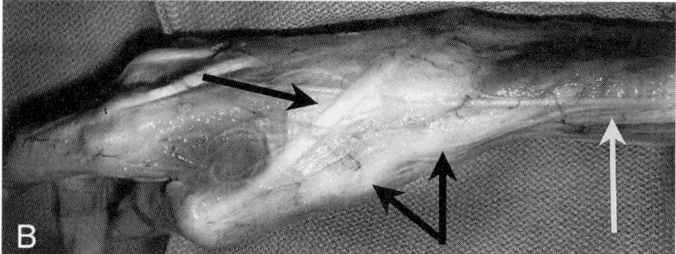

FIGURE 7. **A,** Branching of the radial nerve at the distal forearm and wrist. **B,** The proximal radial nerve (*white arrow*) divides into several sensory branches proximal to the anatomic snuff box, which is formed dorsally by the extensor pollicis tendon (*black arrow*) and volarly by the tendons of the first extensor compartment (*double arrows*).

should be slowly withdrawn until it is no longer in the tendon (1–2 mm). Avoiding the tendon is particularly important, for example, when infiltrating steroids into the carpal tunnel. Infiltration of steroids directly into a tendon can cause attenuation and rupture. When the physician is satisfied that the needle is in the carpal tunnel, 3–5 ml of 1% lidocaine without epinephrine is slowly infiltrated, and the needle is withdrawn.

RADIAL NERVE BLOCK

The radial nerve splits into several sensory branches at the wrist level (Figure 7). To completely block all of these branches, a subcutaneous infiltration of 4–5 ml of lidocaine is administered from the volar aspect of the anatomic snuffbox to the dorsal-radial aspect of the hand (Figure 8).

ULNAR NERVE BLOCK

The flexor carpi ulnaris tendon can be easily palpated proximal to the pisiform bone on the volar-ulnar border of the wrist. The ulnar nerve travels just dorsal to this tendon at the distal forearm and wrist (Figure 9). A 25- or 27-gauge

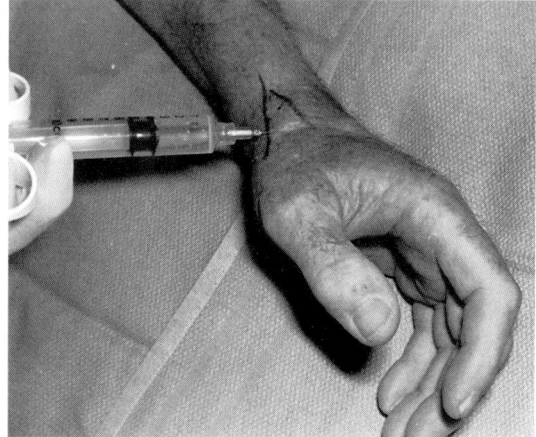

FIGURE 8. Wrist block—radial nerve. Begin the injection slightly volar to the tendon of the abductor pollicis longus, which forms the volar border of the anatomic snuff box (*marked lines*). Advance in a dorsal direction to anesthetize all of the branches of the radial nerve, and slowly infiltrate the subcutaneous tissue.

needle is inserted on the lateral aspect of the wrist, dorsal to the flexor carpi ulnaris, and advanced until past this tendon. Aspiration of the syringe is performed to confirm that the ulnar artery has not been entered and prevent intra-arterial injection of the lidocaine. Once proper

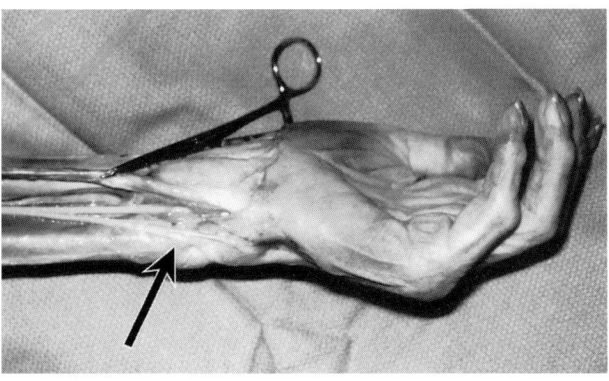

FIGURE 9. Relative positions of the ulnar nerve and the flexor carpi ulnaris (FCU) tendon. The FCU is pulled radially by a hemostat clamp. Note that the ulnar nerve travels just dorsal and radial to this tendon. This knowledge can be exploited when performing an ulnar nerve block. Also notice the proximal takeoff of the dorsal sensory branches of the ulnar nerve (*arrow*).

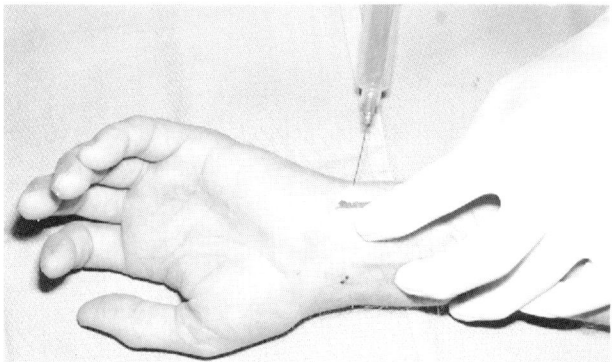

FIGURE 10. Wrist block—ulnar nerve. Recall that the ulnar nerve sits immediately dorsal and radial to the flexor carpi ulnaris tendon (*marked*). While palpating the tendon, place the needle at the ulnar side of the wrist and slowly advance the syringe dorsal to the tendon.

position is confirmed, 3–5 ml of lidocaine is injected at this level (Figure 10).

A word of caution about the technique of placing and advancing the needle: Most hyperdermic needles have a 1- to 2-ml razor-sharp edge on either side of the bevel (Figure 11). This bevel functions as a sharp blade when moved in a lateral direction and is capable of lacerating some vitally important structures—such as the very nerve you are looking to block. The safest method for any kind of injection or infiltration is the direct placement of a needle straight in, and then its withdrawal straight out. During infiltration, if the physician decides to change the location of the needle, it must be completely withdrawn and repositioned at the precise point desired, rather than moved laterally.

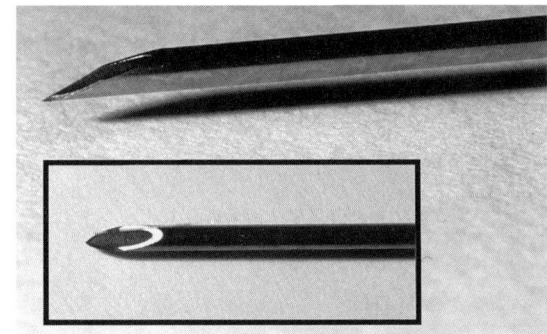

FIGURE 11. The tip of most hyperdermic needles comprises two razor-sharp edges. Lateral movement after the needle has been placed under the skin can cause transection or injury to the deep structures. The safest method is direct placement of a needle straight in, followed by withdrawal straight out.

Hematoma Block

The hematoma block is an effective way to provide local anesthesia prior to the reduction of

metacarpal fractures. Using a 25-gauge needle, the area immediately dorsal to the fracture is infiltrated with approximately 4–5 ml of 1% lidocaine with or without epinephrine. This technique does not specifically block any particular major nerves, but sufficiently anesthetizes the tissues around the fracture so that manipulation and reduction of the fracture can be performed (Figure 12).

Bier Block

The Bier block technique allows prolonged anesthesia of the entire hand, forearm, and distal arm and is relatively simple to perform. It offers the added benefit of markedly reduced bleeding due to tourniquet application, facilitating visualization of injured structures, exploration, and surgical repair. Another advantage of the Bier block is that since the entire limb is completely anesthetized, extensive lacerations can be repaired using a single anesthetic (often requiring less lidocaine than if infiltrating locally around such wounds). This technique can be effective for 60–90 minutes, with the limiting factor being the patient's tolerance of the tourniquet pain at the upper arm. Only one piece of specialized equipment is necessary: a double pneumatic tourniquet.

A drawback of the Bier block is that it entails a substantial bolus of intravenous lidocaine. If proper attention is not paid to the status of the tourniquet prior to infiltration, this bolus of lidocaine may be injected systemically, and potential toxicity may develop.

Perform this technique in the following manner. Place cast padding around the patient's upper arm, as close to the axilla as possible (Figure 13A), and fit the double pneumatic tourniquet snugly over the padding. Each cuff should have its own separate air supply; confirm at this point that each can be independently inflated to 250 mmHg pressure, with no leaking. Once you are satisfied that both cuffs are in good working order, cannulate a vein of the hand or forearm with a standard IV (heparinlock) and tape it into position. This is a good time to clarify with assistants the nomenclature and identity of the proximal and distal cuffs. There is a specific sequence to be followed when using the double pneumatic tourniquet.

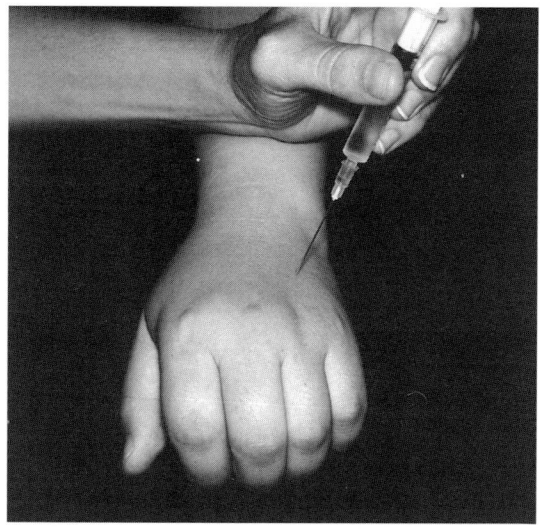

FIGURE 12. Hematoma block. Lidocaine infiltrated dorsal to the fractured metacarpal sufficiently anesthetizes the tissue around the fracture to allow manipulation, reduction, and splinting.

Appropriate use of the proximal and distal cuffs can alleviate the common problem of significant tourniquet pain threatening to curtail a procedure (Figure 13B).

Next, exsanguinate the upper extremity by elevating the patient's arm 1–2 minutes to allow venous outflow (Figure 13C). This can be augmented by squeezing the blood from distal to proximal by grasping the hand and forearm firmly (if the patient can tolerate it). Inflate the distal cuff to 250 mmHg. Once the distal cuff is up, inflate the proximal pneumatic cuff to 250 mmHg, and release the distal cuff. It is helpful to inflate the distal tourniquet first because it further squeezes the blood from the arm.

Lastly, inject 50 ml of 1% lidocaine plain (with no preservatives) into the IV catheter. The patient will rapidly experience a feeling of warmth and anesthesia in the entire upper extremity. This amount of lidocaine may have to be reduced for smaller adults. Note that this technique is not appropriate for use in children. After 3–4 minutes, a dense anesthesia that permits surgical exploration and repair is achieved. The tourniquet should be inflated for a minimum of 30 minutes to ensure that the lidocaine

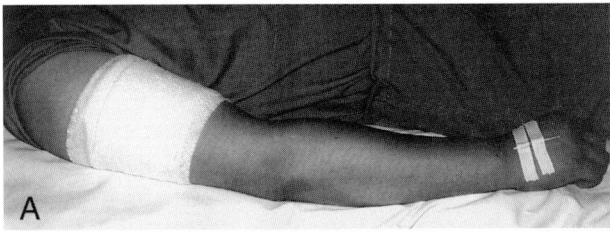

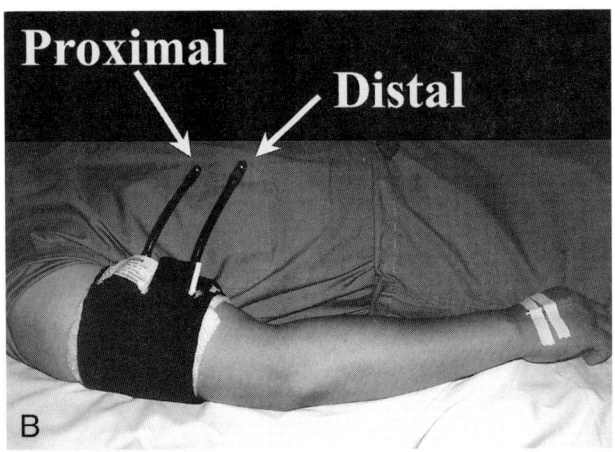

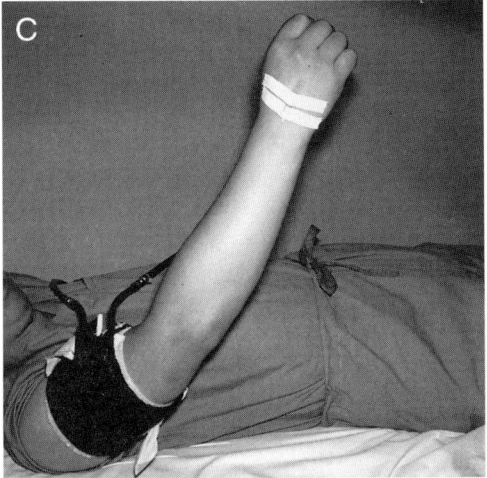

FIGURE 13. Bier block. **A,** Place cast padding circumferentially around the upper arm as close to the axilla as possible. Then place a heparin-lock IV in a dorsal hand vein to allow infusion of the lidocaine after the tourniquet is inflated. **B,** Fit a double pneumatic tourniquet over the cast padding, checking that each individual cuff can be independently inflated to 250 mmHg, with no leaking. When exsanguinating the upper extremity, inflate the distal cuff first, followed by the proximal cuff. After inflation of the proximal cuff, release the distal cuff and inject the lidocaine into the heparin-lock catheter. By leaving the distal cuff uninflated during infusion of the lidocaine, the soft tissues underneath this cuff are rendered insensate by the anesthetic. If the patient is having significant tourniquet pain after an hour or so of tourniquet ischemia, the distal cuff can be inflated and the proximal cuff released (in that order). This maneuver decreases the patient's discomfort from the tourniquet, due in part to the fact that the distal cuff is inflated over anesthetized tissues, and allows the physician to continue working. **C,** Exsanguinate the patient's arm by elevating it for 1–2 minutes.

is sufficiently bound to the tissues of the arm and prevent a systemic lidocaine bolus after tourniquet release.

Should the patient begin to complain of tourniquet pain when work still needs to be done, inflate the distal cuff to 250 mmHg, and release the proximal tourniquet. The tissue underneath the distal cuff is anesthetized; therefore, the patient can more easily tolerate the remaining tourniquet time.

An important feature of the Bier block is that the limb remains anesthetized *only as long as*

the tourniquet remains inflated. Within 60 seconds of tourniquet release, the patient regains sensation of the entire limb. Therefore, if the distal tourniquet has been inflated already, but the patient complains of discomfort and more work remains to be done, a different anesthetic technique must be applied. One approach to this situation is to directly infiltrate the tissues to be worked on, prior to release of the tourniquet. Thus, the patient does not have to suffer through an injection of the injured tissues, and the physician is able to finish the work.

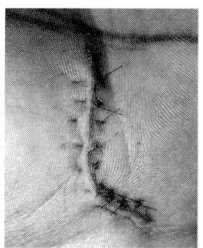

4 Treatment of Lacerations

Lacerations are the most common injuries that the primary care physician is faced with in the outpatient and emergency department setting. Care of hand lacerations usually is straightforward, and the following guidelines provide general approaches, management strategies, and treatments.

The first order of business when evaluating a patient with a skin laceration is to determine whether deeper structures also have been injured. A thorough history—providing an understanding of the mechanism of the injury—and physical examination guides the clinician to a pointed evaluation allowing exclusion or confirmation of other injuries.

After the history and physical assessment have been completed, and a treatment plan has been formulated for the patient, an anesthetic technique appropriate to the clinical situation can be selected (see Chapter 3). Multiple lacerations of the hand and forearm, for example, may be better managed using a regional anesthetic technique such as a Bier block, whereas a small, isolated laceration of the forearm may best be dealt with using local infiltration of lidocaine. Remember, local anesthetic should *not* be administered if you anticipate consultation with a hand surgical specialist, unless specifically approved by the specialist. Nerve blocks and local anesthesia can make physical examination of the nerves impossible for subsequent examiners.

Note that every patient with a laceration should be questioned about **tetanus status.** Depending on the type of injury and the individual's tetanus immunization history, he or she may require an immunization or booster (Table 1).

Wound Preparation

After the anesthetic has been administered and the patient is resting comfortably, the wound can be examined at leisure and thoroughly cleaned. It is extremely important to remove all dirt and foreign debris from the wound prior to closure. In some emergency departments, a pulsed irrigation system is available; it is quite effective at cleansing large wounds. An alternative irrigation system for smaller wounds can be easily constructed using a standard, one-liter, plastic bottle of saline (Figure 1). Another method for cleaning wounds prior to closure entails the judicious use of a surgical scrub solution (such as Betadine) in conjunction with a scrub brush (found at the sinks of all operating rooms). If you do choose to use a surgical scrub solution, be sure to rinse the wound out thoroughly prior to closure.

In wounds that are contaminated with tar or tar-based materials, rinsing with saline is not very efficacious, and it can be difficult to completely remove all the debris from the wound. A helpful trick is to apply a petroleum-based antibiotic ointment, such as Bacitracin, which acts

History of Adsorbed Tetanus Toxoid	Tetanus-Diphtheria Toxoid*	Tetanus Immune Globulin
Clean/Minor Wounds		
Unknown	Yes	No
< 3 doses	Yes	No
≥ 3 doses	No (unless >10 years since last dose)	No
Contaminated/Dirty Wounds		
Unknown	Yes	Yes
< 3 doses	Yes	Yes
≥ 3 doses	No (unless > 5 years since last dose)	No

TABLE 1. Tetanus Dosing for New Wounds

* For children less than 7 years old, diphtheria, pertussis, and tetanus (DPT) is used instead of tetanus-diphtheria (Td).
Adapted from Centers for Disease Control: Tetanus—United States, 1987 and 1988. MMWR 39:37, 1990.

as a solvent to dissolve the tar and makes its removal much easier.

Once the wound has been irrigated and cleared of all dirt and foreign debris, avail yourself of this excellent opportunity to complete your examination of the laceration and ensure that no injuries have been missed. Partial tendon lacerations often give no clues to their existence on physical examination, except for pain with attempted movement. If the laceration overlies the tendons, move the fingers and wrist through a gentle range of motion, examining these underlying tendons for partial lacerations (Figure 2). If not addressed, a partial tendon laceration may ultimately manifest itself by rupturing while the patient is attempting forceful activity, or by "triggering" when the lacerated edges become attached to adjacent tissues. Of course, a third possibility is that the partial laceration is not large enough to structurally compromise the tendon and is small enough to heal without displaced edges limiting excursion.

Remember that there are areas in which it is difficult to precisely isolate the function of a single muscle unit. For example, radial deviation of the hand can be accomplished at the wrist by the abductor pollicis longus, extensor pollicis brevis, flexor carpi radialis, or extensor carpi radialis longus. A transection of one or two of these may not be immediately obvious on wrist movement examination, but may be discovered when exploring the wound after irrigation and cleansing.

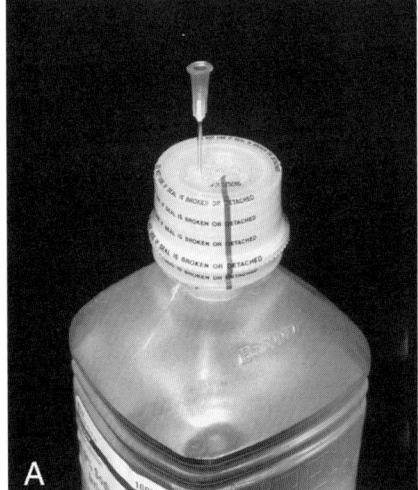 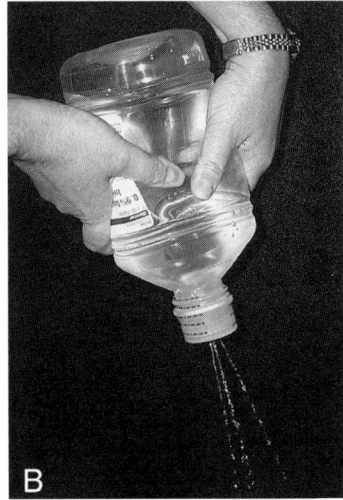

FIGURE 1. Simple construction of an irrigation device. **A,** The top of a standard, disposable, one-liter saline bottle is punctured three or four times with an 18-gauge needle. The seal is not removed, nor is the cap taken off. **B,** The saline bottle is then inverted and used to spray-irrigate the wound.

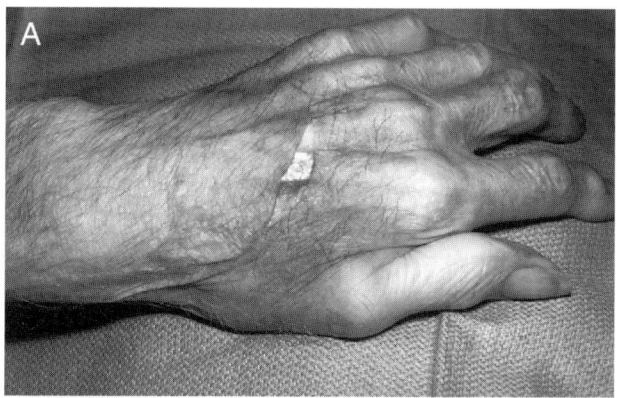

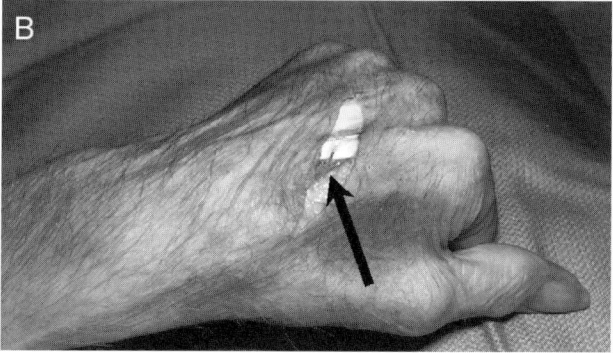

FIGURE 2. A partial tendon laceration. **A,** Inspection of the wound does not immediately demonstrate this injury, and full extension is possible because it is a *partial* transection. **B,** The tendon is drawn forward with finger flexion, exposing the partial tendon laceration. Always inspect underlying structures prior to closure of skin lacerations.

DEBRIDEMENT

Complete cleaning allows evaluation of the skin edges to determine if debridement is necessary. The purpose of debridement is to remove from the wound all **nonviable tissue** (dead or destined to die) because it can provide a nidus of infection. The caveat in this setting, however, is for *judicious* trimming of the skin edges, removing only what is necessary. Quite commonly there is an adjacent area of abrasion in which the epithelium has been scraped off but the dermis remains intact. Abraded skin does *not* need to be debrided. It will re-epithelize (assuming that it remains viable). Any areas of skin that are of questionable viability can be left intact and, if required, debrided by a hand surgeon at a later date.

The main question to ask when determining whether tissue needs to be debrided or not is: Is the area **viable?** Tests of vascularity are also tests of viability. Does the area bleed when stuck with a needle? Tissue requiring debridement often is dark blue or black in color and has tenuous attachments remaining. Additionally, it does not bleed when cut.

Wound Closure

After examination, irrigation, final evaluation, and debridement if necessary, the wound is ready for closure. Nearly all lacerations of the hand and forearm can be adequately repaired with a 4–0 or 5–0 nylon suture. Closure in layers (i.e., placing absorbable sutures in the deep tissues) is rarely necessary, particularly in an emergency setting. The most important aspect of closing the wound with sutures is obtaining good eversion of the wound edges. This is even more critical, as well as being doubly difficult to achieve, in the thick skin of the palm of the hand. The best suture technique, particularly on

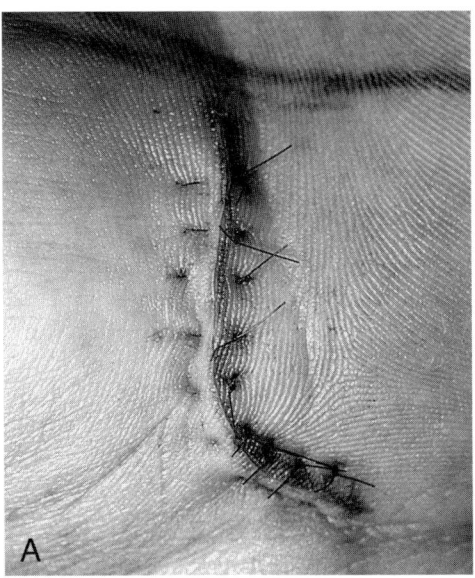
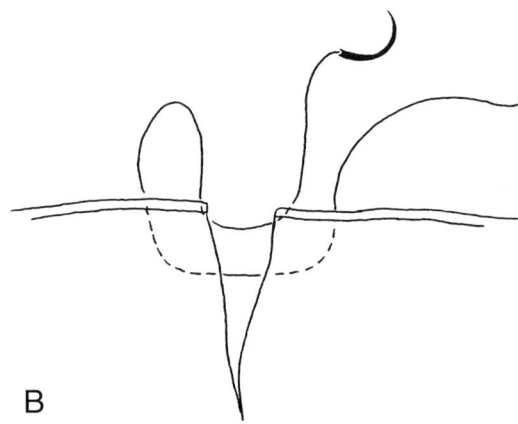

FIGURE 3. **A,** Mattress sutures result in good skin eversion, which is particularly difficult to obtain in the thick skin of the palm of the hand (as here). Note that these sutures are "interrupted," meaning that each suture is individually tied rather than running together in a row. **B,** To place a mattress suture, perform the first pass in the normal fashion. However, instead of tying the knot at this point, pass the suture approximately 1 ml back from each skin edge. Then tie the knot.

the palm of the hand, is the judicious placement of **mattress sutures** (Figure 3).

Sutures can be "interrupted," meaning that each stitch is individually tied (Figure 4). Al-

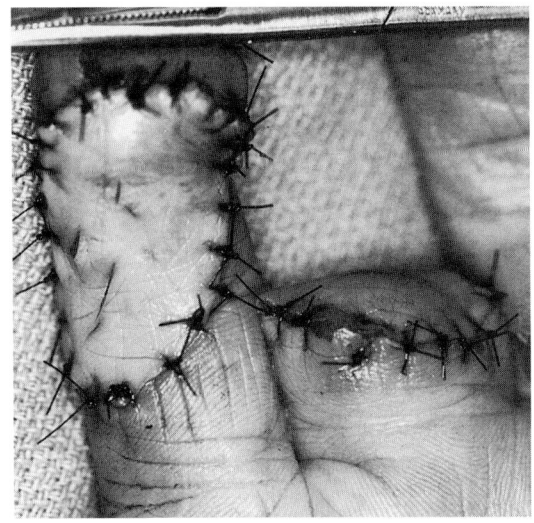

FIGURE 4. Interrupted sutures. Each suture is placed individually and tied.

though it takes more time to place interrupted sutures than "running" sutures, the interrupted method allows easier eversion of the skin edges. In addition, one or two sutures can be easily removed during the recuperation period, if necessary, without undoing the entire repair. Finally, the placement of an occasional mattress stitch between simple sutures is easier. A running suture entails placing several stitches in a row before tying a knot (Figure 5). Running sutures are somewhat quicker to place because you are not tying multiple knots.

Sutures in the hand and forearm should be left in place for 2–3 weeks. Schedule at least two post-injury visits: the first should be 3–5 days after the repair for a "wound check." The purpose of this early check is to verify that no signs of infection or early cellulitis are evident. The second appointment is scheduled 2–3 weeks after the repair for suture removal.

After the laceration has been repaired, give the patient prescriptions for an antibiotic and an analgesic. The antibiotic choice is tailored to the type of injury (and therefore aimed at certain pathogens) and the patient's allergies (Table 2). The analgesic is selected based on the amount of pain the patient is expected to have. For minor injuries, a nonsteroidal anti-inflammatory drug (NSAID) may be appropriate. For more severe injuries, acetaminophen with codeine (Tylenol #3), acetaminophen with oxycodone (Percocet), or meperidol (Demerol) are other options (Table 3).

Dressing and Post-Injury Care

Antibiotic ointment should be applied to the repaired incision and sutures, and the sutures should be covered with a nonadherent dressing (such as Adaptic or Xeroflo) and then wrapped in a soft dressing such as Kerlex. Depending on the size or nature of the injury, various types of splinting may be advisable for the patient's comfort in the first 48–72 hours after injury. If only a single digit is involved, immobilization with an alumifoam splint may be appropriate (Figure 6). If the injury is more proximal or more extensive, place the patient in a volar supportive splint in a "safe position" (Figure 7). The patient is much more comfortable in the post-injury period if the hand is immobilized and elevated (especially at night). If there are no other underlying injuries, discontinue the immobilization after 72 hours, and encourage the patient to begin gentle motion of the hand and digits. While immobilization is useful in reducing pain (particularly pain due to swelling), prolonged immobilization can lead to stiffness of

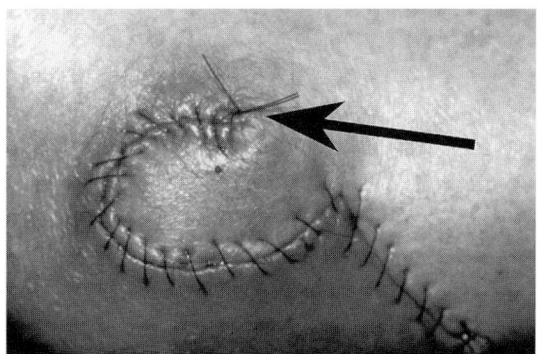

FIGURE 5. A running suture. Multiple sutures are placed after the first knot (*arrow*). The final tie is not visible here.

the hand, wrist, and digits. Stiffness usually is not an issue for a patient splinted for only a week or two, but longer periods can lead to trouble down the road. In addition, gentle active and passive range of motion can be beneficial, particularly in reducing swelling of the injured part, which will also go a long way toward limiting pain.

Deep Structure Involvement

The question will arise as to when is it acceptable to repair a laceration in the acute setting if there is deep structure involvement. For example, the examining physician may diagnose the transection of several flexor tendons in a patient with a volar wrist laceration. When is hand surgical consultation emergently required, and at

TABLE 2. Common Antibiotics Given After Laceration Repair		
Antibiotic	**Usual Adult Dose**	**Usual Child Dose**
Cephalexin	500 mg qid	40 mg/kg/day divided qid
Amoxicillin	500 mg tid	40 mg/kg/day divided tid
Amoxicillin/clavulanate (Augmentin)	500/125–800/125 bid	25 mg/kg/day divided bid
Erythromycin	333 mg tid	40 mg/kg/day divided qid
Ampicillin/clavulanate (Unisyn)	1.5–3.0 g IV q 6hr	100–200 mg/kg/day divided q 6hr

qid=four times daily, tid=three times daily, bid=twice daily

TABLE 3. Common Analgesics for Treating Hand Injury Pain	
Analgesic	**Usual Adult Dose**
Ibuprofen	800 mg po tid with meals
Tylenol #3	1 or 2 tablets q 4 hr prn
Percocet	1 tablet q 6 hr prn
Demerol	50–100 mg q 4 hr prn

Note: the level of analgesia increases from ibuprofen to Demerol
prn = as required

what point can it be deferred for repair on an elective basis? With the exception of acute arterial injuries, lacerations in which deep structures are involved usually can be closed acutely, with definitive treatment of the other injuries deferred. This course of action *must* be discussed and confirmed with the ultimate treating surgeon prior to execution, to ensure that all parties agree with the treatment plan. Surgical treatment of in-

juries is easiest and most efficacious in the acute setting. However, the reality of current practice may dictate that treatment be delayed for several days due to practical considerations such as operating room staffing and physician availability. For most of these injuries, in an uncomplicated setting, deferral of definitive treatment of the deep structures does not compromise patient care and results.

DAMAGE TO EXTENSOR TENDONS

If a patient presents with a dorsal hand or forearm laceration in which the underlying extensor tendons have been cut, the skin laceration can be repaired and the patient splinted in extension until definitive treatment of the tendons can be performed electively (Figure 8). This repair should be *scheduled* to occur within

FIGURE 6. **A,** The alumifoam splint for immobilization of a single digit is easily malleable and well padded. **B,** Place the foam padding against the skin, remembering to keep the finger and the wrist in the "safe" position, with the interphalangeal (IP) joints extended, the metacarpophalangeal (MCP) joints slightly flexed, and the wrist slightly extended. It is much easier to hold the apparatus in position when the entire splint is used. Take care not to pinch the finger tip when folding the alumifoam splint over on itself (*single arrow*). By leaving the splint long (*double arrows*), it is more easily held in place with an overlying ace bandage.

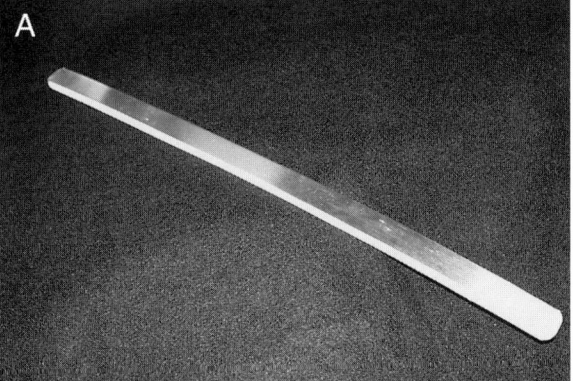

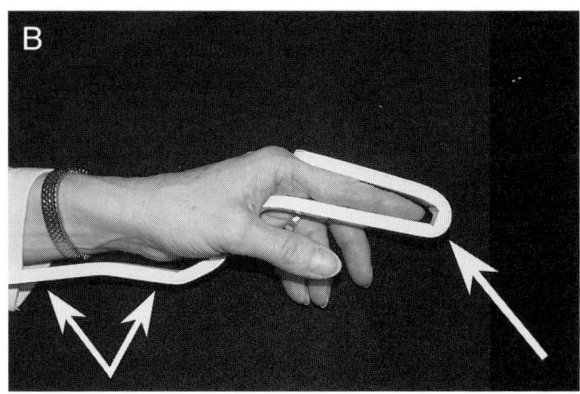

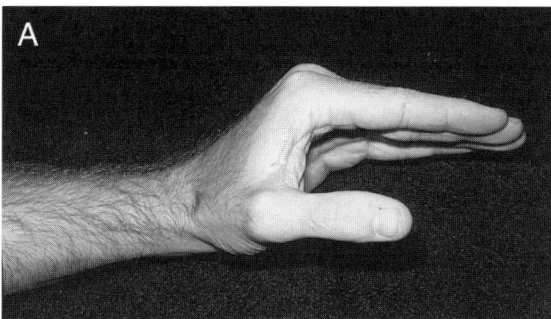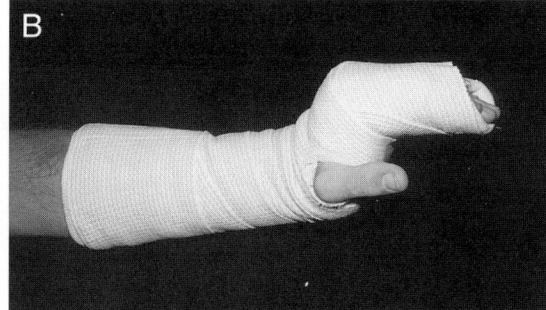

FIGURE 7. **A,** The safe hand position, in which prolonged immobilization does not result in irretractable joint stiffness. The wrist is dorsiflexed approximately 20 degrees; the MCP joints are flexed approximately 70 degrees; and the IP joints are fully extended. The thumb is abducted to prevent contracture of the first web space. **B,** A hand splinted in the safe position. For instructions on splint construction, see Chapter 6.

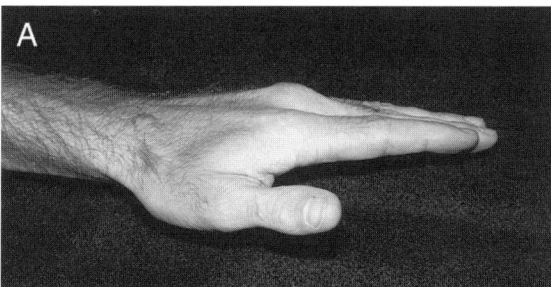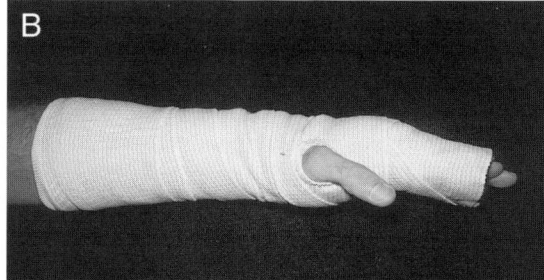

FIGURE 8. **A,** Desired hand position when splinting a patient with an extensor tendon injury prior to surgical repair. The wrist is extended to approximately 20 degrees, and the MCP joints are in neutral or slightly flexed 10–20 degrees, with the fingers in full extension. This position safeguards the extensor tendons from excessive tension. **B,** A hand in a volar splint after an extensor tendon injury.

1–2 weeks after injury. See Chapter 6 for specific instructions on splint construction.

DAMAGE TO FLEXOR TENDONS

If flexor tendon injury is diagnosed, the skin laceration can be repaired in the emergency department, with definitive treatment of the flexor tendon(s) deferred. In contrast to extensor tendon injuries, the fingers and wrist should be splinted in flexion (Figure 9). Splinting in flexion puts the finger flexors at a mechanical disadvantage and blocks powerful contraction of these muscles, thereby avoiding displacement of the proximal tendon which could make ultimate repair more difficult. In contrast to other splinting methods, maintaining the fingers and

wrist in a flexed posture is most easily accomplished with a *dorsally based* splint.

Injuries to extensor or flexor tendons should be evaluated by a hand surgeon as soon as possible, within a week at most; surgical repair should be performed within 2–3 weeks of injury. See Chapter 6 for specific instructions on splint construction.

FRACTURES

If a fracture is relatively nondisplaced, the presence of an overlying laceration does not confer urgency to reduction and/or fixation. The extensive literature concerning "open fractures" applies mainly to severely comminuted fractures of the lower extremities with associated massive

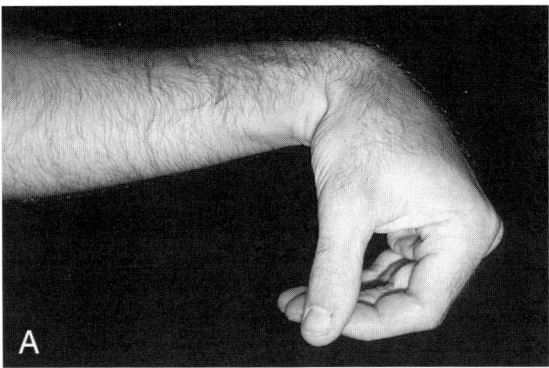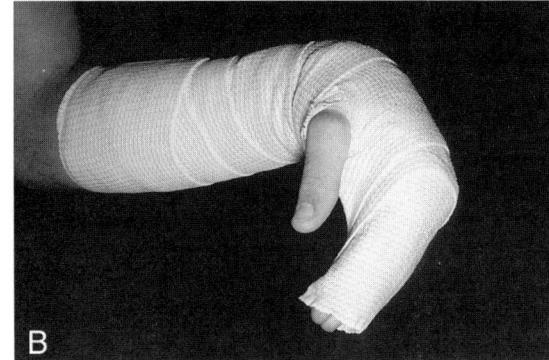

FIGURE 9. **A,** Desired hand position for immobilization after flexor tendon injury. Note that the wrist, MCP joints, and fingers are flexed. Wrist flexion should be at least 20 degrees *less* than full flexion to minimize patient discomfort. **B,** A hand splinted for flexor tendon injuries.

soft tissue damage. In these injuries of the lower extremity, serial irrigation and debridement are necessary prior to wound closure, while in the hand delayed closure usually is not required unless massive contamination is present. It is incorrect to extrapolate data concerning lower extremity fractures and apply it to the hand. A relatively nondisplaced phalangeal or metacarpal fracture can be splinted after repair of any associated lacerations, and fixation (if necessary) can be deferred. However, in a severely comminuted open fracture, or in a fracture that is displaced through the laceration, urgent hand surgical consultation usually is required.

DAMAGE TO NERVES OR ARTERIES

A laceration that involves a major nerve often has injured other structures as well. Remember that many of the nerves of the upper extremity are closely associated with an adjacent artery (e.g., the ulnar artery and nerve, the neurovascular bundles of the fingers). Evidence of injury to these nerves on physical exam should raise the level of suspicion of an occult arterial injury (if not already diagnosed).

If the artery has been *completely* transected, vasospasm can temporarily stop the hemorrhage, making the diagnosis of arterial injury more difficult to ascertain. In addition, collateral flow may

sufficiently perfuse the tissues distal to the injury, leaving no evidence of vascular insufficiency. An example is complete perfusion of the hand (via the ulnar artery) after radial artery thrombosis. However, vasospasm can reverse, causing significant bleeding later if not addressed. An *incomplete* transection of one of the major arteries of the forearm represents one of the few truly life-threatening injuries to the upper extremity: because the cut ends cannot seal by vasospasm, the hemorrhage persists until it is occluded.

When an arterial injury is suspected or diagnosed, urgent evaluation by a hand surgeon is mandated. If arterial injury is excluded, the presence of a nerve injury does not demand emergent surgical treatment. A laceration overlying a nerve transection can be closed and the patient splinted in a safe position (see Figure 7).

As most trauma surgeons realize, treatment of a traumatic injury is easiest immediately after the occurrence. However, certain real-life pressures may preclude immediate, definitive care. When that is the case, the treatment plan should be balanced with an eye towards optimal patient care at all times.

Antibiotics

Most patients should receive antibiotics for at least several days after repair of a laceration of the hand or forearm. The duration of antibiotic administration may be lengthened in those injuries that are at a higher risk for developing an infection (i.e., contaminated or dirty wounds). The choice of antibiotic is tempered by the patient's allergies (if any), as well as the mechanism or etiology of the injury. In general, good coverage against gram-positive organisms is required. A third-generation cephalosporin, such as cephalexin, provides adequate coverage in most circumstances. If the patient has a documented allergy to this drug, alternatives such as erythromycin, amoxicillin, or augmentin can be considered (see Table 2).

Bite Wounds

ANIMAL BITES

Since there is a wide variety of both gram-negative and gram-positive organisms in the normal oral flora of animals, broader antibiotic coverage is necessary. Typically, *Pasteurella multocida,* a facultative anaerobe, is the offending organism in post-bite cellulitis. For these reasons, amoxicillin/clavulanate (oral) or ampicillin/clavulanate (parenteral) is currently the drug of choice when treating dog or cat bites.

Diligent irrigation and cleansing of these wounds is mandatory. If a patient presents with multiple small puncture wounds, suture repair usually is not indicated. Due to the heavily contaminated nature of the inoculum (saliva), it is the better part of valor to allow multiple small lacerations to heal by secondary intention, with the patient applying antibiotic ointment a few times a day and taking oral antibiotics. If the patient presents with a larger laceration, the wound can be loosely closed with interrupted sutures after thorough irrigation.

Cat bites can be particularly aggressive in terms of infection, rapidly progressing to a severe cellulitis requiring parenteral antibiotics and hospitalization (Figures 10, 11). These

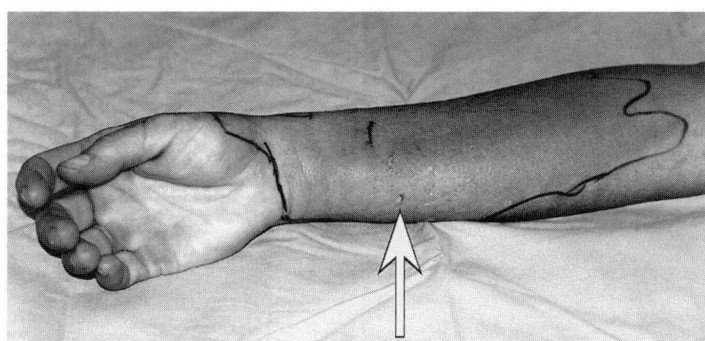

FIGURE 10. This patient presented 24 hours after suffering a cat bite on the volar mid-forearm. The degree of erythema is *outlined;* the *arrow* points to the puncture wound. Cat bites can be particularly aggressive, with rapid progression of cellulitis. Prompt administration of antibiotics and very close observation is mandatory.

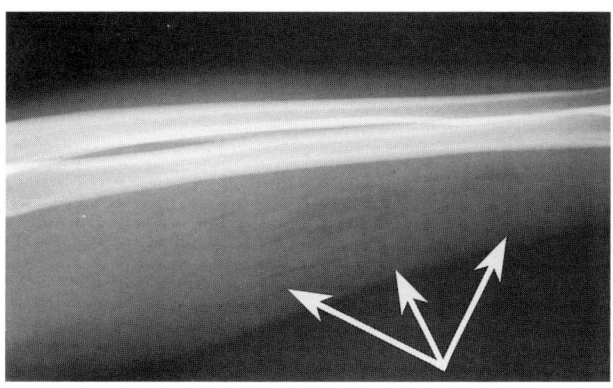

FIGURE 11. Radiograph of the injury in Figure 10, demonstrating subcutaneous air within the soft tissues of the forearm (*arrows*). The presence of soft tissue air (diagnosed either by radiograph or by palpation of crepitance on physical exam) represents a surgical emergency, mandating prompt exploration and debridement in the operating room.

wounds (if treated in the outpatient setting) *must be closely followed* (at least once a day) until the erythema begins to resolve. Maintain a very low threshold for admitting these patients to administer parenteral antibiotics: cat bites have a propensity for rapid advancement of cellulitis even after antibiotics have been started.

HUMAN BITES

Human bites have the reputation of being one of the dirtiest types of wound encountered. In the setting of hand injuries, it is rare to see a formal bite. Much more common (and less obvious as a human bite to the uninitiated) is an injury resulting from fisticuffs, in which the

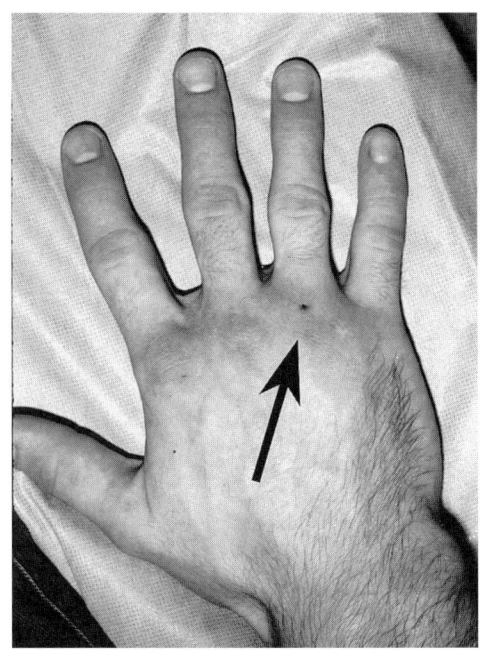

FIGURE 13. A patient who suffered a small cut (*arrow*) near an MCP joint from striking his opponent in the mouth. He complained of localized tenderness and intermittent drainage. Therefore, despite minimal erythema and swelling, emergent surgical exploration was undertaken (see Figure 14).

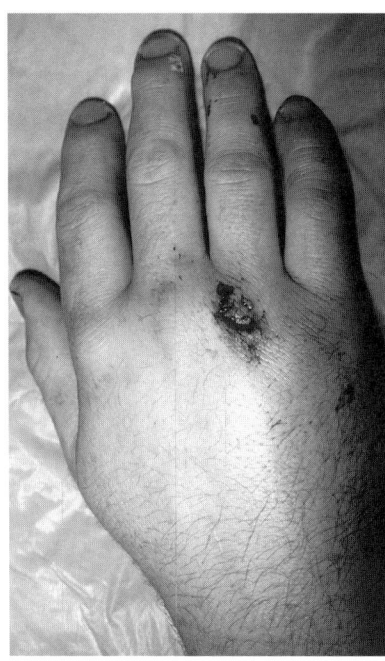

FIGURE 12. This patient presented to the emergency department with a cut over the metacarpophalangeal (MCP) joint of his ring finger, suffered in a fight the night before. Note the diffuse hand swelling. He complained of pain and tenderness around the inoculation site. This wound is considered a human bite because it was created on the opponent's teeth.

assailant (now your patient) has struck an opponent in the mouth and cut his or her hand on the opponent's teeth (Figures 12, 13). This type of injury (by definition) is a human bite; it should be treated aggressively with irrigation, cleaning, and antibiotics. The drug of choice is the same as for animal bites: amoxicillin/clavulanate or ampicillin/clavulanate. Human bites, regardless of location, are rarely closed with sutures. Closing (suturing) a wound that likely still contains organisms risks converting a simple wound into an abscess. The dirtier the wound, the less likely simple suture closure (at least in the acute setting) is appropriate.

Injuries of this nature commonly occur at and around one of the MCP joints of the dominant hand. If this is the case, urgent referral to a hand specialist is indicated: inoculation or penetration of the MCP joint must be explored

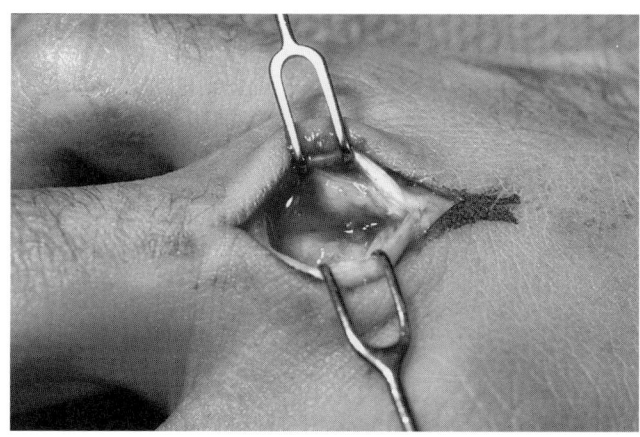

FIGURE 14. Intraoperative view of injury in Figure 13. Exploration demonstrated purulence within the MCP joint. Treatment consisted of thorough irrigation and debridement of the joint area, closure of the wound by secondary intention, and administration of parenteral antibiotics.

and irrigated emergently in the operating room (Figure 14). Failure to recognize and refer this type of injury can lead to the formation of a septic, infected joint at the MCP level. Pyogenic arthritis of the joint can result in severe deformity and disability. While referral and prompt surgical intervention may not prevent an infection at the joint, failure to recognize and aggressively treat this type of injury can expose the primary care physician to liability.

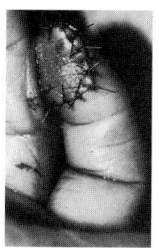

Amputations and Soft Tissue Loss

5

A spectrum of tissue loss presents to the physician in the emergency department setting, ranging from loss of a small piece of fingertip skin to amputation of an entire finger to loss of the whole hand. Since some distal amputations of the finger are essentially treated as soft tissue loss (i.e., treatment focuses on coverage or closure of the wound rather than replantation), both topics are discussed together in this chapter.

Replantation

The microsurgical ability necessary to replant an amputated finger or hand was developed in the 1960s. Refinements in techniques and tools have lead to a uniformly high survival rate of the digit after replantation. The early criterion of "biologic survival" as a measure of success has now been tempered by a more critical analysis of **function** after replantation. Patients require myriad hospital-based resources following surgery, and the rehabilitation process is lengthy. If a replanted digit has poor sensation or cannot move because of scarring around the tendons, the hand's function is decreased, and the patient would have been better served with simple wound closure. Revision amputation (i.e., revising the amputation to allow primary closure) offers the benefits of little or no hospitalization and a quicker return to work. Therefore, patients are screened more carefully prior to replantation today than in the 1970s and 1980s.

RELATIVE INDICATIONS AND CONTRAINDICATIONS

There are several relative indications and relative contraindications for replantation. The term "relative" is used because every situation is unique, and each patient's circumstances should be carefully evaluated and taken into account. The suggestions that follow are only *general guidelines*—they are not meant to be absolute criteria. All patients with an amputation should have the opportunity to meet and discuss their injury with a hand surgeon so that they can make informed decisions about their medical treatment. Thus, the patient who chooses replantation (even if relative contraindications exist) is fully informed preoperatively about the length of surgery and hospitalization required and (even more importantly) the extent of postoperative therapy necessary.

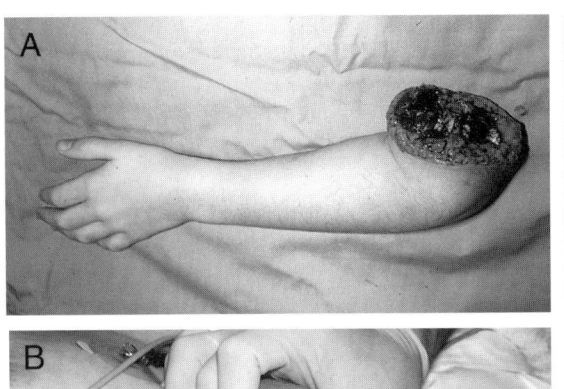
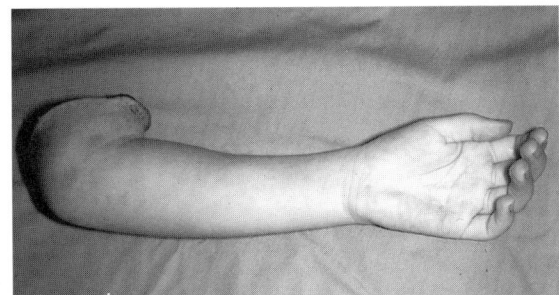
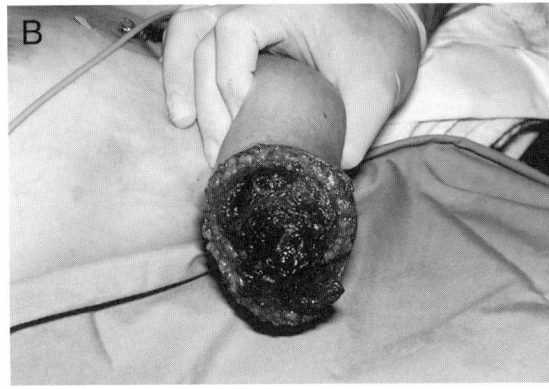
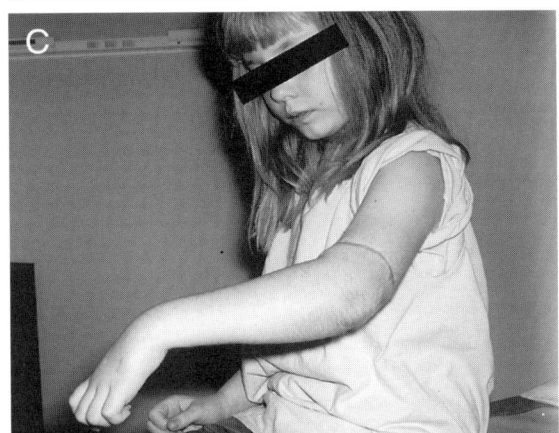
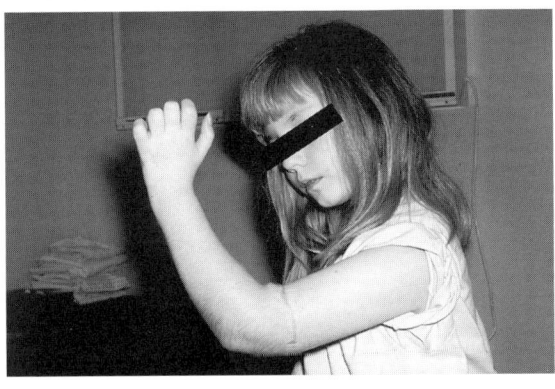

FIGURE 1. **A,** Amputated arm at the mid-humerus of an 8-year-old girl. Due to the large amount of muscle tissue in an amputation at this level, the child was rushed to a replantation center to re-establish perfusion as quickly as possible. **B,** The proximal stump. Reperfusion of the arm was accomplished approximately 6 hours following amputation. **C,** Postoperative result 6 months after major limb replantation, demonstrating wrist and elbow flexion and extension. A year after replantation, she had regained sensation in her hand and fingers (although to a lesser degree than her noninjured hand) and was able to perform independent, isolated finger flexion and extension. This case underscores the principle that children generally experience excellent recovery after replantation. An adult would not be expected to have such a dramatic return of neural function after the same injury.

Any amputated part on a child is a **relative indication** for replantation, because children tend to enjoy favorable results after replantation (Figures 1, 2). Any type of thumb amputation is a relative indication for replantation (Figure 3). The thumb contributes so much to the function of the hand, and its loss is so devastating, that every possible effort should be made to preserve it. Additionally, the thumb has such a high

degree of mobility that joint stiffness typically does not impair function as much as it does in the fingers. Moreover, unlike finger joint stiffness, thumb joint stiffness does not impair movement of adjacent digits because the thumb's flexor and extensor tendons have a different origin.

Multiple digit amputation also is a relative indication for replantation, because the loss of

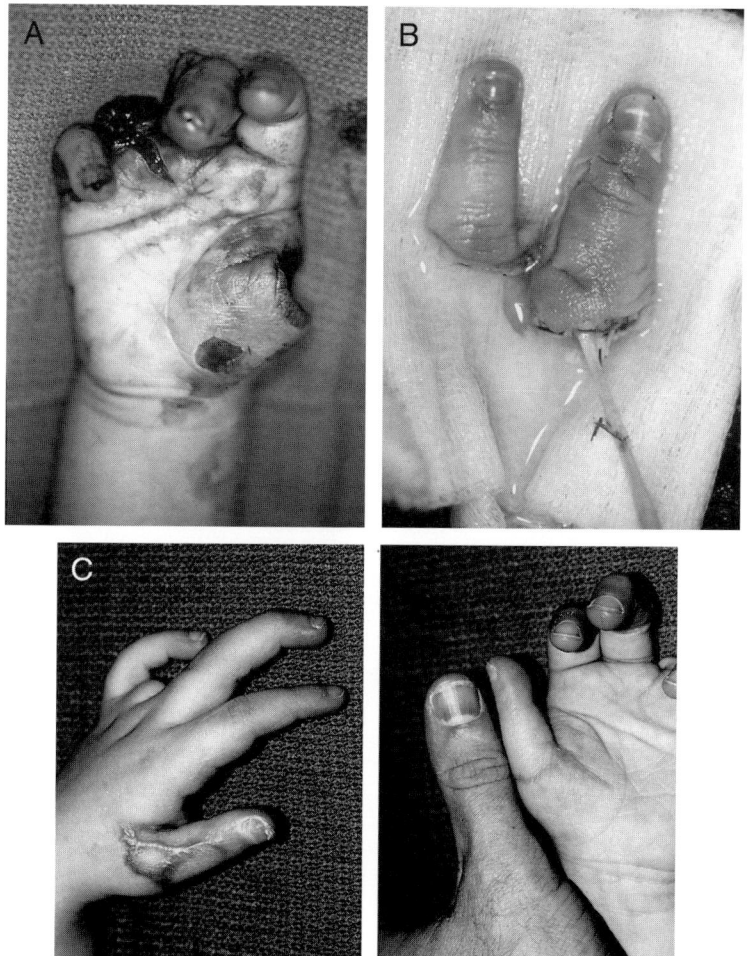

FIGURE 2. **A,** The hand of a two-year-old with amputation of the thumb and ring finger after the child fell from a riding lawn mower driven by his father. **B,** The thumb and ring finger after retrieval from the riding mower's mulching attachment (note the grass clippings and debris). **C,** Seven months after successful replantation of the thumb. The ring finger was too badly damaged in the mulcher and could not be replanted. The author's thumb is shown for size comparison.

function after the loss of several digits can be devastating to overall hand function (Figures 4, 5). A final relative indication for replantation is any amputation distal to the insertion of the flexor digitorum superficialis (zone 1; Figures 6, 7). These replanted digits tend to do well, have good return of sensation, and usually don't have problems with finger stiffness. There is only one flexor tendon to repair, eliminating the potential for scarring between the tendons, which can block motion.

Two of the strongest **contraindications** to replantation are crush and avulsion injuries (Figures 8, 9). Avulsion injuries are, unfortunately, a common mechanism of finger amputation. A typical scenario is one in which a glove gets caught in machinery and is pulled off, along with part or all of the hand. A subtype of

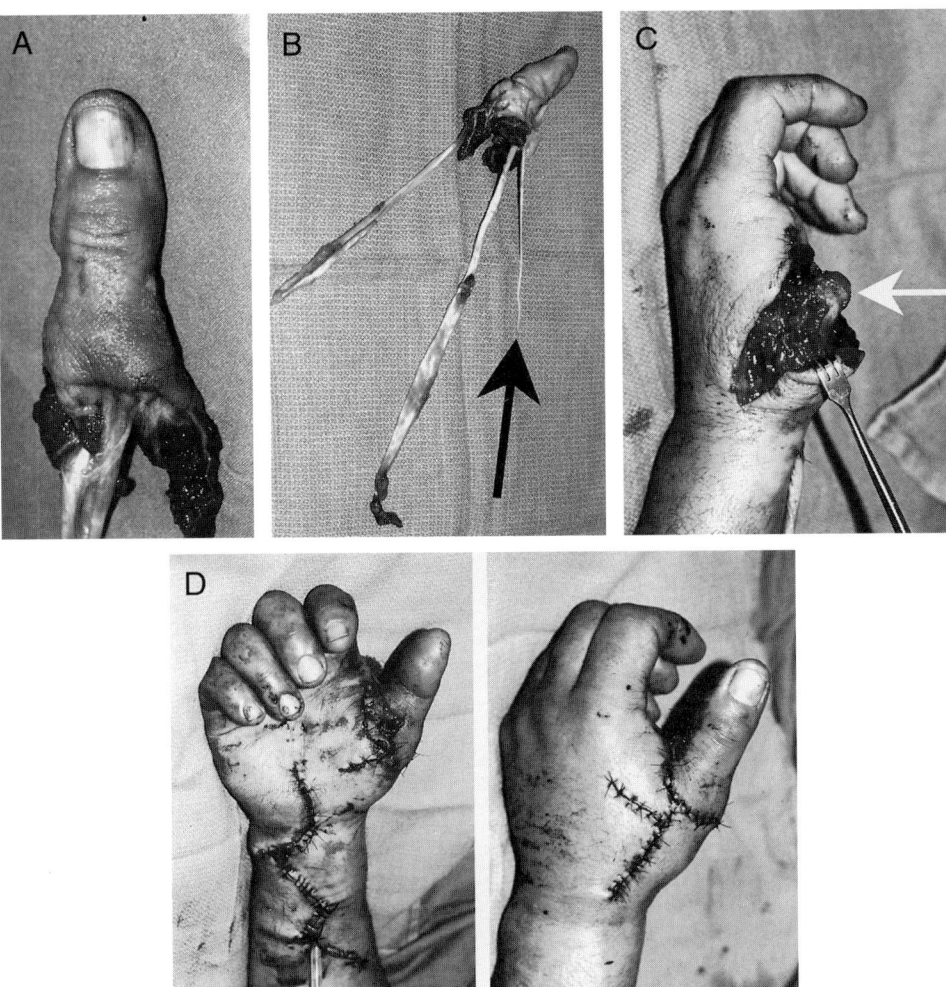

FIGURE 3. **A,** Thumb amputation from an avulsion injury. **B,** The mechanism of the injury is demonstrated by the fact that the extensor and flexor tendons have been pulled from the proximal forearm and separated from their musculotendinous junctions. In addition, the digital nerves (*arrow*) also have been avulsed from the median nerve proximal to the wrist. There is a relative indication for proceeding with replantation (thumb), as well as a relative contraindication (avulsion-type injury). **C,** Exposed distal metacarpal (*arrow*) demonstrating the level of amputation. **D,** Immediate postoperative views show successful replantation of the avulsed thumb.

this injury is "ring avulsion," in which the patient's ring is caught on some object and the finger is pulled off or degloved of its soft tissue (Figures 10, 11). Avulsion injuries have a much poorer prognosis than amputations that occur as a result of a clean cut, due to the severe damage sustained by the vasculature. Avulsion injuries are extremely destructive to the arteries, be-

cause the intimal layer becomes stretched and severely damaged both proximally and distally until the vessel is actually transected. Even a successful microvascular anastomosis in this setting is doomed to thrombose if the damaged portion of the artery is not resected and replaced with vein graft.

If there are multiple levels of injury within

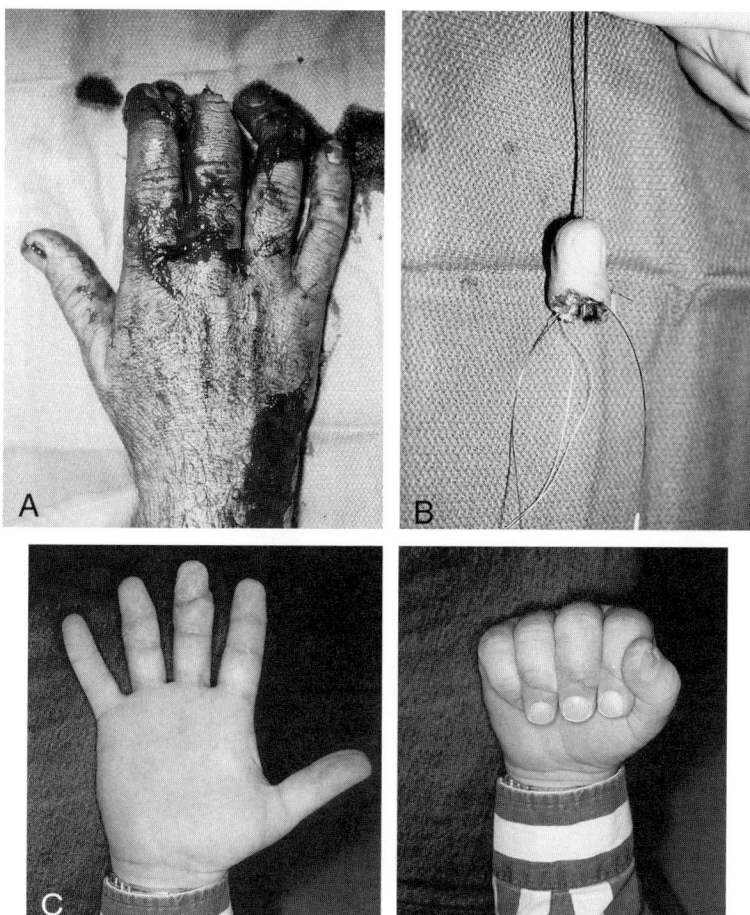

FIGURE 4. **A,** Construction worker who suffered amputations of his long, ring, and index fingers at the distal interphalangeal level. During the history taking in the preoperative setting, the patient related that he was an amateur guitarist. If revision amputation had been the procedure selected, he most likely would have been unable to resume that avocation. **B,** Amputated segment of the long finger after preparation for replantation. **C,** One year after multiple finger replantation, demonstrating full extension and flexion.

the amputated part, or multiple amputations of the same part (for example, a finger amputated at both the distal and proximal interphalangeal joints), replantation is contraindicated. Typically, injuries as severe as these are unlikely to gain a reasonable amount of function, and the digits are destined to be stiff and insensate. Another relative contraindication is the replantation in an adult of a single digit within zone 2 (Figure 12). Zone 2 runs from the metacarpophalangeal joints to the mid-level of the

middle phalanges (see Figure 6). In this area, the flexor digitorum superficialis and flexor digitorum profundus are both transected within the fibro-osseous tunnel. Fingers replanted at this level often are troubled with recurrent tendon adhesions between these two tendons, making the finger stiff and limiting the function of the adjacent (uninjured) fingers. Remember that the tendons of the flexor digitorum profundus have a common origin and do not provide independent finger flexion. If one finger is stiff, it af-

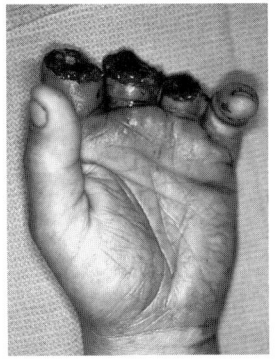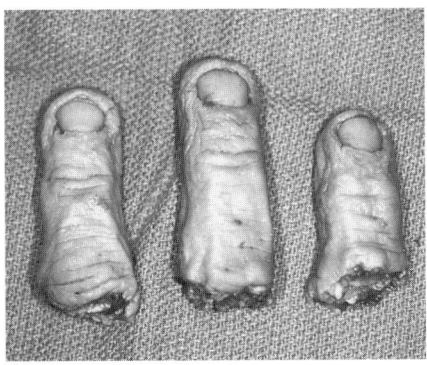

FIGURE 5. Circular saw injury. The fact that multiple digits are amputated is a relative indication for proceeding with replantation, but the location within zone 2 is a relative contraindication. Although replantations within zone 2 (see Figures 6 and 12) are prone to stiffness, the loss of three fingers is not an acceptable alternative.

fects and limits the flexion of the other fingers, as well.

A long ischemia time also is a relative contraindication to replantation. An amputated digit is relatively resistant to ischemia because there is no muscle tissue present, and skin, bone, and tendon tissues can survive for extended periods. Case reports exist of successful replantation after 24–36 hours (as long as the digit is properly stored; see next section). However, injuries to the hand proximal to the wrist require prompt restoration of blood flow, or the replantation or repair effort will fail due to muscle and soft tissue necrosis from the prolonged ischemia time.

A final relative contraindication to replantation involves the patient's general health and habits. Smoking is a notorious vasoconstrictor, and replants in smokers are prone to profound vasospasm, which can lead to loss of the replanted part. Brittle diabetics and individuals with severe cardiac or pulmonary disease may not be able to tolerate the prolonged operative procedure. In situations where pre-existing medical problems exist, consultation between the surgeon, anesthesiologist, and primary care physician is advisable to ascertain the perioperative risks and gain a consensus on the best course of action.

FIGURE 6. Zones 1 and 2 in the hand refer to flexor tendons and are commonly used to describe the level of flexor tendon injury. Zone 1 refers to the finger distal to the insertion of the flexor digitorum superficialis (FDS) tendon. Zone 2 refers to the section of the finger where the FDS and flexor digitorum profundus tendons travel closely together within the fibro-osseous tunnel (see Chapter 1, Figures 38–43). Injury location in one zone or the other has ramifications for outcome after tendon repair or replantation. Zone 2 used to be referred to as "no man's land" due to the universally poor prognosis after tendon transection at that level. However, aggressive and labor-intensive hand therapy (specifically, early controlled motion) has dramatically improved results, but the process is long, difficult, and painful for the patient.

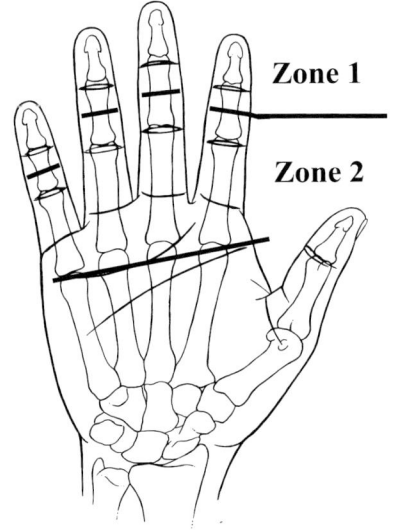

Zone 1

Zone 2

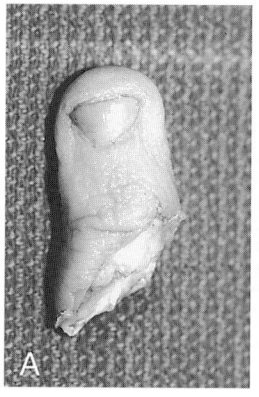
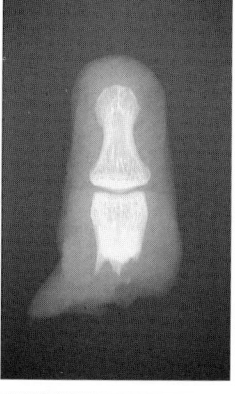

FIGURE 7. **A,** Digit amputated in zone 1 (distal to the insertion of the FDS). Amputation at this level is a relative indication for replantation due to the good prognosis for return of sensation and function. **B** and **C,** Postoperative result at 2 months showing active extension and flexion.

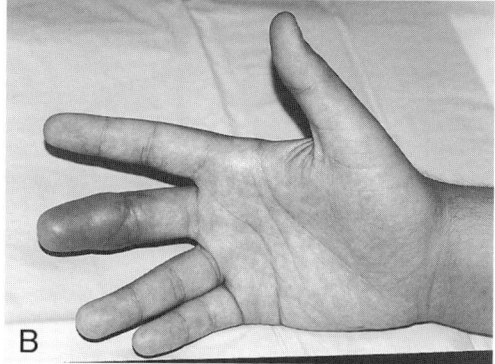
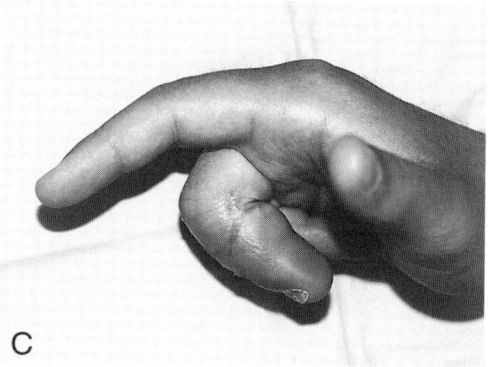

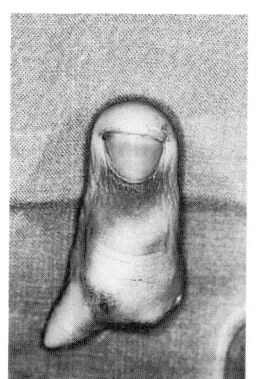
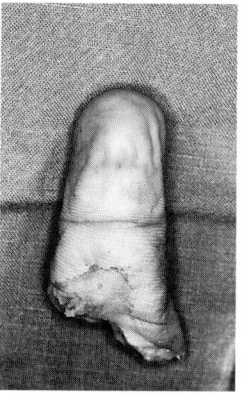

FIGURE 8. Amputated digit with severe crush injury. The mechanism is indicated on physical examination by extensive ecchymosis on the dorsal and volar aspects of the digit. The history portion of the evaluation can reveal the type of injury, as well.

PRESERVING THE AMPUTATED PART

If a patient presents with an amputated digit, proper care should be directed toward preserving the finger's viability for as long as possible (Figure 13). This is vitally important in the interval before the replantation team arrives or in preparing the patient for transport to another facility. The amputated part should be wrapped in one or two gauze sponges that are soaking wet with normal saline. The wrapped finger is then placed into a small, plastic specimen bottle (such as a urinalysis specimen cup). The container is closed and placed in a plastic bag containing an ice and water slush, with care taken to maintain a tight seal on the specimen bottle's lid. This arrangement accomplishes several things: it prevents a secondary frost-bite injury resulting from direct exposure to ice; it protects from prolonged exposure to a hypotonic solution (ice water), which also could be damaging;

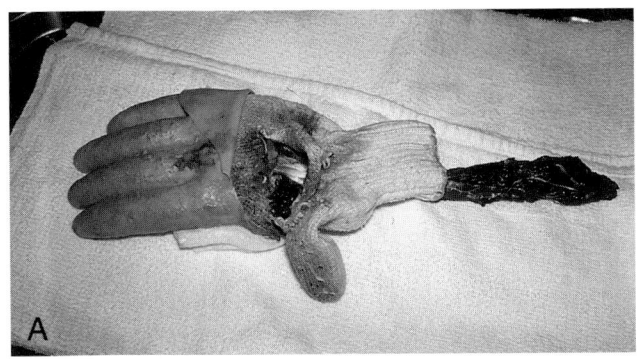

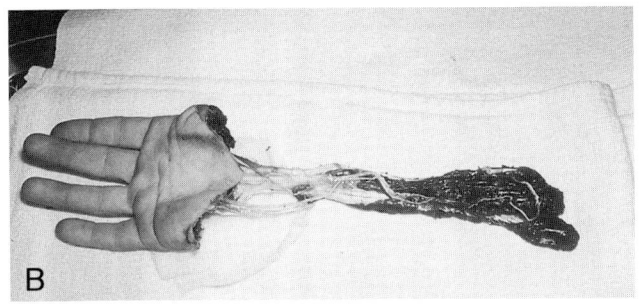

FIGURE 9. Hand avulsion injury. **A,** The glove worn by the worker is still in place over the amputated hand. **B,** The etiology of this injury is easily recognized by the attachment of the proximal flexor and extensor muscles and tendons, which were avulsed (or pulled from) the proximal forearm during the accident.

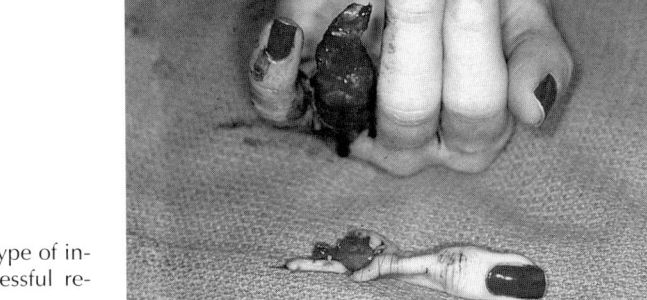

FIGURE 10. Ring avulsion. This type of injury has a poor prognosis for successful replantation.

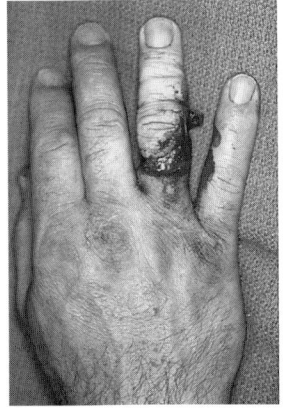
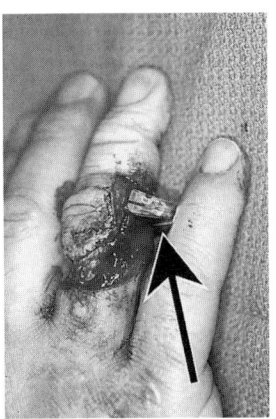

FIGURE 11. Ring avulsion (partial). This gentleman's ring caught on a hook as he was trying to remove a soccer goal net. He fell and sustained a circumferential laceration at the base of his ring finger. Although difficult to ascertain here, the finger is pale and ischemic secondary to the injury. The lateral view demonstrates that the ring remains in place on the finger (*arrow*).

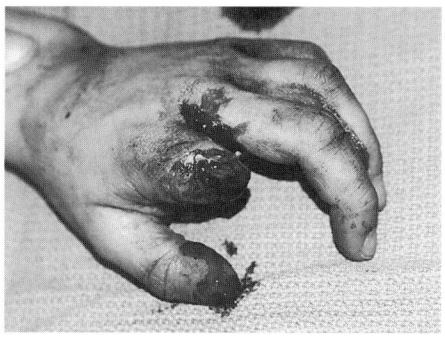
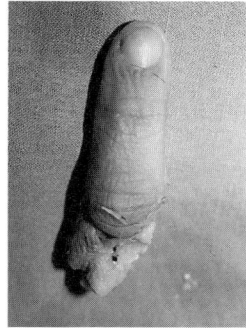

FIGURE 12. An amputation in zone 2 of the index finger. Isolated amputations at this level are a relative contraindication to replantation due to the high incidence of tendon scarring and digit stiffness. A reasonable approach to this injury may involve revision amputation.

and it maintains the amputated part in an isotonic solution at a consistently cold temperature (4°C).

A moist gauze (soaked with saline) should be placed next to and around the open wounds on the hand, and the hand should be splinted with a volar splint in a position of comfort. Keep the arm elevated to decrease any blood loss and make the patient as comfortable as possible. Consider prescribing a parenteral analgesic, such as morphine.

SUBTOTAL AMPUTATION

A subtotally amputated digit can range from a laceration with an underlying fracture, to a complete amputation attached by only a small skin bridge. The question arises as to the best way to protect and preserve these digits prior to definitive treatment. If the patient is a candidate for replantation, it may be tempting to complete the amputation, allowing the amputated part to be placed in a cold saline container to protect it from warm ischemia. However, this action is not advisable. The best way to manage this injury is to dress the hand with a soft, bulky dressing (such as a gauze wrap) and place the whole hand and forearm in a volar splint, taking care to keep the extremity in an elevated position. This management protects the finger from additional injury and maximizes patient comfort by immobilizing the hand.

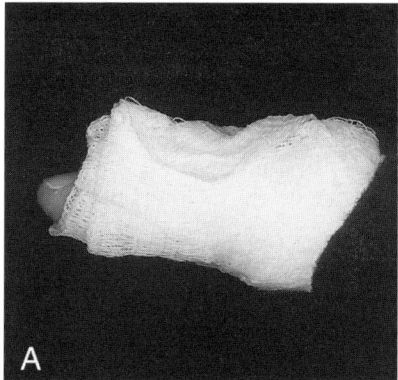
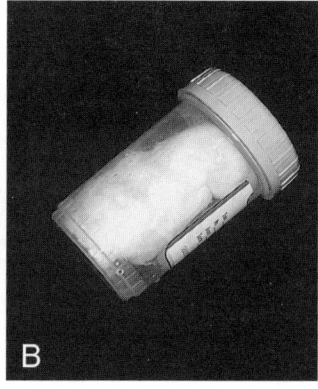
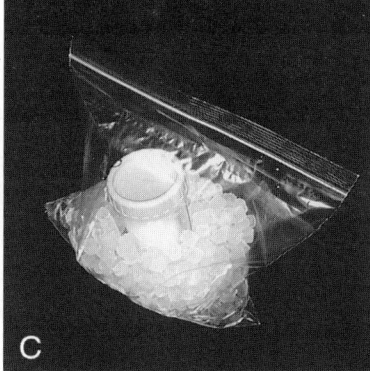

FIGURE 13. Preserving an amputated digit prior to replantation. **A,** First, wrap the digit in several gauze sponges soaked with saline. **B,** Next, place the digit and saline-soaked sponges in a container with a sealable cap. **C,** Lastly, place the sealed container in a zip-lock bag containing ice and water. This arrangement maintains the digit in contact with an isotonic solution while avoiding a secondary hypotonic injury and eliminates the possibility of secondary frost bite.

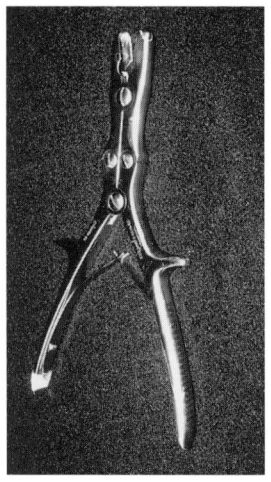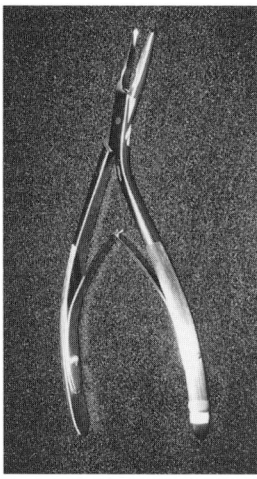

FIGURE 14. Bone rongeurs are used to slightly trim back any bone that may be protruding, to allow primary coverage of the injured digit. They are found in all operating rooms and are helpful when performing a revision amputation in the emergency department.

REVISION AMPUTATION

Patients who present with fingertip amputations and are not candidates for replantation require soft tissue coverage. Soft tissue coverage also must be addressed in patients who are not interested in replantation. In these situations, treatment often can be performed in the emergency department.

Revision amputation is a procedure for patients who are not undergoing replantation. It is relatively simple and straightforward, and can be performed in the emergency department. The goal of revision amputation is to maximize the useful length of the digit while providing good soft tissue coverage of the remaining distal bone. The procedure varies somewhat depending on the level of the amputation, but it usually entails slightly trimming the exposed bone (if necessary) so that the overlying soft tissue and skin of the finger can be closed primarily with a 4–0 or 5–0 nylon suture. Trim-

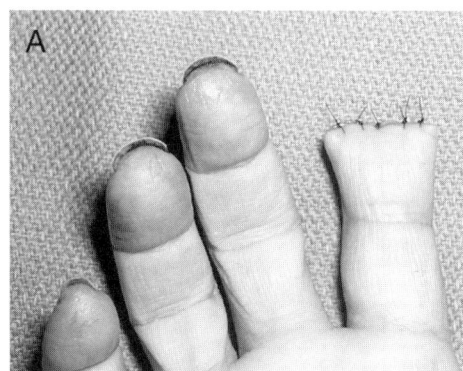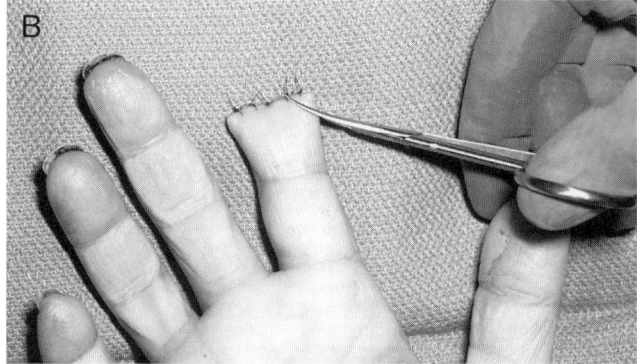

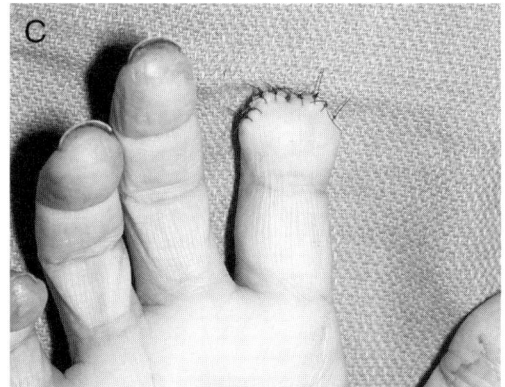

FIGURE 15. **A,** "Dog ears" or "hammer head" deformity. In a revision amputation, there often are volar and dorsal flaps which can be sutured together to obtain primary closure. The flaps must be trimmed to avoid this technical error. **B,** Following closure of the central portion of the revision amputation, the finger should be reassessed to determine if further debridement of soft tissue is necessary to avoid lateral fullness. If a dog ear is present, it is easily corrected by obliquely cutting the corner with a curved, sharp scissors. **C,** After excising the dog ear deformity, the skin edges can be reapproximated primarily.

ming may require the use of a bone rongeurs (Figure 14).

Remember that the neurovascular bundles travel on the volar lateral aspect of the fingers; therefore, they are encountered in almost all revision amputations. Care must be taken to avoid entrapment of the digital nerve within the scar of the distal fingertip, because this can be exquisitely painful for the patient. The nerves should be trimmed back and, if possible, directed away from the finger wound to avoid a sensitive posttraumatic neuroma. The cut end of the digital artery can be ligated (if necessary) with a small absorbable suture, such as a 4–0 Vicryl.

Occasionally both the flexor and extensor tendons are visible at the base of the wound. It may be tempting to attach these tendons to each other or to the distal bone. Such attachments are not a good idea: they inhibit postoperative motion not only of the affected digit, but the adjacent digits as well. If the flexor and extensor tendons are sutured together, they will block each other's action, making active flexion or extension difficult. The best course is to leave the tendons alone, and allow them to seek their own position in the postinjury setting.

After trimming the bone to the desired position, quite often the skin presents dorsal and volar flaps that can be sutured together to cover the bone. A common error in this technique is insufficient trimming of the radial and ulnar edges of these flaps, creating a "dog ears" or "hammer head" deformity (Figure 15A). Take care to trim this excess tissue at the time of the revision amputation (Figure 15B and C), because this redundancy *will not* smooth out postoperatively, and patients tend to be disturbed by the broad, flat appearance of their fingertip.

Soft Tissue Loss

Soft tissue loss from a finger is a common injury, most frequently occurring as damage to the distal tip (Figures 16, 17). For example, a patient presents to the emergency department with the end of their finger sliced off and loss of skin and underlying soft tissue. There are several treatment options available, depending on the level and amount of tissue loss:

1. Conservative management (no surgical treatment, dressing changes only)
2. Skin graft
3. Local flap coverage
4. Distant flap coverage.

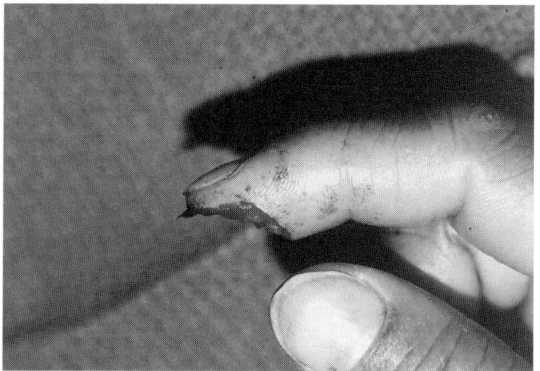

FIGURE 16. Loss of the volar skin and pulp of an index finger. Revision with primary closure will most likely result in a hooked nail deformity (see Figure 19). Revision of the wound with bone resection to allow primary closure would involve unneccessary shortening of the finger and loss of the nail. Local flaps and/or skin grafts should be considered in this situation.

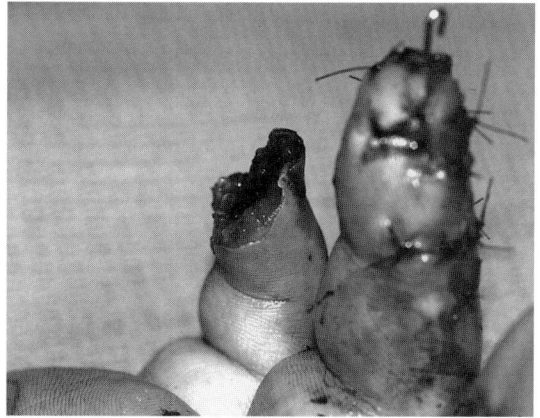

FIGURE 17. Loss of the volar surface of the fifth finger. Flap coverage of this type of deformity is necessary to prevent a hook nail deformity and to restore the pulp of the digit.

CONSERVATIVE MANAGEMENT

Wounds that are 1 centimeter in diameter or smaller without bony protrusion at the base of the wound usually heal nicely with conservative measures, allowing the wound to heal by secondary intention (Figure 18). This is particularly true for injuries in the young and the elderly, and in some circumstances the recommendation can be expanded to include wounds up to 1½ centimeters in diameter. For conservative management to be effective there should be no exposed bone, because even though a defect with bone exposure *might* heal by secondary intention, there will not be **adequate soft tissue coverage** of the fingertip, which will cause problems later. Another requirement is that the patient be able to manage the dressing changes, and do so reliably, during the healing phase.

If there is loss of a portion of the distal phalanx, which supports the nailbed matrix, a potential problem in conservative management is the development of a "parrot beak deformity" (Figure 19). This deformity also can be caused by over-aggressive suturing at the fingertip; primary closure of a wound at the tip when there is a significant amount of skin loss results in tight sutures that can "pull down" the nail matrix. The parrot beak (or hooked nail) deformity is very disturbing to the patient, and difficult to repair secondarily. It is best avoided by recognizing that when loss is significant (distal tip skin, pulp, and/or distal phalanx > 1 centimeter in diameter) it may be necessary to perform closure with a local flap to prevent late contracture.

Advantages of conservative management include: easy implementation in the emergency department; no requirements for spe-

FIGURE 18. A, Amputation of the distal tip of the ring finger. There is loss of the distal skin and a portion of the distal nail bed, but no protruding bone. This patient was treated with conservative management (dressing changes), because sufficient soft tissue was present at the base of the wound. If the patient had brought in the amputated tip, another reasonable option would have been a skin graft, which might afford quicker healing. **B,** Late results after conservative management. The wound healed with virtually no deformity of the distal skin and excellent sensation. The residual nail deformity most likely reflects injury to the nail matrix during the original amputation, but also may be partially due to scarring of the nail bed secondary to wound contracture.

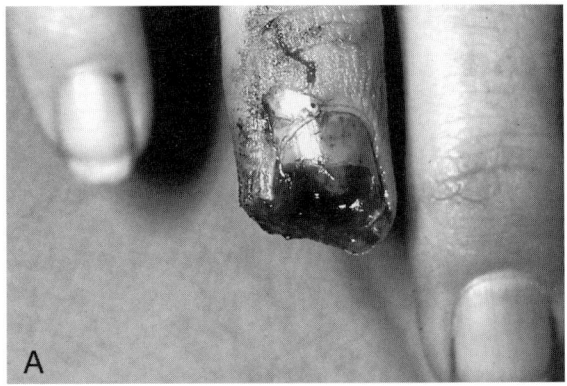

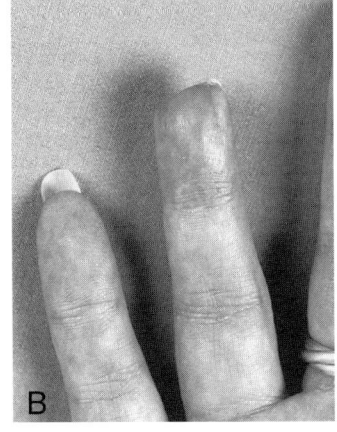
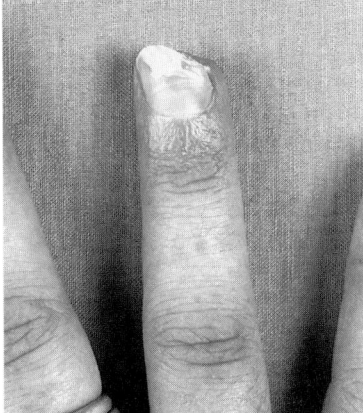

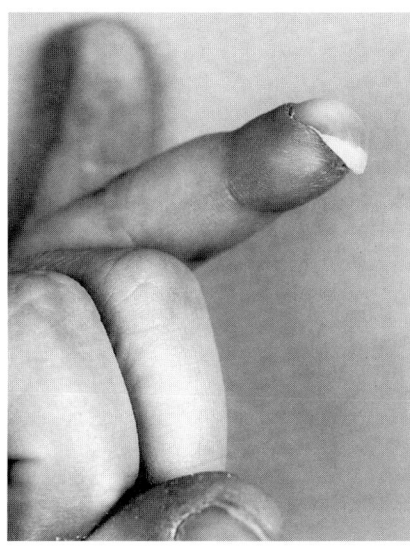

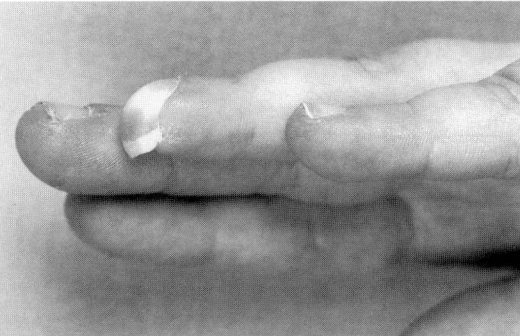

FIGURE 19. The "parrot beak" (hooked nail) deformity is extremely troubling to patients because there is clicking whenever they use their fingertip.

cial surgical training or techniques; no need for donor tissue; and excellent return of sensation. In contrast, some of the other local flap options (such as a crossfinger flap) provide good padding but may offer inferior return of sensation.

SKIN GRAFTS

When the physician is concerned that the wound is too large to heal by secondary intention, but there is good padding, the placement of a skin graft over the area may speed the healing process and prevent potentially disabling scar contracture (Figure 20). A skin graft is a particularly attractive option when the fingertip has been sliced off and the patient brings in the amputated portion (Figures 21, 22). A skin graft can be derived from the amputated part and, after the remaining fat is trimmed from the undersurface of the skin, sutured over the wound. It may be tempting when a patient brings in an amputated part (such as a distal fingertip, which has skin and a significant amount of pulp tissue remaining) to simply suture the entire piece back in place as a "composite graft," with the hope that the entire part will survive. In reality, composite grafting usually is unsuccessful and should not be undertaken in most situations.

Skin Grafting Method

If the patient has brought in the amputated part, prepare it by trimming the fat from the skin using a curved, sharp scissors (see Figure 25). This is vitally important: the fat will act as a barrier to skin revascularization and make graft

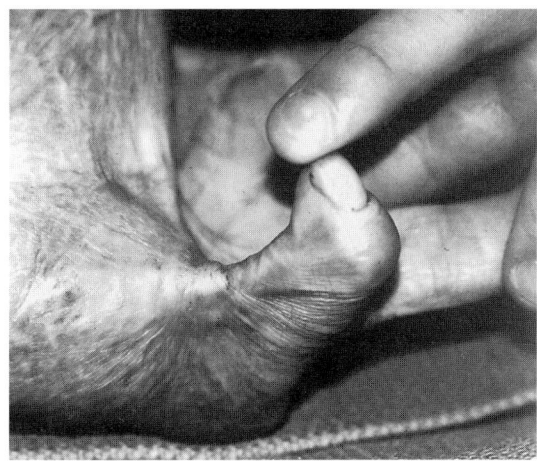

FIGURE 20. Severe contracture of the small finger after a burn. Despite the fact that insufficient skin was present, the wound was allowed to heal secondarily (by contraction). Compare this result to that achieved in Figure 23. Significant defects of skin > 1 cm in diameter on the volar aspect of the hand and fingers must receive soft tissue coverage to avoid late scar contracture.

failure likely. Once all the fat and pulp tissue has been sharply excised leaving only the skin, place the graft in saline-moistened gauze until needed. Thoroughly clean the fingertip and debride all nonviable tissue. Now suture the skin graft into place circumferentially, using nylon sutures to hold it in position.

The most important determinant of success is

firm adherence of the skin graft to its recipient site, to allow vascular ingrowth of the graft. If (for example) the skin graft is "tenting" upward in the middle because the skin is too thick to be positioned correctly, it should be trimmed to allow direct contact with its underlying bed. The main goal when fashioning the dressing is to provide soft compression that will hold the skin

FIGURE 21. **A,** Volar soft tissue loss of the index finger at the distal tip. The amputated part was brought in with the patient, and there was no protruding bone at the base of the wound. Due to the large amount of skin loss, healing by secondary intention (conservative measures) would entail risk of a hooked nail deformity. Skin grafting was

deemed appropriate. **B,** The skin side of the amputated part (*left*) and the residual pulp attached to the underside of the skin (*right*). The pulp was excised tangentially with a sharp curved scissors, leaving only the dermis and skin to be placed as a graft. Failure to remove all of the pulp jeopardizes the survival of a graft, because the pulp will act as a barrier to revascularization of the skin. **C,** Full-thickness skin graft approximately 3 weeks later. The thick skin of the volar finger often darkens and hardens after skin grafting. However, this phase only represents the dessication of the outer keratinized skin layers. Underneath (assuming that the graft has survived), the dermis and basal layers are viable. The hardened outer covering can act as a biologic dressing during recuperation. **D,** Demonstration of maintenance of the fingertip contour, with no evidence of scar contracture.

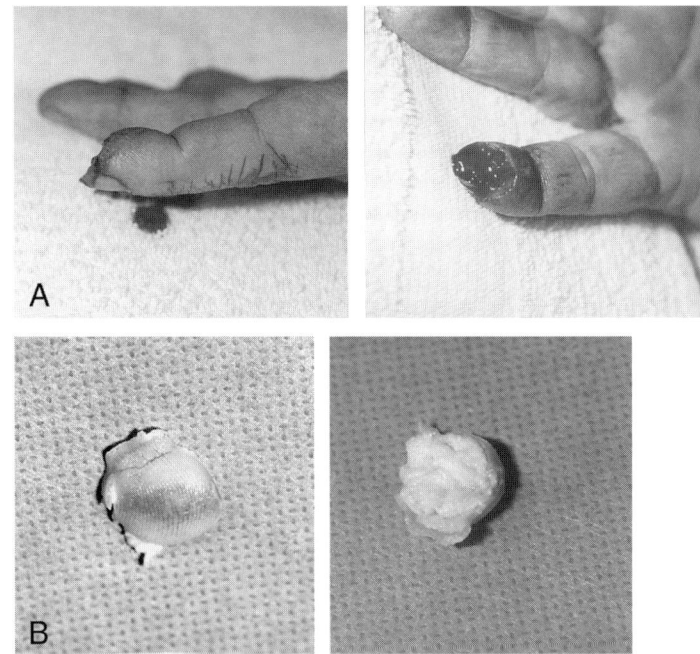

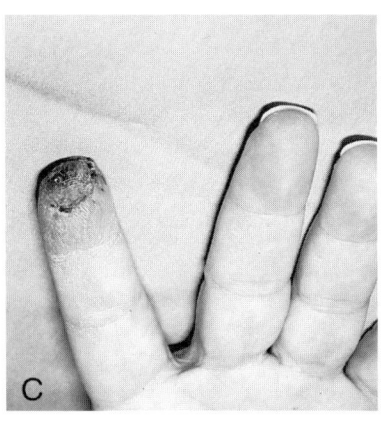

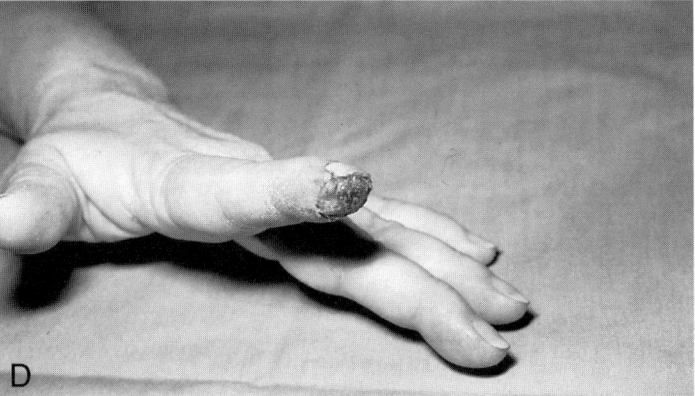

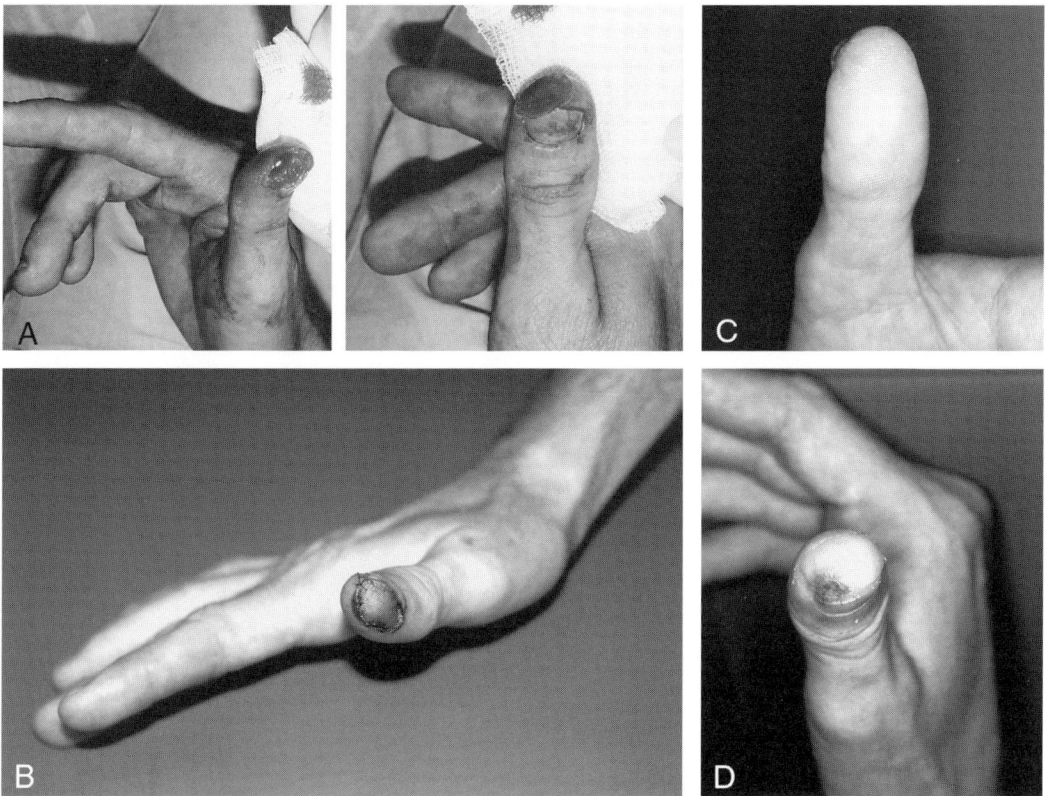

FIGURE 22. **A,** Knife injury to the radial aspect of the thumb. The patient lost a section of skin > 1 cm in diameter, which was retrieved and used as a skin graft after removal of the fatty tissue on the underside. **B,** Skin graft 3 weeks after placement demonstrating typical discoloration. **C** and **D,** Late (6-month) follow-up demonstrating normal contour.

graft in position and prevent any movement that could shear off new capillary blood flow.

If a segment of autologous skin from the amputated fingertip is not available (either because the distal tip was too badly damaged or the patient did not retrieve it), skin can be harvested from other areas (Figures 23, 24). Salvaging tissue from an amputated part carries different donor-site consequences than harvesting skin from a normal area. Harvest of uninjured skin should be performed only by physicians comfortable with minor surgical procedures. Although skin can be harvested from almost anywhere, the proximal forearm is a good location because of skin laxity (allowing primary closure) and proximity to the injury. However, the patient should be warned of a propensity for

widened scars at this location. Other donor sites that are favored because of their relatively hidden positions include the groin crease (Figure 24A) and the retroauricular area. The volar wrist is discouraged as a donor site, because the resultant scars can look like a failed suicide attempt.

After obtaining the donor skin, the procedure is similar to that when using skin from the amputated part. If harvesting the skin from the groin crease, infiltrate the skin and subcutaneous tissue with 1% lidocaine with epinephrine to achieve anesthesia and assist with hemostasis. Outline a lenticular-shaped excision, which will allow primary closure after harvest (Figure 24B). Defat the skin in the same way as an amputated part, trimming all the fat from the

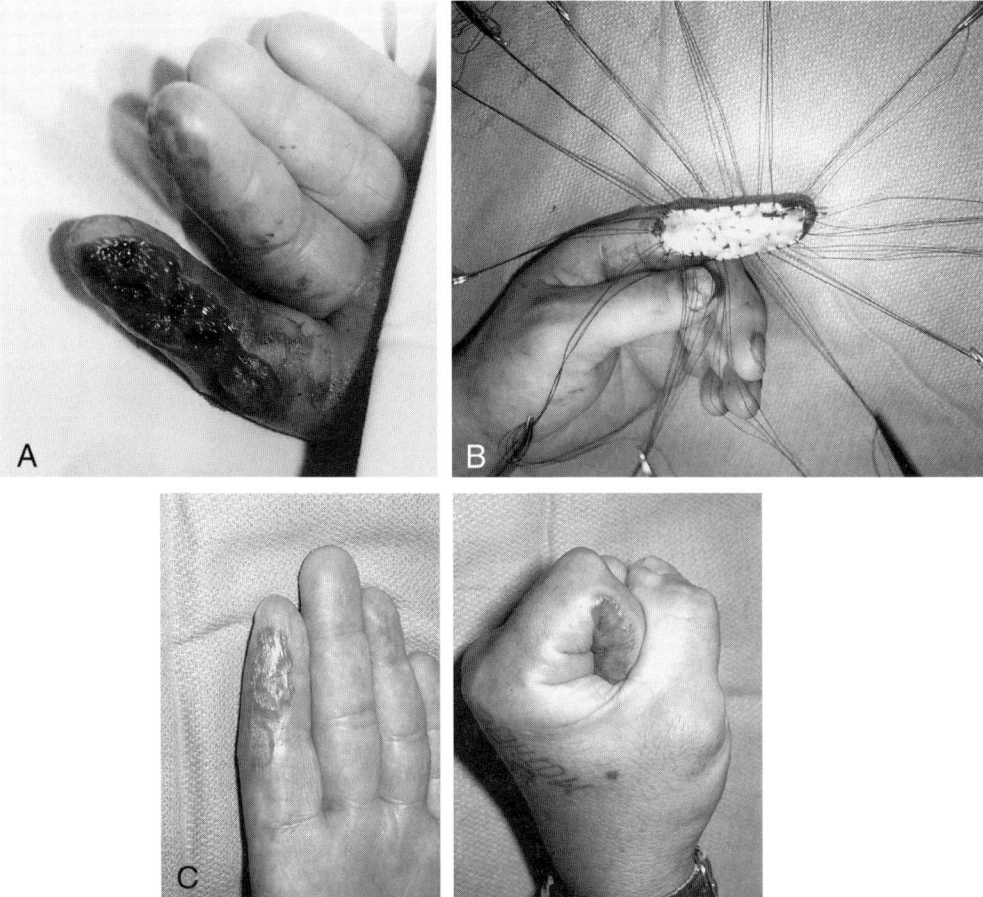

FIGURE 23. **A,** Skin loss over the entire radial aspect of the index finger. Underlying structures were not damaged. The large wound size necessitated skin coverage to prevent secondary flexion contracture (see Figure 20). The presence of viable soft tissue and pulp at the base of the wound made skin grafting a good option. **B,** A skin graft (after harvest from the groin; see Figure 24) along the entire radial-volar aspect of the index finger wound. The graft will only survive if neovascularization occurs between it and the underlying wound bed. Any movement of the graft will disrupt this neovascularization and predispose to graft failure. Therefore, in patients with skin grafts, the hand and fingers must be immobilized completely, with mild compression on the graft to maintain adherence to its bed. **C,** Late result showing full active extension and full active flexion.

underside of the graft until only the dermis and epithelium remain (Figure 25).

Since the main determinant of graft survival is successful revascularization of the graft via capillary ingrowth, anything that blocks or impedes vascular ingrowth can cause the graft to fail. The most common cause of graft failure is **hematoma or seroma formation** below the graft. The fluid collection lifts the graft off the underlying bed, making revascularization impossible. Therefore, to improve graft survival, it is a good idea to make several small holes in the graft (prior to insetting) with a #11 blade ("pie-crusting"). These holes allow any fluid accumulation to leak out around the graft rather than lift it from its bed (Figure 26).

LOCAL FLAP COVERAGE

Another option available to patients with distal tip amputation is local flap coverage. Local flaps are required when there is a significant

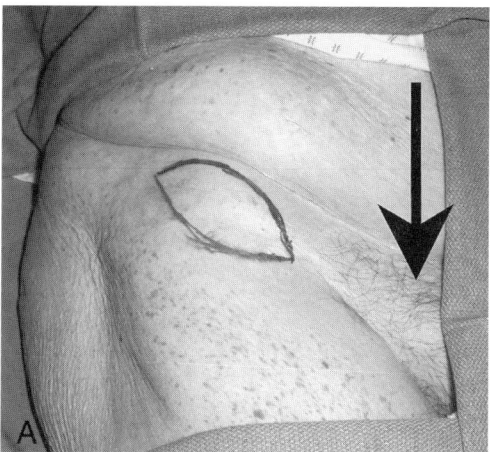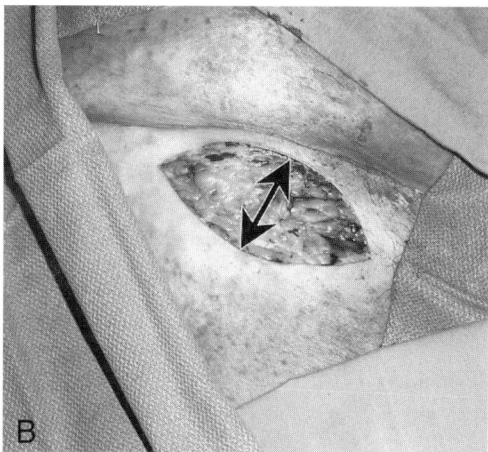

FIGURE 24. Harvest of skin from the groin crease. **A,** A lenticular-shaped incision is planned parallel and within the groin crease (for orientation, the *arrow* points medially, at the pubis). **B,** The resultant wound can be closed primarily (*arrows*), using several absorbable stitches in the deep tissue and 4–0 nylon at the cutaneous portion, with minimal donor site morbidity.

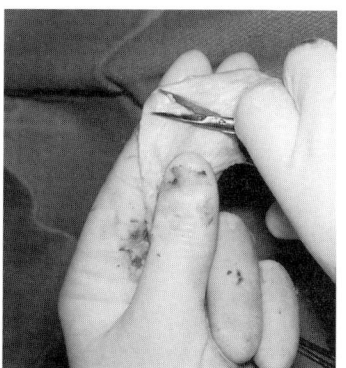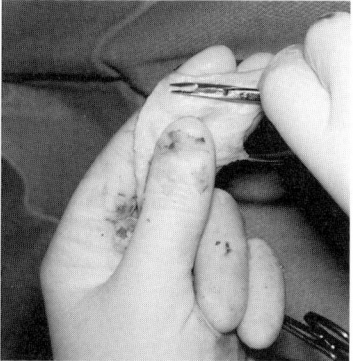

FIGURE 25. Elimination of *all* subcutaneous fat is essential prior to placement of a skin graft, whether the graft is from an amputated part or from donor (noninjured) skin. The excess fat deep to the dermis is excised using a curved, sharp scissors.

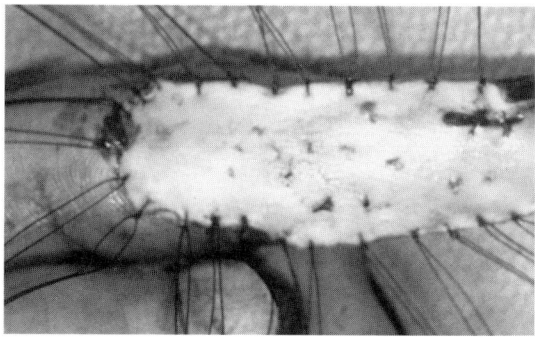

FIGURE 26. The most common cause of graft loss is fluid formation between the graft and the bed, which lifts the graft up and prevents the capillaries from reaching it. Punching several small holes in the skin graft ("pie crusting") allows any fluid accumulation to seep out. Note: hole-punching is done *prior* to placement; if done after insetting, underlying tissue may be cut, promoting excessive bleeding.

amount of soft tissue loss and tip padding needs to be restored. Depending on the exact configuration of the defect, adjacent tissue can be moved from the same finger (such as in a V-Y advancement flap, Figure 27); from adjacent fingers (such as in a crossfinger flap, Figure 28); or from the palm (hypothenar or thenar flaps, Figure 29). Crossfinger flaps should be elevated in an operating room under tourniquet control and loupe magnification: if incorrectly

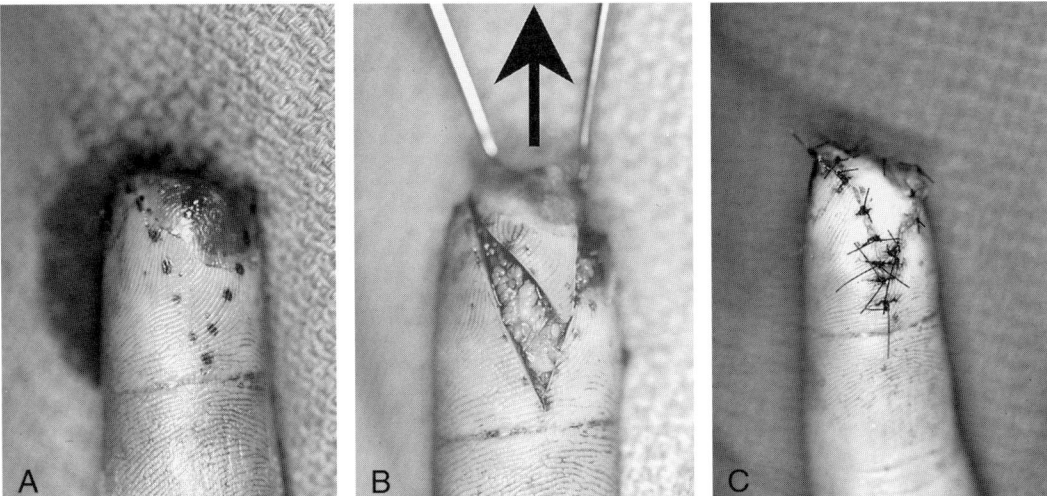

FIGURE 27. The **V-Y flap** often is appropriate for local flap coverage of distal tip amputation. **A,** A V-shaped flap is outlined. When designing the flap, *never* go beyond the DIP flexion crease. To do so would likely result in a late complication of flexion contracture at the DIP joint. **B,** The flap is incised sharply through the skin and dermis, and the septal attachments along both sides are gently released. The lateral attachments of the septae are divided, but the central attachments (directly underneath the flap) are left intact to preserve the flap's vascularity and viability. The flap is then advanced distally to provide coverage of the tip. **C,** The donor section (the most proximal aspect of the flap harvest) is closed primarily, resulting in a "Y" shape. Since this type of flap comprises tissues from the volar aspect of the finger, it is useful in distal fingertip injuries; however, the V-Y flap does not supply enough tissue for volarly angulated injuries, in which a significant amount of volar tissue is missing (see Figures 28 and 29).

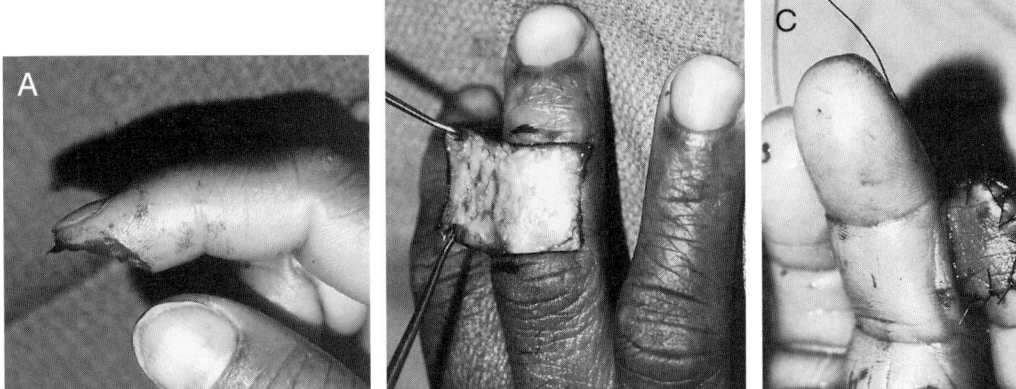

FIGURE 28. **A,** Amputation of most of the pulp and skin of the volar and distal index finger. Conservative treatment is inappropriate due to significant pulp loss, and a skin graft would provide poor coverage of the underlying bone because the volar padding is missing. Therefore, the best choice is some type of flap. Since most of the volar tissue of the finger is gone, a local advancement (V-Y) flap is not possible. **B,** A **crossfinger flap** is harvested from an adjacent finger. This procedure requires meticulous dissection under tourniquet control and loupe magnification. Failure to preserve the paratenon over the extensor mechanism can create a significant donor site deformity. Here, the flap is elevated and ready to inset onto the index finger. After flap elevation, the donor site is skin grafted with a full-thickness skin graft, usually harvested from the groin. **C,** Once inset, the crossfinger flap is left in place for at least 3 weeks, during which time vascular connections are made between the flap and its bed so that it can survive without being attached to the donor finger. Finally, the flap is divided from the donor finger.

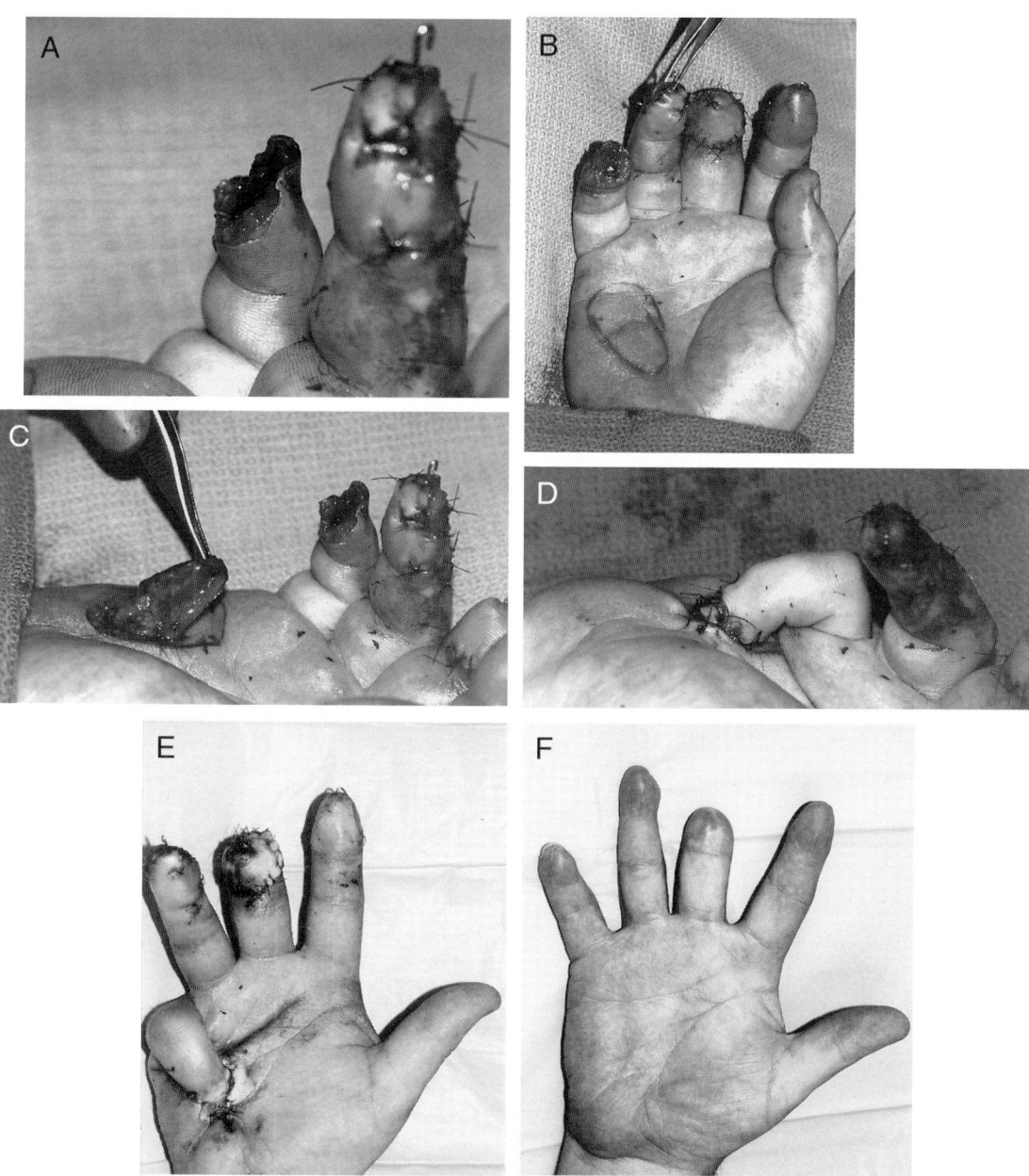

FIGURE 29. **A,** Loss of most of the volar tissue, including the tip, of the fifth finger. The underlying distal pha-lanx is intact. A flap is needed for pulp replacement, but due to multiple finger injuries, the adjacent finger is too badly damaged to serve as a donor for a crossfinger flap. A local V-Y advancement flap also is inappropriate be-cause most of the volar tissue is missing. Therefore, for this patient a **hypothenar flap** is the best choice. **B,** The hy-pothenar flap outlined on the volar-ulnar aspect of the palm. **C,** Elevation of the hypothenar flap prior to flap inset. **D,** Fifth finger immediately after insetting of the hypothenar flap. **E,** Two weeks later. The fingers must be held in position for at least 3 weeks to allow sufficient neovascularization to occur between the finger and flap, so that the flap will survive after division of its base. The prolonged flexion of the finger required in hypothenar and thenar flap procedures can result in an unacceptably stiff finger that is unable to extend. Aggressive hand therapy is nec-essary. **F,** After division of the hypothenar flap and aggressive range-of-motion exercises, the full length of the fifth finger was salvaged, and full active extension was achieved.

elevated significant donor site problems, such as extensor tendon exposure and loss, can result. Note, too, that *prior to undertaking* hypothenar and thenar flap procedures, aggressive hand therapy for rehabilitation after flap division must be discussed and planned.

DISTANT FLAP COVERAGE

Distant flaps also can be used for volar finger coverage. They are easily raised from the trunk or chest area, but remember that these flaps are completely insensate. Even with intact digital nerves, very little reinnervation of the skin can be expected due to the relative thickness of the flaps (Figure 30).

A flap remains viable because its base (and therefore its vascularity) is left intact. The flap receives vascular ingrowth from the base of the finger or hand wound over a 3-week period. After this time, it will survive completely on its new vascular supply, and it can be divided from

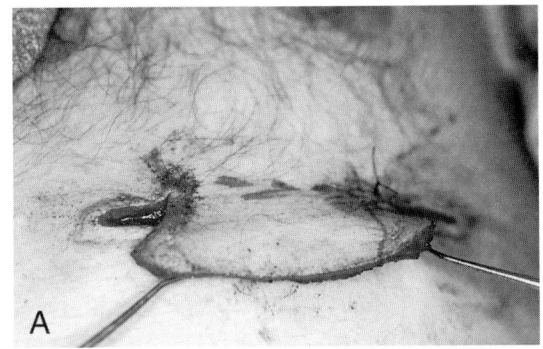

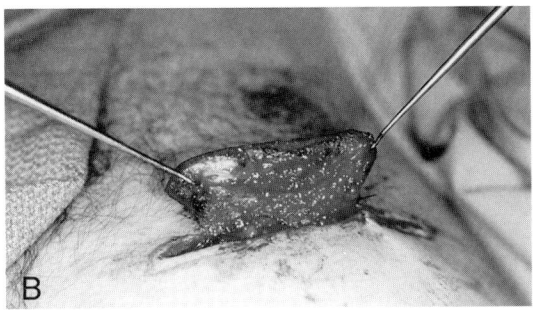

FIGURE 31. **A,** In men, the area directly underneath the nipple is the least hirsute and is most appropriate for harvest of a distant flap. **B,** The flap is designed with a wide base to preserve as much vascularity as possible and should be at least 0.5-centimeter thick distally and up to 1-centimeter thick at the base.

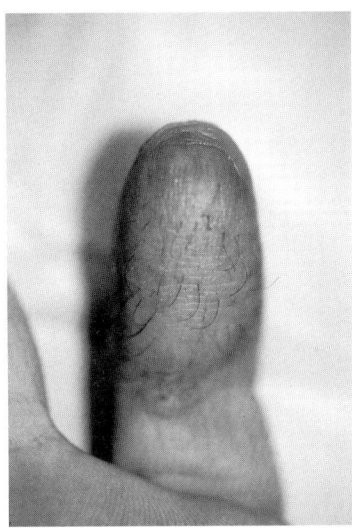

FIGURE 30. Distant flaps remain insensate, even if the underlying digital nerves are intact. In addition, normal volar skin has septal connections between the underlying bone and the skin that prevent shearing when grasping or lifting heavy objects. These connections do not exist between the flap and the underlying tissue, and patients may complain of difficulty in performing these activities. Finally, in hirsute individuals the flap may continue to grow hair, which is troubling to patients.

its attachment to the chest. Obviously, it is a considerable inconvenience for the patient to be "sewn to themselves" for a period of 3 weeks. However, if this technique allows preservation of a digit that otherwise would not be salvageable, most patients agree it is worth it.

In males, the area directly below the nipple has the least amount of hair and is most appropriate for volar finger coverage. For positioning ease, the area *contralateral* to the injured hand is prepared for flap elevation. A digital block (as appropriate) is applied to the injured finger, and 1% lidocaine (no epinephrine) is used to achieve local anesthesia of the chest area. Remember that these flaps are "random" (i.e., they do not have a defined vascular pedicle). Elevating them on a base that is too narrow could destroy the vascular supply. Be generous when designing the flap base, and do not make it too thin (usually 0.5–1 centimeter thick; Figure 31A). After

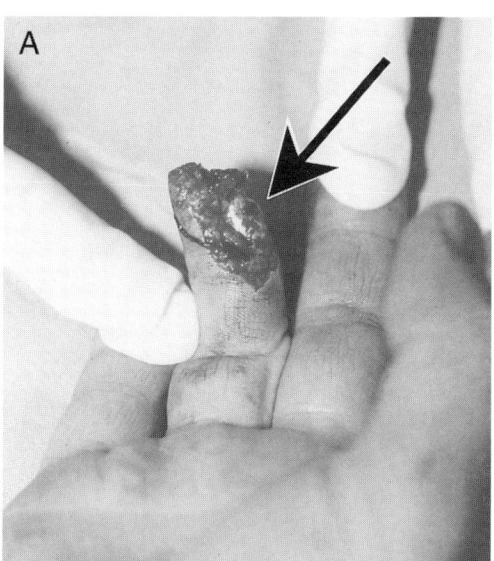
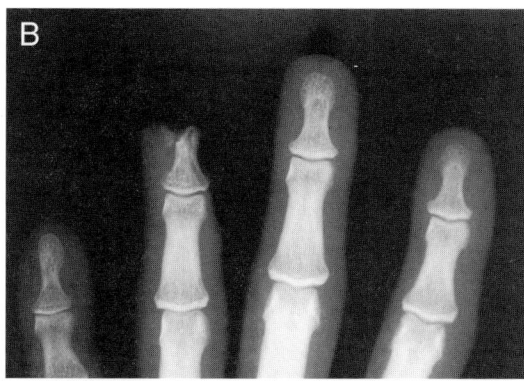
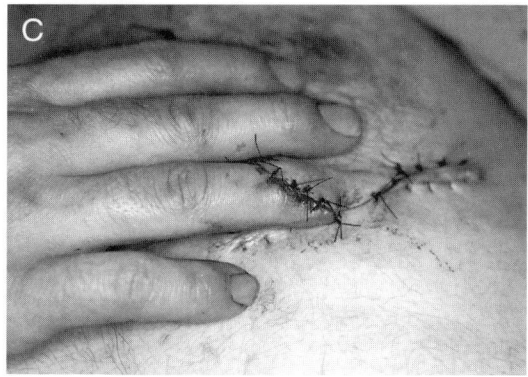

FIGURE 32. Same patient as in Figure 31. **A,** Loss of the radial aspect, including the distal tuft of the distal phalanx (*arrow*), of the ring finger. Due to wound size, exposed bone, and loss of padding, both conservative management and skin grafting are inappropriate. A local flap, such as a crossfinger or hypothenar flap, would not provide enough soft tissue for coverage. Therefore, coverage is provided with a distant flap (a random chest flap). **B,** Radiograph demonstrating loss of the distal tuft of the ring finger, as well as soft tissue loss. **C,** After inset of the flap. In 3 weeks, enough neovascularization will have occurred between the flap and the underlying finger that the flap can be divided from its base.

raising a flap of skin and soft tissue (Figure 31B), suture it directly to the finger (Figure 32). It is usually a good idea to admit the patient to the hospital, at least overnight, to ensure they are comfortable with their hand and arm position. Watch that proper hand positioning is maintained: if the patient pulls too much on the flap, or holds their arm in a way that kinks or impinges on the flap, the vascular supply can be compromised and the flap lost. Rolled towels can be placed between the arm and the patient's side, and 6-inch ace bandages can be gently wrapped around the patient's trunk and arm to help maintain the hand and arm in the correct position.

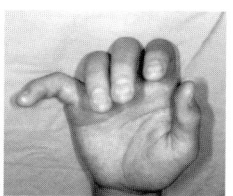

6 Fractures & Dislocations

Dislocations

The interphalangeal joints and metacarpophalangeal joints of the hand are extremely well supported by their surrounding joint capsules and collateral ligaments. These ligamentous structures lend stability to the joints, allowing controlled motion while maintaining the positions of the bones in the hand. External deforming forces of sufficient magnitude can rupture or tear these supporting ligaments, resulting in a dislocation. The following section discusses the different types of dislocations (and their treatments) at the proximal interphalangeal (PIP) joint, the distal interphalangeal (DIP) joint, and the metacarpophalangeal (MCP) joint.

PROXIMAL INTERPHALANGEAL JOINT DISLOCATIONS

Due to its position in the hand and the lever-type forces that it can be subjected to, the PIP joint is the most commonly dislocated joint in the hand. It is a hinged-type joint that is extremely stable to external stresses because of support by three major ligamentous structures: the collateral ligaments on the radial and ulnar sides of the joint and a strong fibrous structure on the volar aspect of the joint called the "volar plate." The volar plate connects the proximal phalanx to the middle pha-

lanx: by virtue of its volar position, it prevents hyperextension of the PIP joint. The collateral ligaments support the joint on either side of the finger and prevent radial and ulnar deviation of the finger. Typically, any dislocation of the PIP joint involves disruption of the volar plate and at least one of the collateral ligaments, if not both.

There are three types of dislocations possible at the PIP joint. The most common is the dorsal dislocation: the middle phalanx is dislocated *dorsal* to the proximal phalanx (Figures 1, 2). A lateral dislocation is possible with complete rupture of one of the collateral ligaments and at least some disruption of the volar plate (Figure 3). The third possibility is a volar dislocation, in which the middle phalanx is dislocated *volar* to the proximal phalanx (Figure 4). Volar dislocations are rare.

Dorsal PIP Dislocation

Dorsal PIP dislocations are common athletic injuries that typically involve hyperextension of the proximal interphalangeal joint in combination with a compressive force. The force pushes the middle phalanx over the proximal phalanx (Figure 5).

The diagnosis of dorsal PIP joint dislocation usually is obvious from the patient's presentation. The finger is somewhat shortened and

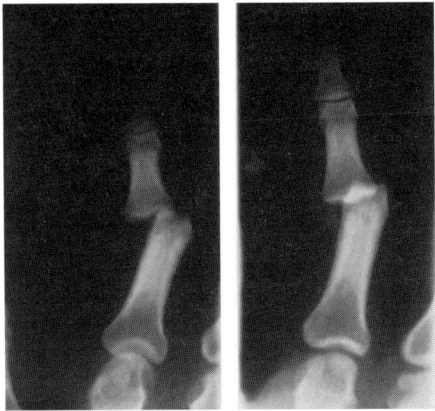

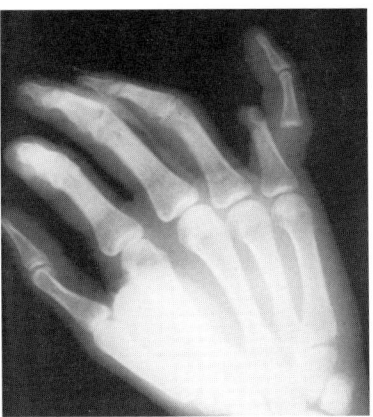

FIGURE 1. Dorsal dislocation of the PIP joint, in which the middle phalanx is dislocated dorsal to the proximal phalanx.

FIGURE 2. Dorsal dislocation of the PIP joint, fifth finger.

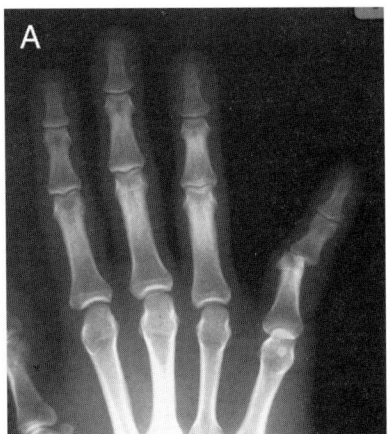

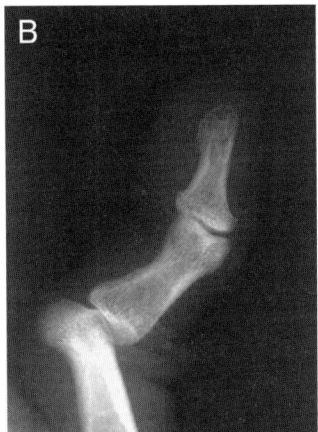

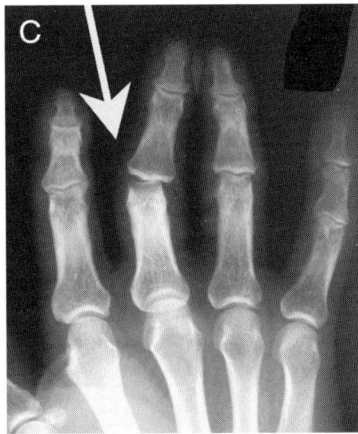

FIGURE 3. **A** and **B,** Lateral dislocation of the fifth finger PIP joint, with complete disruption of the radial collateral ligament and at least some disruption of the volar plate. **C,** Lateral dislocation of the long finger PIP joint, with injury to the radial collateral ligament (*arrow*). Due to loss of this support, the distal digit is ulnarly inclined.

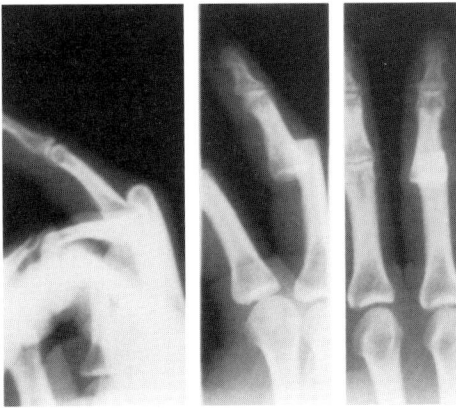

FIGURE 4. Volar dislocations of the PIP joint are rare. They occur when the middle phalanx is dislocated volar to the proximal phalanx.

swollen over the proximal interphalangeal joint, and the patient is unable to flex it. The typical presenting complaint is: "Doc, I jammed it."

It is advisable to obtain anteroposterior and lateral films of the finger *prior* to manipulation, to rule out associated fractures (Figure 6). If a fracture is revealed, obtain a hand surgeon's advice, and defer attempts at relocation. Similarly, a laceration overlying the dislocation (an "open joint") also requires urgent operative intervention, and a hand surgical consultation should occur promptly. If there are no fractures, a dislocated joint with an overlying laceration can be reduced while waiting for the hand surgeon to arrive, to make the patient more comfortable.

If the x-rays reveal no associated fractures and the skin is intact, treatment is relatively straightforward. Local anesthesia is applied (typically with a digital block), and when the finger is *completely* anesthetized, a gauze 4 × 4 sponge is gently wrapped around the distal

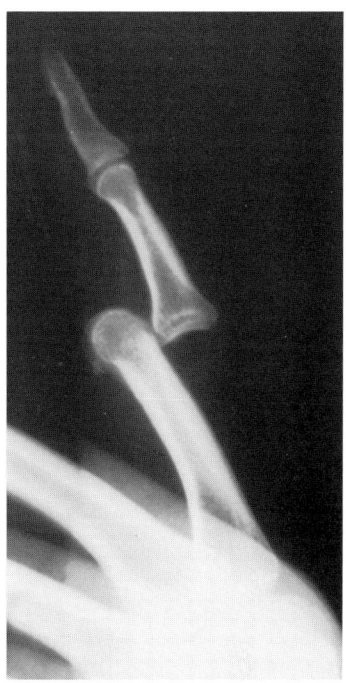

FIGURE 5. Lateral view of a dorsal PIP dislocation, the most common dislocation of this joint.

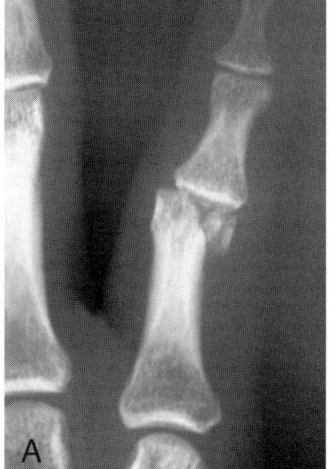 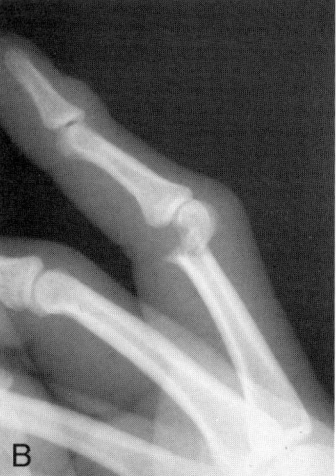

FIGURE 6. **A,** Intra-articular fracture of the proximal phalanx at the PIP joint. This patient's presentation was typical for a PIP joint dislocation. Attempts at reduction prior to radiographic examination could have made treatment of the fracture more difficult by displacing the bony fragments. **B,** Fracture of the proximal phalanx. This patient suffered an injury while playing basketball, and the clinical presentation was consistent with dorsal PIP joint dislocation. Premanipulation x-rays demonstrated the fracture, which necessitated a hand surgery consultation and deferral of manipulation.

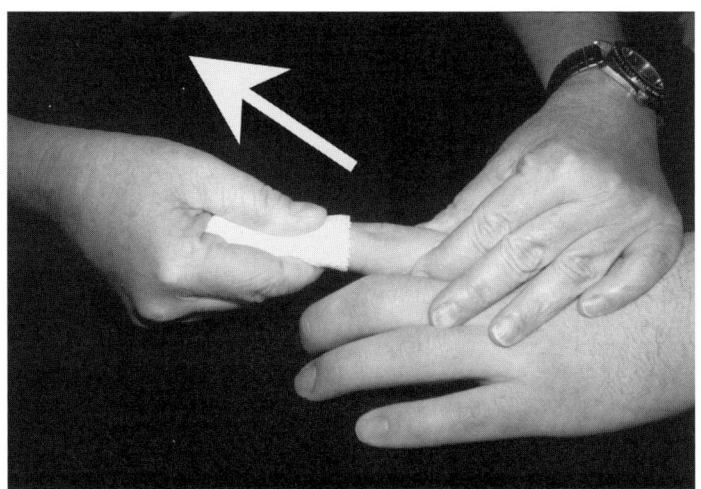

FIGURE 7. Reduction of PIP joint dislocation. After obtaining complete digital block, wrap a 4 × 4 gauze sponge around the distal finger. While stabilizing the patient's hand and proximal phalanx, apply firm traction by pulling the injured digit outwardly (*arrow*).

finger and middle phalanx (Figure 7). The gauze is helpful to maintain traction when attempting joint reduction. The physician then uses his or her nondominant hand to stabilize the patient's proximal phalanx and hand and applies gentle outward traction to the middle phalanx with the dominant hand (holding onto the gauze). With adequate anesthesia, this maneuver is easily performed. Successful reduction is confirmed by gentle active and passive range of motion of the joint and post-reduction radiographs (Figure 8).

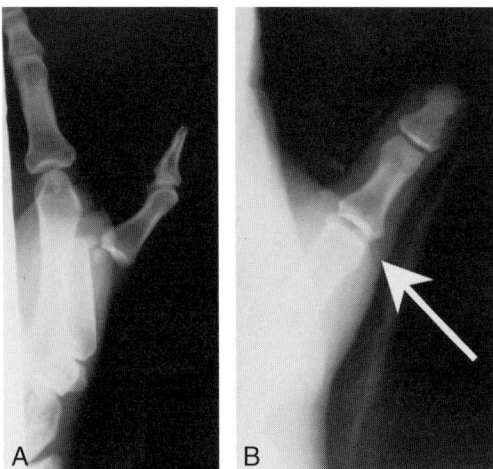

FIGURE 8. **A,** Dislocation of the thumb MCP joint. **B,** Post-reduction films demonstrate normal joint space (*arrow*). Post-manipulation films are *mandatory* to insure that reduction has been obtained.

After reducing the joint, splint the finger with the PIP joint in approximately 20 degrees of flexion, and instruct the patient to see a hand surgeon for follow up within 1 week.

An alternative post-reduction option is to "buddy-tape" the middle and proximal phalanges of the injured digit to an adjacent uninjured finger (Figure 9). There are several advantages to this technique. The intact volar plate and collateral ligaments of the uninjured digit prevent hyperextension and radial/ulnar deviation and block redislocation of the injured joint. Buddy-taping allows early mobilization, which can avoid problems with late joint stiffness (a risk when hand therapy services are inadequate or patient compliance is questionable). Finally, a finger that is buddy-taped is more functional than one that is immobilized in a splint, allowing the patient to return to regular activities more quickly (with limitations on amount of force, e.g., no heavy lifting). Buddy-taping is only successful when the fingers are approximately equal in length. Buddy-taping of the fifth and ring fingers is not advisable, because the joint positions are not at the same level (Figure 10).

Occasionally, reduction is not possible in the outpatient setting. After one (or at most two) attempts at reduction have failed (usually manifest by the inability of the patient to regain joint range of motion after manipulation, but confirmed by radiograph), no further attempts

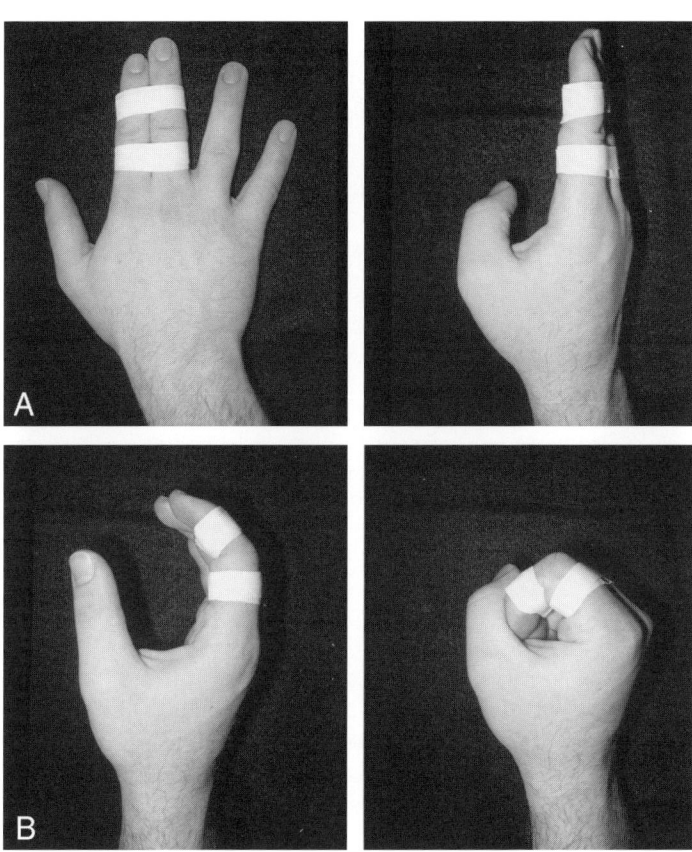

FIGURE 9. "Buddy taping": an alternative method for protecting a finger after successful PIP joint reduction. **A,** The uninjured finger's intact volar plate and collateral ligaments stabilize the PIP joint of the injured finger. **B,** Demonstration of the degree of motion possible when digits are buddy-taped. Redislocation and hyperextension, which are potential hazards if the finger is not splinted, are prevented.

should be made, and a hand surgeon should be consulted promptly. Closed reduction failure is *not* due to inadequate technique, but almost always is due to an interposing anatomic structure (e.g., volar plate) making closed reduction *physically impossible* (Figure 11). If this occurs, op- erative intervention is necessary to physically remove the obstruction from the joint space and replace it in its proper anatomic position.

PIP joint stiffness, due to prolonged immobilization or injury, is extremely difficult to overcome and can be quite problematic and disabling.

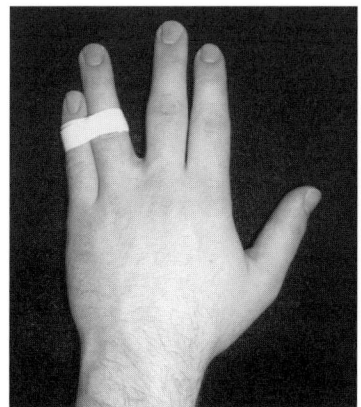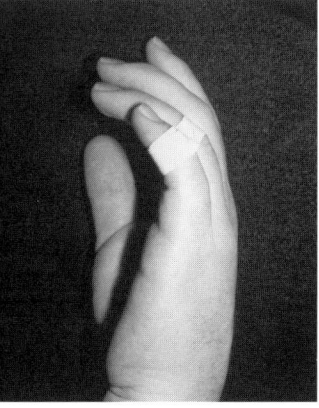

FIGURE 10. Buddy taping is only an option when there is an adjacent finger of approximately equal length to the injured finger. When there are discrepancies in phalangeal length, the PIP joints rotate on different axes, and the noninjured joint cannot protect the dislocated joint from nonanatomic stresses.

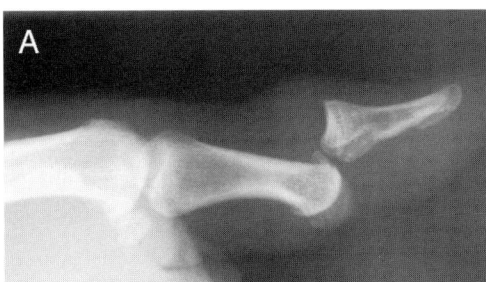
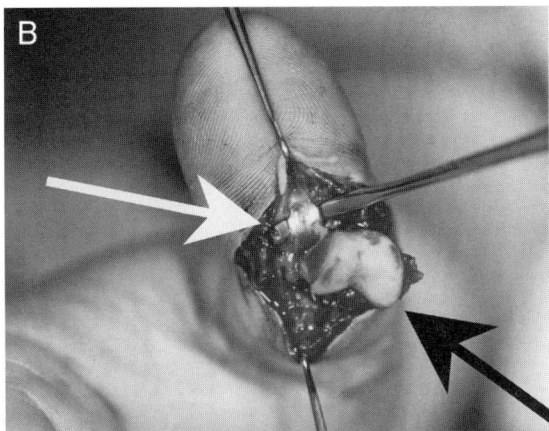

FIGURE 11. **A,** Dislocation of the thumb DIP joint. Despite several attempts at manipulation, reduction was unsuccessful in the outpatient setting, and a surgical consultation was scheduled. **B,** Reduction failure was due to an anatomic structure (the flexor pollicis longus tendon, *white arrow*) trapped within the joint space, blocking reduction. The distal end of the proximal phalanx is seen at the base of the wound (*black arrow*).

The best treatment is prevention. Therefore, even for those patients with PIP joint dislocations that have been successfully reduced in the outpatient setting, referral to a hand specialist for follow-up and supervision of therapy is recommended.

Lateral PIP Dislocation

A lateral PIP dislocation is manifest by laxity of the joint in either the radial or ulnar direction, and represents a partial or complete tear of either the radial or ulnar collateral ligament and usually the volar plate. The diagnosis is definitively confirmed by greater than 20 degrees of angulation in either the radial or ulnar direction on gentle traction (Figure 12). The patient is very tender over the affected side. For example, a patient complains of pain and swelling of the index finger PIP joint after playing basketball. The radial aspect is markedly tender (more so than the ul-

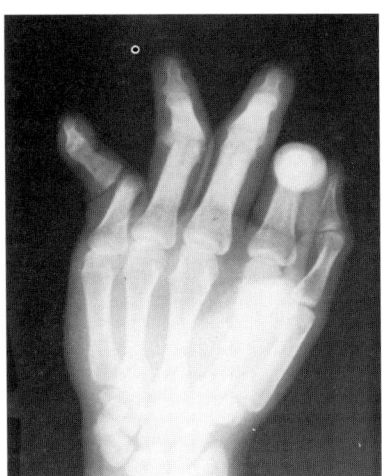
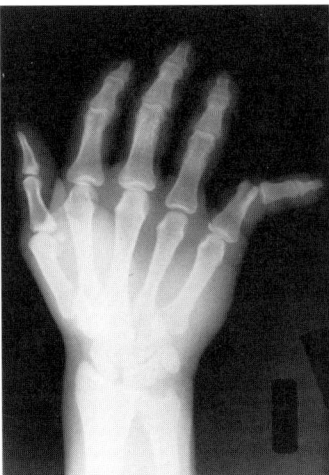
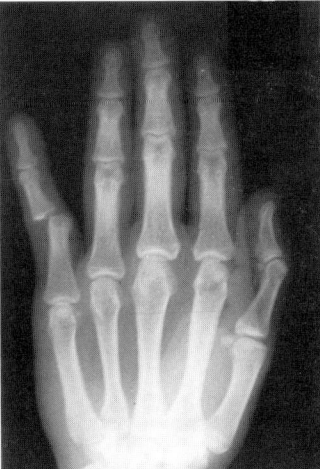

FIGURE 12. Three examples of lateral PIP dislocation of the fifth finger. The injury in the middle image involves the radial collateral ligament and the volar plate.

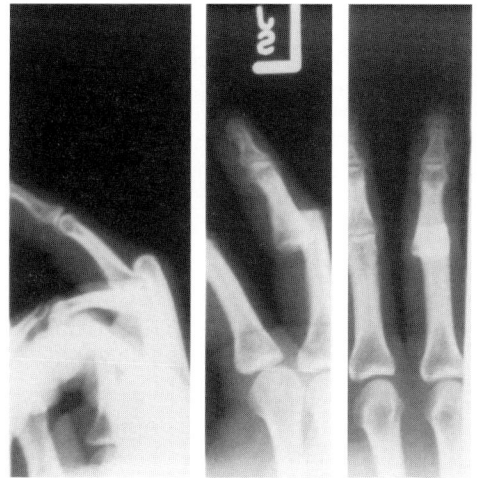

FIGURE 13. Volar PIP joint dislocation, in which the middle phalanx is dislocated volar to the proximal phalanx and pushed through the volar plate. These injuries are rarely reducible in the outpatient setting.

nar aspect), and gentle traction by the examiner demonstrates a 25 degree angulation in an ulnar direction, with no associated laxity in a radial direction. In this case, the ruptured radial collateral ligament cannot limit ulnar deviation.

If these patients have stable active and passive range of motion post-reduction, then an urgent hand surgical consultation is not required, and the treatment is essentially the same as for a dorsal dislocation. The finger is splinted in slight flexion or buddy-taped, and the patient is referred to a hand specialist for follow-up within 1 week. However, if the finger maintains an angulated posture after attempted reduction, then the collateral ligament may be interposed. As for dorsal PIP dislocations, this situation requires surgical consultation for retrieval of the ligament from the joint space and direct repair.

Volar PIP Dislocation

Volar PIP dislocations, in which the middle phalanx is projected volar to the proximal phalanx, are rare. They usually represent the middle phalanx traveling *through* the volar plate (Figure 13). These injuries usually are not reducible without surgical management; therefore, manipulation in the acute setting should be deferred, and an urgent hand surgical consultation should be scheduled.

DISTAL INTERPHALANGEAL JOINT DISLOCATIONS

The anatomic configuration of the DIP joint is similar to that of the PIP joint. However, DIP joint dislocations are less frequent than PIP, probably due to the smaller moment-arm of the finger at the DIP level. Patients presenting with acute injuries and deformation at the DIP joint are more likely to have suffered a "mallet finger" (Figure 14) or a fracture of the distal phalanx (Figure 15).

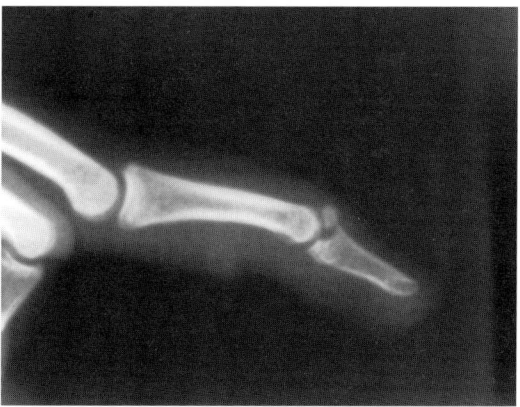

FIGURE 14. A mallet finger injury involves disruption of the terminal extensor tendon from the distal phalanx, and a bony chip may be present (as shown here). Patients are unable to actively extend the distal phalanx (see Figure 20).

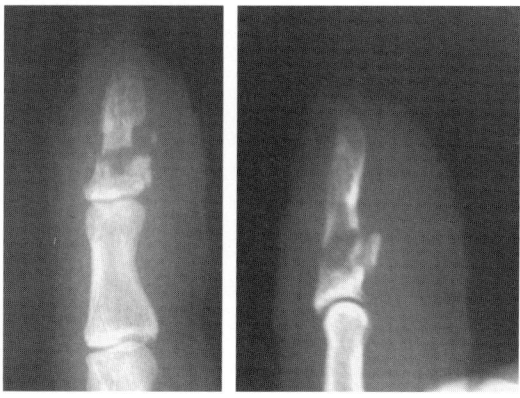

FIGURE 15. Fracture of the distal phalanx.

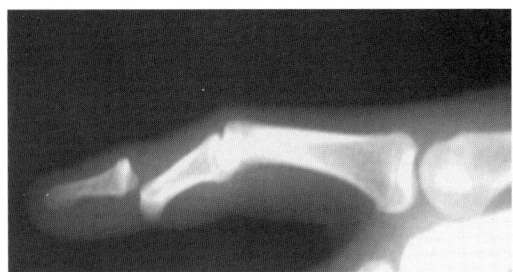

FIGURE 16. Dorsal dislocation of the index finger DIP joint.

A mallet finger represents rupture or disinsertion of the extensor tendon from the distal phalanx, with a resultant inability to actively extend the finger at the DIP joint.

If a dislocation is discovered (Figure 16), treatment remains largely the same as for dorsal and lateral PIP joint dislocations. A 4 × 4 gauze is used to prevent the physician's grip from slipping, and gentle traction is applied after application of digital anesthesia. As with all joint dislocations, failure to obtain reduction after one or two attempts probably represents an anatomic interposition, and a hand surgical consultation is indicated (see Figure 11). Treatment of mallet fingers is discussed in detail on pages 108–109.

METACARPOPHALANGEAL JOINT DISLOCATIONS

Dislocations of the MCP joints are relatively infrequent, due to their strong ligamentous support and protected positions within the hand. Dorsal dislocations are more common than volar (similar to the interphalangeal joints of the hand). However, because of the complex anatomic configuration at the MCP joint, there is a much higher likelihood that closed reduction is not possible. The metacarpal head can become trapped between the lumbrical muscle and the flexor tendons. Applying traction in an attempt to reduce the joint only serves to further tighten the "sling" formed by the lumbrical and flexor tendons, making reduction impossible. Repeated attempts at closed reduction can damage the surrounding structures, increase edema, and confound surgical correction. Therefore, in the situation of an acute MCP joint dislocation, urgent hand consultation is the best option, and manipulation by the primary care physician is best deferred.

Gamekeeper's Thumb

"Gamekeeper's thumb," more commonly referred to today as "skier's thumb," deserves

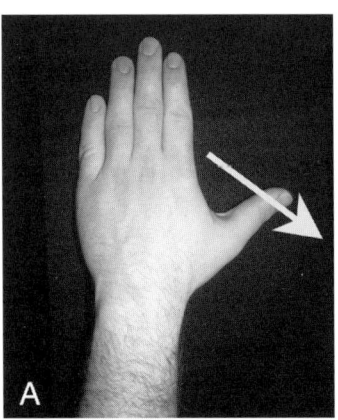
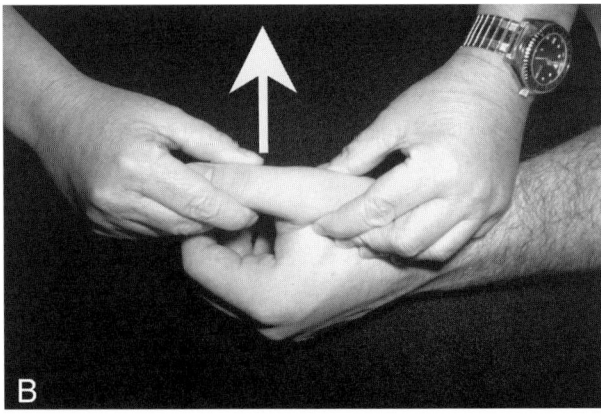

FIGURE 17. **A,** Mechanism of injury in gamekeeper's thumb. Excessive stress on the thumb (*arrow*) disrupts the ulnar collateral ligament of the thumb MCP joint. **B,** The diagnosis is established by noting excess laxity in a radial direction (30 degrees more than the contralateral side). These patients are tender and usually do not tolerate stress on the thumb without anesthesia; therefore, infiltrate 1% lidocaine prior to manipulation. While stabilizing the patient's thumb metacarpal, apply pressure (*arrow*) on the proximal phalanx to determine the degree of laxity. Repeat on the uninjured thumb and compare.

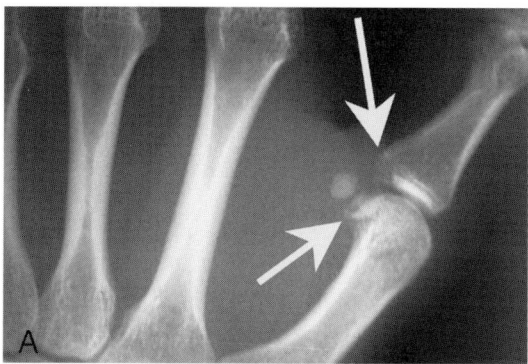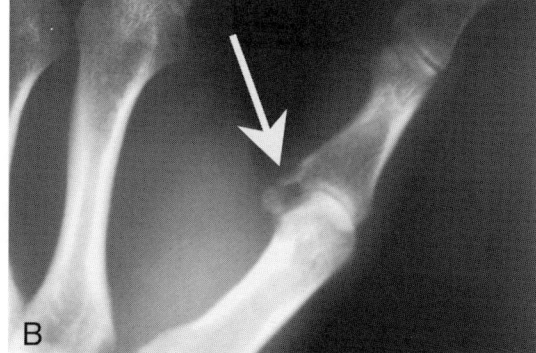

FIGURE 18. Patients with gamekeeper's thumb may or may not have abnormal x-rays. Note that if a bone chip is present, it remains attached to the insertion of the ulnar collateral ligament (UCL), avulsed from the base of the proximal phalanx. Thus, the chip gives a precise indication of the UCL's position (i.e., displaced or nondisplaced). **A,** Defect of the proximal phalanx (*top arrow*) and a proximally displaced bony chip (*bottom arrow*). The sesamoid bone is visible directly above the bone chip. **B,** Mildly displaced bone chip (*arrow*) in a patient with gamekeeper's thumb.

special mention. This injury involves the disruption of the ulnar collateral ligament of the thumb MCP joint, caused by acute radial deviation of the thumb (Figure 17A). It is common in skiing because falls often occur while the ski pole is held incorrectly. Patients present complaining of pain at the ulnar aspect of the thumb MCP joint and a decrease in strength when making a fist. The diagnosis is confirmed by demonstrating greater than 30 degrees of radial deviation of the thumb proximal phalanx on application of gentle outward traction, *as compared to the contralateral side*. This diagnostic maneuver is assisted by local infiltration of lidocaine, which makes the patient more comfortable and allows gentle radial traction (Figure 17B).

Radiographs *may* show a small avulsion chip fracture from the proximal phalanx of the thumb at the attachment of the ulnar collateral ligament (Figure 18). It is important to realize that disruption of the ulnar collateral ligament can occur in the absence of a bony chip and with normal x-rays. If the patient is tender on the ulnar aspect of the MCP joint and demonstrates increased laxity with radial traction (but less than 30 degrees of the uninjured thumb), then probably the ligament is only *partially* torn.

Greater than 30 degrees of radial instability represents a complete rupture.

Treatment of gamekeeper's thumb involves immobilization in a thumb spica splint, with the thumb adducted slightly toward the palm, for a period of 4–6 weeks. If the ligament is completely disrupted, treatment may be more complicated. The goal is for the ulnar collateral ligament to heal in its anatomic position, allowing it to provide support for the thumb MCP joint. However, if the ligament has been completely disrupted, it is possible for it to be held away from its anatomic position by the adductor pollicis aponeurosis, forming a **Stener lesion.** Operative repair is necessary in this situation, because as long as the ligament is held away from its insertion, it will not heal properly. Determining whether a Stener lesion is present (and thus whether operative intervention is necessary) is sometimes difficult. If there is a bone chip but it is not displaced, a Stener lesion probably *is not* present (Figure 19A). If the chip is displaced away from the base of the proximal phalanx (remember, it remains attached to the ulnar collateral ligament), a Stener lesion probably *is* present, and surgical intervention is indicated (Figure 19B).

When a Stener lesion complicates the injury,

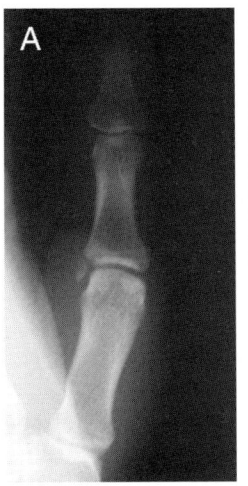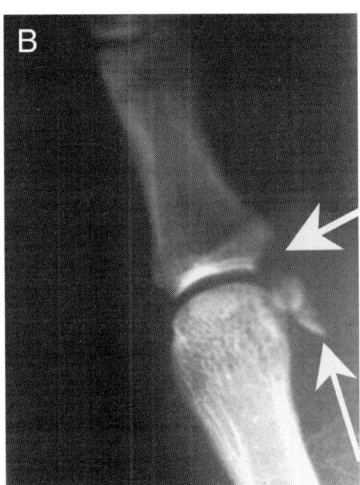

FIGURE 19. **A,** A nondisplaced bony chip at the base of the proximal phalanx. This radiographic evidence also indicates that the UCL is in anatomic position, because it remains attached to the bony chip. Such injuries heal properly with immobilization; operative intervention is unnecessary. **B,** A displaced bony chip (*bottom arrow*) in a patient with gamekeeper's thumb. The sesamoid bone is present between the defect (*top arrow*) and the chip. The extreme proximal displacement of the chip suggests that it is being held out of position by the adductor pollicis aponeurosis, and operative intervention is required to repair the ligamentous insertion.

the thumb should be placed in a slightly adducted position in a spica splint, and the patient should see a hand specialist within 1 week. When operative repair is indicated, it is easier to accomplish and achieves better results if done immediately, rather than several months later. Expedited consultation with a hand surgeon is important.

Mallet Finger

The "mallet finger" deformity occurs after disruption of the distal extensor tendon from its insertion at the distal phalanx. Patients present with the inability to actively extend the finger at the DIP joint (Figure 20A). Radiographs are normal, or reveal a chip fracture from the distal phalanx (Figure 20B). In the latter case, the extensor tendon is still attached to the bony chip.

Treatment of mallet finger involves prolonged immobilization in full extension or slight hyperextension of the DIP joint for 12 weeks (Figure 21). After this time the patient need only wear the splint at night, for an additional 4

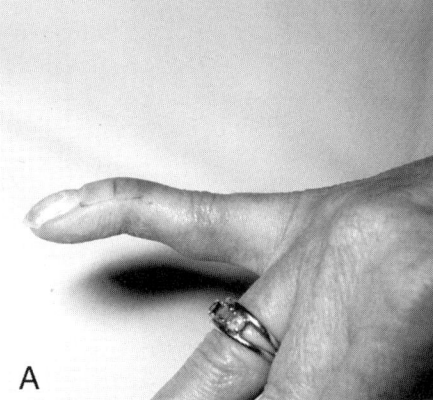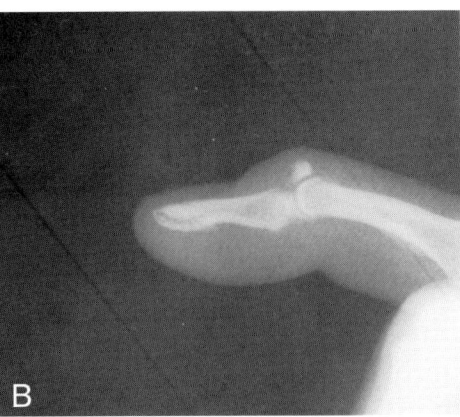

FIGURE 20. **A,** Mallet finger deformity of the fifth finger, preventing active extension of the distal phalanx. This injury results from disruption of the extensor tendon insertion from the distal phalanx. **B,** A small bony chip, which remains attached to the distal extensor tendon, is evident on x-ray.

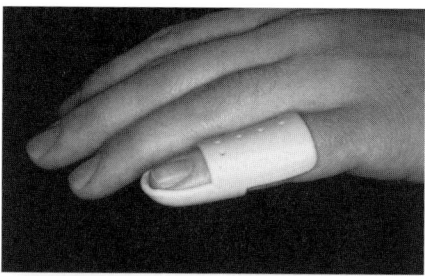

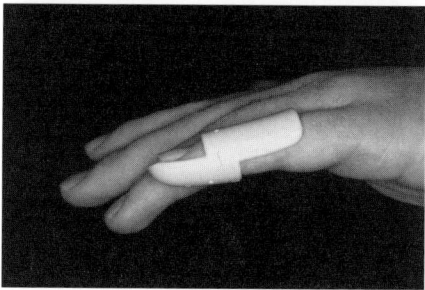

FIGURE 21. Treatment of mallet finger involves immobilization of the DIP joint for a minimum of 12 weeks. The Link, or stack, splint (*shown here*) is a convenient immobilizer. An alternative product is the alumifoam splint (see Figure 44B).

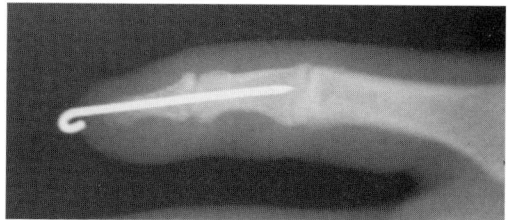

FIGURE 22. Surgical placement of a K-wire across the DIP joint can help maintain the finger in an extended position during the time that is required for the extensor tendon to heal.

weeks, but he or she is cautioned that continual splinting must resume if any "extensor lag" (recurrent drooping at the DIP joint) develops.

In those injuries in which there is no bony avulsion component, the tendon usually is frayed and attenuated, making direct surgical repair difficult to achieve. Surgical placement of a K-wire (Figure 22) through the DIP joint can help maintain the extended position of the finger during the healing phase. If there is a large bony chip, direct surgical repair can achieve gratifying results, with less immobilization required for healing (Figure 23). If the bony fragment is not significantly displaced, excellent healing often can be achieved through splinting alone (as described above).

Fractures

Hand fractures are relatively common injuries, but they typically heal without difficulty due to the hand's excellent vascular supply. Importantly, the bone must heal in an acceptable position, because an angular or rotational deformity can limit or alter hand function. The following section reviews fractures of the wrist, metacarpals, and phalanges.

WRIST (CARPAL) FRACTURES

Fractures of the **scaphoid bone** are the most common wrist fractures. Like distal radius fractures, the typical presenting history is a "fall on

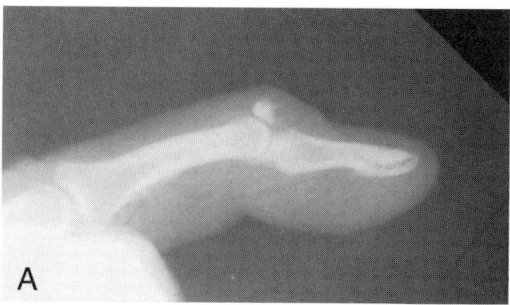
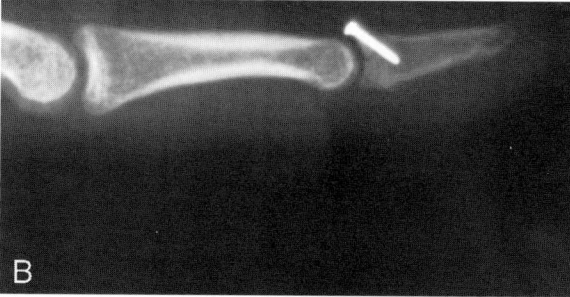

FIGURE 23. **A,** Mallet finger with a relatively large bony fragment that is significantly displaced. In injuries such as these, direct repair of the bone fragment may be possible. **B,** Direct repair using a microscrew to fix the bone chip and its attached tendon into anatomic position.

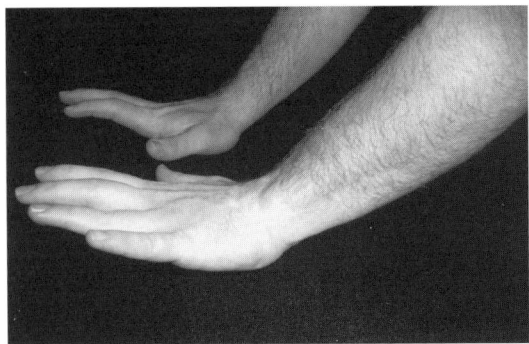

FIGURE 24. Mechanism of scaphoid fractures. Patients with this injury often give a history of a fall on an outstretched hand.

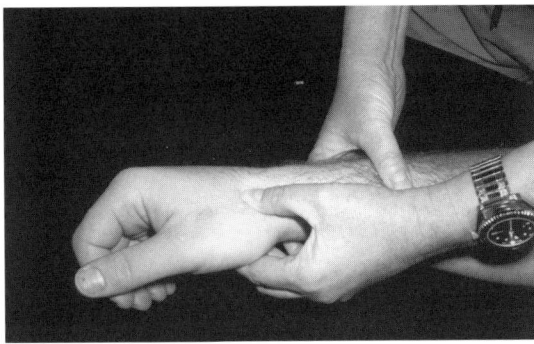

FIGURE 25. Tenderness within the anatomic snuff box is suspicious for a scaphoid fracture.

an outstretched hand" (Figure 24). The physician should have a high index of suspicion for scaphoid fractures, because in the acute setting they often are *not visible* on plain radiographs. Therefore, when a patient presents complaining of wrist pain after a fall or other trauma, a scaphoid fracture should be ruled out. Palpate the scaphoid by applying pressure at the base of the anatomic snuff box (Figure 25). If there is tenderness in this area, a scaphoid fracture is possible (even if x-rays are negative), and the best course of action is to make the presumptive diagnosis of "possible scaphoid fracture" and treat the patient accordingly.

Treatment of scaphoid fractures involves the placement of a thumb spica splint that extends

above the elbow, with the elbow flexed at 90 degrees. The wrist should be positioned slightly extended with a small amount of radial deviation; the thumb is held in a neutral position. Referral to a hand surgeon within 1–2 weeks allows re-examination to check for persistent tenderness, as well as radiographic re-evaluation. If a scaphoid fracture is present, it becomes more obvious on plain x-rays and tomograms over time.

It is important to make the diagnosis of scaphoid fracture early, because if not diagnosed and adequately immobilized, there is a higher risk of progression to nonunion. Nonunion can lead to degenerative arthritis of the wrist, a chronic and painful condition that often is disabling. Operative salvage procedures at this

FIGURE 26. Perilunate dislocation. Fractures within the carpus usually are the result of high-energy injuries and often are accompanied by a significant degree of ligamentous injury. Referral to a hand surgeon is advised.

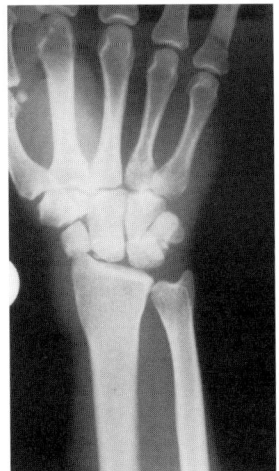
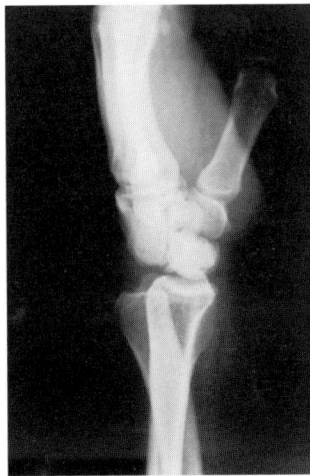

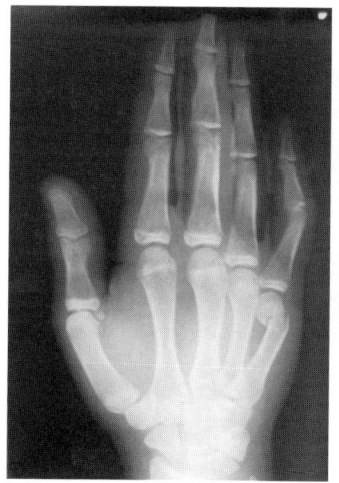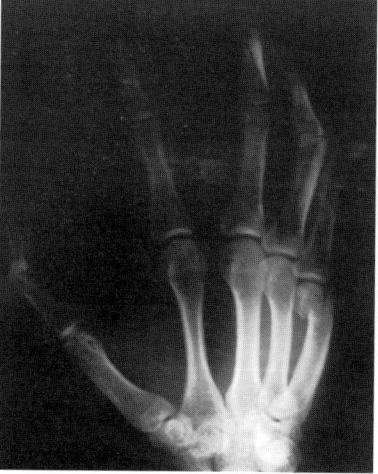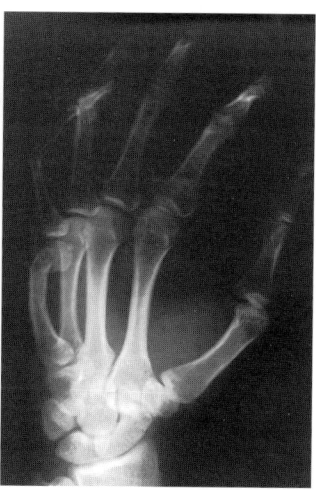

FIGURE 27. A "boxer's fracture" is a fracture of the neck of the fifth metacarpal, usually caused by striking the fist against an immobile object. This term is not applicable to any other type of metacarpal fracture.

point are much less satisfactory than adequate treatment in the acute setting.

Other carpal bone fractures typically result from high-energy events, such as significant falls or vehicular trauma. Unless the injury is nondisplaced and relatively self-limited, consultation with a hand surgeon usually is indicated. Specifically, ligamentous injury must be ruled out, and wrist immobilization should be implemented. In carpal fractures, a perilunate dislocation represents one of the few true emergencies (Figure 26). Volar displacement of the lunate into the carpal tunnel compresses the median nerve, and failure to decompress this nerve operatively can result in serious and permanent neurologic damage. Clues to the presence of a perilunate dislocation are paresthesia and numbness within the median nerve distribution.

METACARPAL FRACTURES

A **boxer's fracture** is an angulated fracture of the neck of the *fifth* metacarpal that is caused by axial loading, such as punching an immobile object with a closed fist (Figure 27). The application of this term to any other type of metacarpal fracture is not appropriate and should be discouraged. Fractures of the other metacarpals

can be produced in the same manner, but the treatment may differ.

The treatment for a true boxer's fracture is relatively straightforward. After the diagnosis is made radiographically and other injuries are excluded, local anesthesia can be obtained using a hematoma block, and reduction and splinting can be performed in the outpatient setting. Reduction is best accomplished by applying pressure on the fractured segment with one hand while pushing upward on the proximal phalanx (Figure 28). The hand is then splinted in an ul-

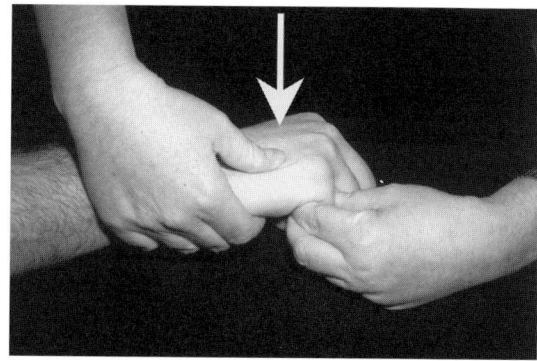

FIGURE 28. One method for reduction of a boxer's fracture after obtaining a hematoma block. While the splint material is curing, place direct pressure (*arrow*) on the fractured metacarpal while pushing upward on the flexed proximal phalanx.

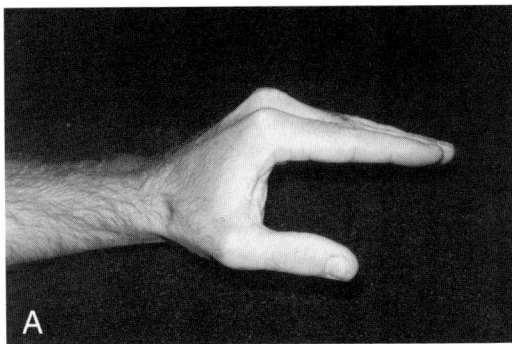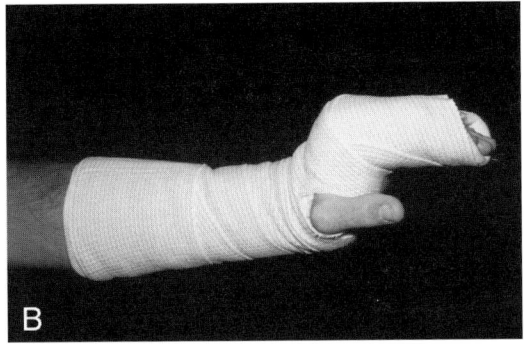

FIGURE 29. **A,** The safe position, in which patients with hand fractures should be splinted (see Figures 53). **B,** Hand immobilized in the safe position after reduction of a boxer's fracture.

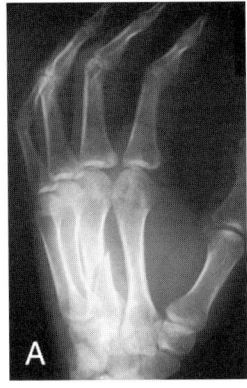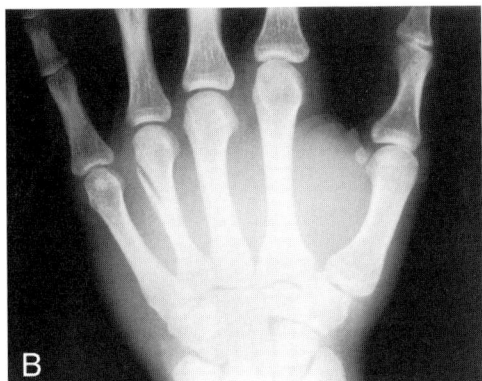

FIGURE 30. Spiral fractures are unstable and are likely to produce finger shortening. **A,** Spiral fracture of the third metacarpal. **B,** Spiral fracture of the fourth metacarpal.

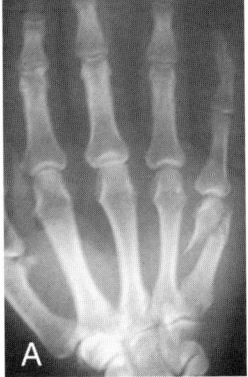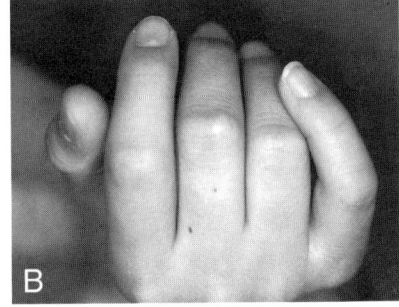

FIGURE 31. **A,** Spiral fracture of the fifth metacarpal. Spiral fractures in border digits are more prone to heal in nonanatomic positions, producing rotational deformities, because they lack supporting ligaments on both sides of the metacarpal. These fractures should be referred to a hand surgeon for reduction and stabilization. **B,** Scissoring of the fifth finger due to a rotational deformity of a proximal phalanx fracture. This fracture was allowed to heal with the finger rotated radially, and when the patient attempts to flex it, the finger bends toward the more radial digits.

nar gutter splint in a **safe position** (Figure 29). Most fractures treated with immobilization alone will need to be splinted for approximately 4–5 weeks. Resolution of tenderness over the fracture site is the single best indicator that immobilization is no longer neccessary.

Current literature suggests that up to 40 degrees of dorsal angulation is acceptable in boxer's fractures. There are several issues to keep in mind. First, this measurement is taken from a direct lateral x-ray of the fracture, which is difficult to obtain. Second, this degree of angulation is ac-

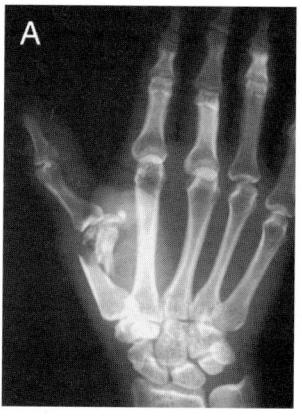
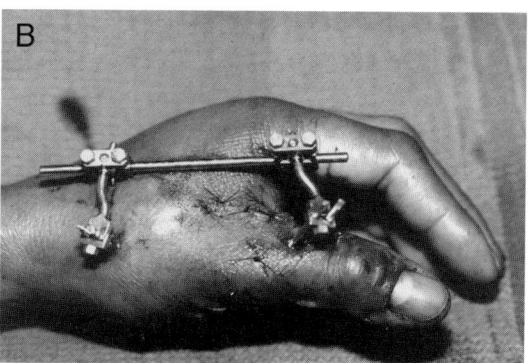

FIGURE 32. A, Severely comminuted fracture of the first metacarpal. Multiple pieces require stabilization. **B,** External fixation to secure the thumb metacarpal in anatomic position during bony healing.

ceptable because most individuals can hyperextend the MCP joint of the fifth finger. Thus, the patient is able to fully extend the finger after bony healing because the MCP hyperextension compensates for the more proximal bony angulation. However, if the patient cannot hyperextend to compensate for this deformity, a corrective osteotomy may be necessary to allow full extension of the small finger. If more than 40 degrees of volar angulation remains after attempted reduction, referral to a hand surgeon is indicated for possible open reduction with internal fixation, or stabilization using percutaneous K-wires.

Metacarpal fractures can limit hand function if not treated properly. In those fractures that

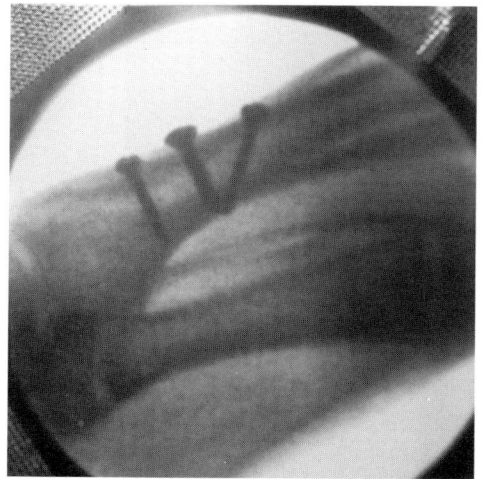

FIGURE 33. Open reduction and internal fixation, using microscrews, of the fracture shown in Figure 30A.

have a spiral or comminuted component, healing may occur with an unacceptable shortening of the bone (Figure 30). The loss of the correct finger length can upset the delicate balance of the flexor and extensor tendons and lead to unacceptable limitation in hand function. In border digits, the surrounding ligamentous support is not available on both sides of the bone; thus, the fractured bones may rotate, causing **scissoring** with flexion if allowed to heal in this position (Figure 31). These issues should be considered when deciding upon the treatment options for metacarpal fractures. A relatively nondisplaced, noncomminuted fracture with no rotational deformity can be adequately treated with immobilization in a splint.

Casting a fracture in the acute setting is rarely indicated. It is likely that the hand will reach maximal edema and swelling 2–3 days after the injury, and the presence of a circumferential cast can cause compression, leading to ischemia of the hand and forearm. In the acute setting, splinting is the best treatment option. A splint does not guarantee avoidance of circumferential pressure problems, but it is much safer and more forgiving than a cast. Still, patients always should be instructed to call or return for evaluation if the splint feels too tight or if neurologic deficits, such as numbness, develop in the splinted upper extremity.

Comminuted fractures (in multiple pieces) and spiral fractures require operative fixation or stabilization (Figures 32, 33). When closed

FIGURE 34. **A,** Transverse fracture of the midshaft of the fourth metacarpal. This type of fracture is responsive to immobilization alone, if anatomic reduction can be achieved. Unfortunately, attempts at reduction were unsuccessful in this patient, necessitating open reduction and internal fixation. **B,** Open reduction and internal fixation using a specialized plate and screw system to maintain the metacarpal in anatomic alignment. One advantage of open reduction and internal fixation techniques is that the hand and fingers can be mobilized much sooner than if splinting alone is used; thus, resultant hand stiffness is reduced and the patient can resume normal activities more rapidly.

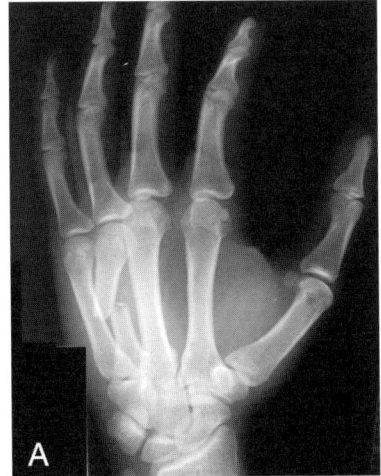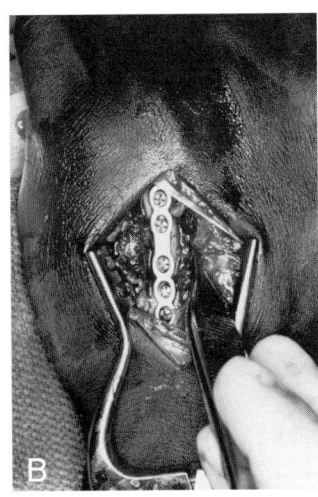

reduction is not possible, open reduction and internal fixation can be achieved using plates and screws (Figure 34). Again, however, placing the patient in a volar splint in a safe position is all that needs to be accomplished in the acute setting, with referral to a hand specialist within the next several days. When closed reduction or simple immobilization is the only treatment necessary, the splint can be changed to a cast after about 1 week if the edema has begun to resolve. The cast should remain in place for 4–5 weeks. The *absence of tenderness* over the fracture site is the single best indicator that the fracture has healed and immobilization is no longer necessary (Figure 35). Note that it is common for radiographic findings to lag behind the clinical situation; the fracture often remains visible on x-ray, even though it has healed.

Fractures of the base of the thumb metacarpal are called **Bennett's fractures** (Figure 36). Because of the thumb's border position on the hand, it is provided less support than the middle metacarpals and therefore is more prone

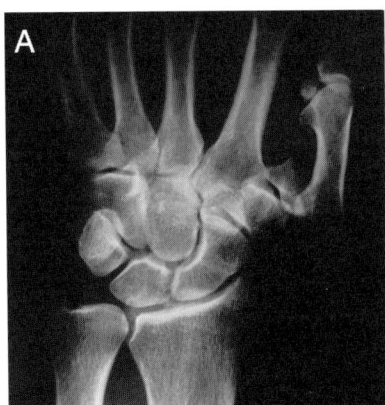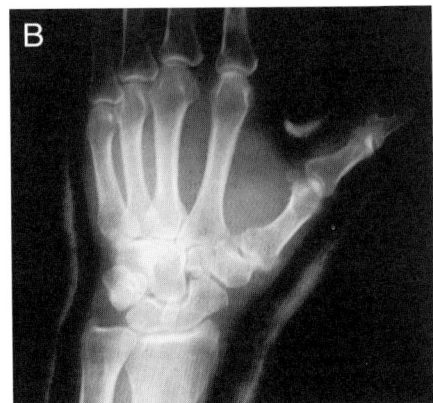

FIGURE 35. **A,** Displaced transverse fracture of the first metacarpal. **B,** After reduction and splint placement, the bone is in precise anatomic position. As long as this position can be maintained, operative intervention is unnecessary. Treatment entails 5 weeks of immobilization; bony healing is confirmed by a complete absence of tenderness over the fracture.

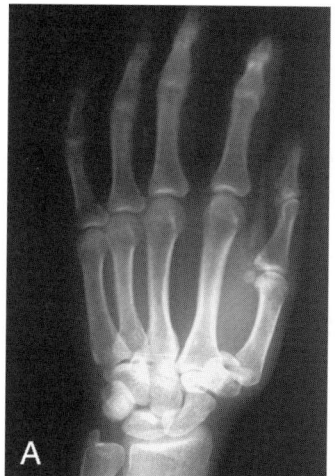
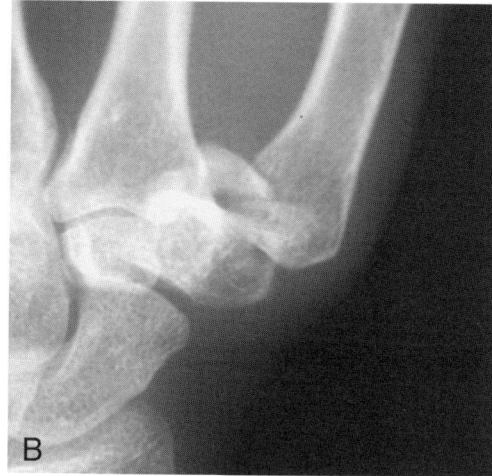

FIGURE 36. **A,** Bennett's fracture (fracture of the base of the thumb metacarpal). **B,** Close-up view. When the base of the first metacarpal is fractured, the distal metacarpal is pulled radially and proximally by the abductor pollicis longus muscle (see Chapter 1, Figure 27). These fractures require referral to a hand specialist for reduction.

to malposition after fracture. Specifically, the thumb metacarpal often is pulled radially and proximally by the abductor pollicis longus muscle. As a result of this tendency for displacement, referral to a hand surgeon is indicated for percutaneous pinning or open reduction and internal fixation of the fracture.

A similar situation exists for **reverse Bennett's fractures,** which are fractures of the base of the fifth metacarpal (Figure 37). As with the thumb metacarpal, due to a tendency for displacement resulting in functional problems, re-

ferral to a hand surgeon for fracture stabilization is recommended.

PROXIMAL AND MIDDLE PHALANGEAL FRACTURES

Phalangeal fractures are much more likely than metacarpal fractures to heal in a nonanatomic position, producing rotational or angular deformities with scissoring (see Figure 31B) if not treated properly. The metacarpals have supportive and stabilizing ligaments be-

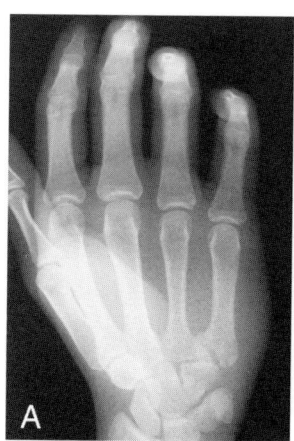
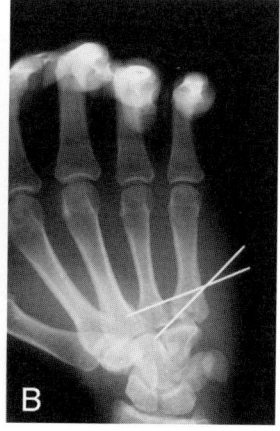

FIGURE 37. **A,** A reverse Bennett's fracture is analogous to a Bennett's fracture, but the base of the fifth metacarpal is fractured. **B,** Due to its position on the border of the hand and the ulnar pull of the attached musculature, this fracture must be reduced with K-wires.

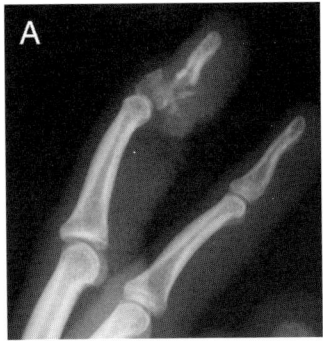
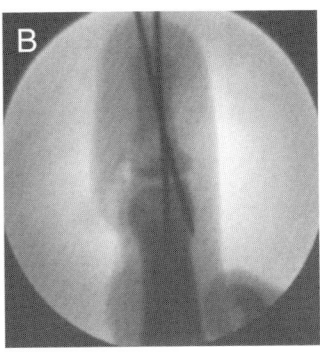

FIGURE 38. **A,** Severely comminuted distal phalanx fracture with volar displacement. **B,** One method of stabilization for this type of fracture is percutaneous K-wires, which are left in place for 5–6 weeks while bony healing occurs. K-wires are invaluable in maintaining the position of the bone while it is healing.

tween them, which the phalanges lack. Treatment options for phalangeal fractures include percutaneous K-wire fixation to maintain anatomic position during healing (Figure 38), and open reduction and internal fixation using microplates and screws (Figure 39). Occasionally, nondisplaced fractures can be treated with immobilization alone. The availability of screws as small as 1 millimeter in diameter have greatly improved the surgeon's ability to reconstruct correct anatomic position in these fractures, allowing good bone healing with minimal

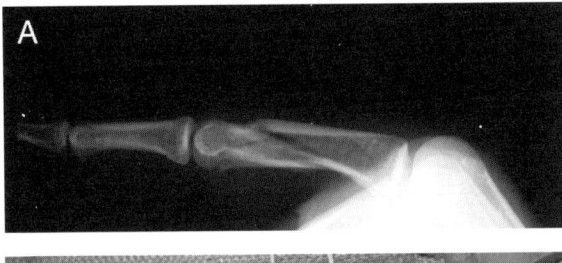
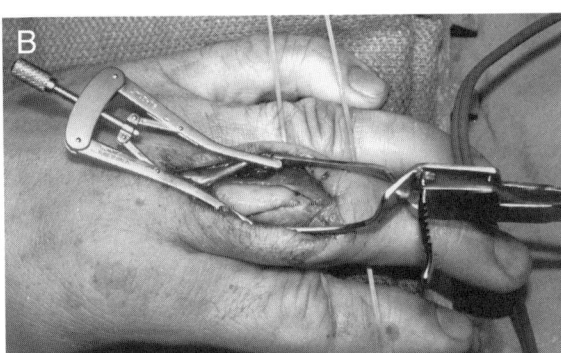
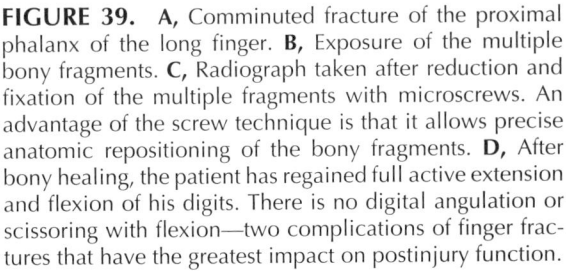
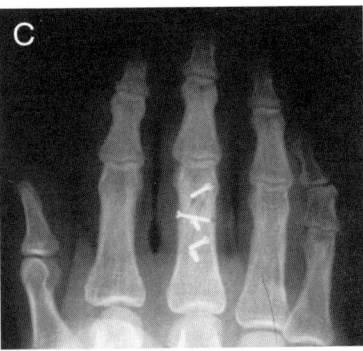
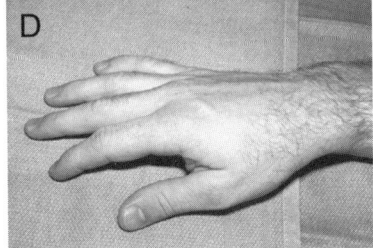
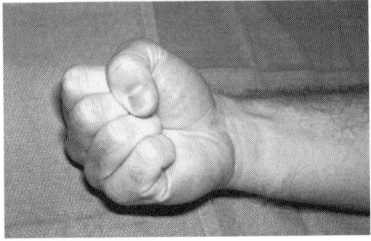

FIGURE 39. **A,** Comminuted fracture of the proximal phalanx of the long finger. **B,** Exposure of the multiple bony fragments. **C,** Radiograph taken after reduction and fixation of the multiple fragments with microscrews. An advantage of the screw technique is that it allows precise anatomic repositioning of the bony fragments. **D,** After bony healing, the patient has regained full active extension and flexion of his digits. There is no digital angulation or scissoring with flexion—two complications of finger fractures that have the greatest impact on postinjury function.

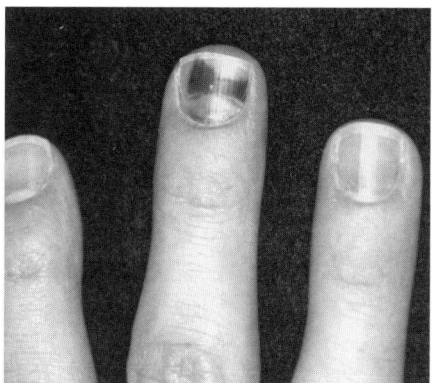

FIGURE 40. A subungual hematoma is a collection of blood underneath the fingernail that puts pressure on the nail matrix and can be exquisitely painful. Drainage usually is indicated for patient comfort. Subungual hematomas can be clues to underlying injuries of the distal phalanx and/or nail matrix.

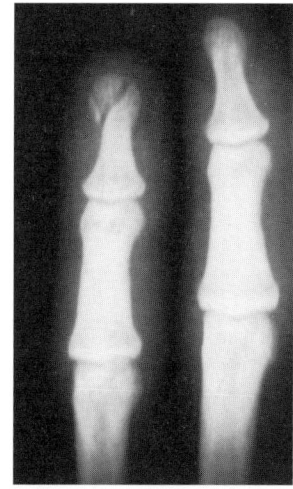

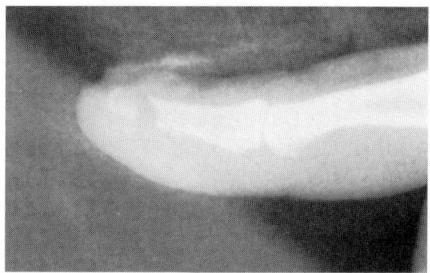

FIGURE 41. Tuft fractures.

deformity. When there is the potential for malunion (fracture healing in a nonanatomic position), the patient should be splinted in a safe position and referred to a hand surgeon for possible operative intervention within 1 week.

DISTAL PHALANGEAL FRACTURES

Fractures of the distal phalanx, tuft fractures, and associated nail bed injuries are common. They generally occur in the longer fingers, which are more likely to be struck by doors and falling objects (typical scenarios). The diagnosis of these fractures usually is straightforward, from the radiographs, but there are several important points to keep in mind.

Distal phalangeal fractures frequently are associated with **nail bed injuries.** If a patient presents with a subungual hematoma, be suspicious of an underlying fracture, and obtain an x-ray (Figure 40). Conversely, if an x-ray reveals a distal phalanx fracture, be suspicious of an underlying nail bed injury (Figure 41). The nail bed (the germinal and sterile matrix that produces the nail) is located directly on the surface of the tuft of the distal phalanx. A *displaced* fracture of the distal phalanx, there-

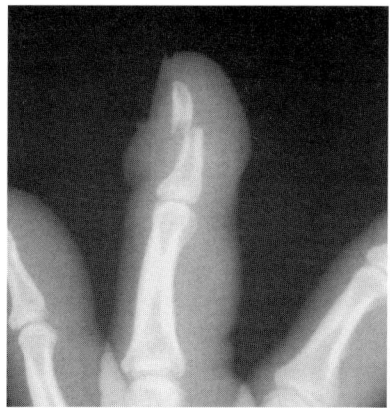

FIGURE 42. Displaced distal phalanx fracture. Note that the distal aspect of this fracture is displaced dorsally. Therefore, there is a high probability of nail bed injury, because the nail matrix lies on the dorsal aspect of the distal phalanx.

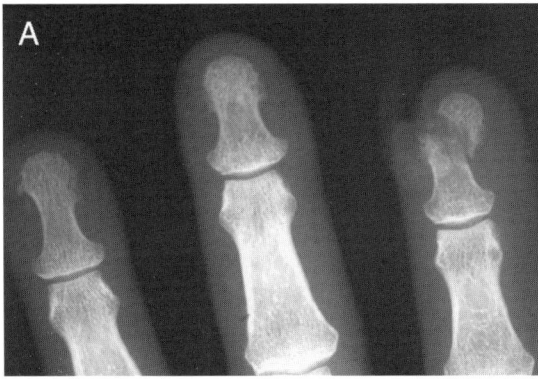 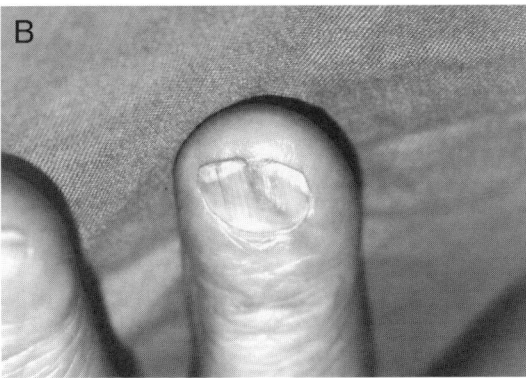

FIGURE 43. **A,** Displaced distal phalanx fracture. The more significant the distal phalanx fracture, the more likely an underlying nail bed injury. **B,** This patient's nail matrix injury went unrecognized. Although the bone healed without difficulty, the damage to the underlying nail matrix resulted in a split nail deformity.

fore, is likely to be associated with a laceration of the overlying nail bed (Figure 42). Nail bed lacerations are especially probable if a subungual hematoma covers more than 50% of the nail surface.

Nontreated lacerations of the nail bed can result in late deformities such as split nail or a nonadherent nail (Figure 43). These deformities are difficult to rectify and typically require a nail bed graft from the great toe. The best treatment option is acute repair, which requires a hand surgical consultation. That is not to say that a consultation is required for all distal phalangeal fractures, but note that ex-

ploration of the nail bed may be warranted if the fracture is displaced.

Nondisplaced fractures of the distal phalanx typically heal without surgical intervention. They are best immobilized using a stack or Link) splint, or an alumifoam splint for a period of 3–5 weeks (Figure 44). Nondisplaced fractures often heal without consequence.

Subungual hematomas can be very painful. When patients present with an acute hematoma, perform decompression in the outpatient setting. The easiest and most efficacious way to do this is with an ophthalmic

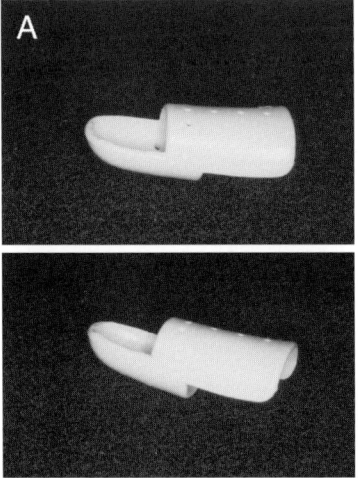 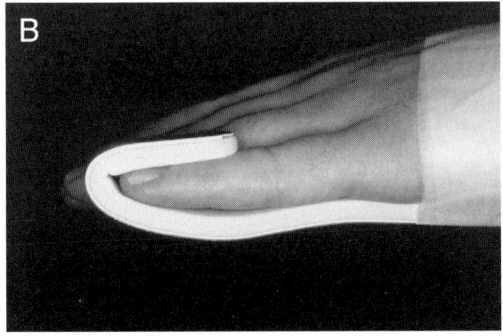

FIGURE 44. **A,** Link, or stack, splints come in a variety of sizes and are quite useful for distal fingertip injuries. **B,** An alumifoam splint can be bent and fashioned to provide support and protection for distal phalanx injuries, as well.

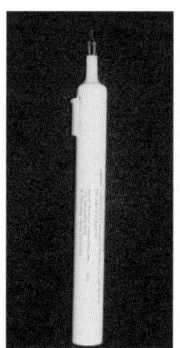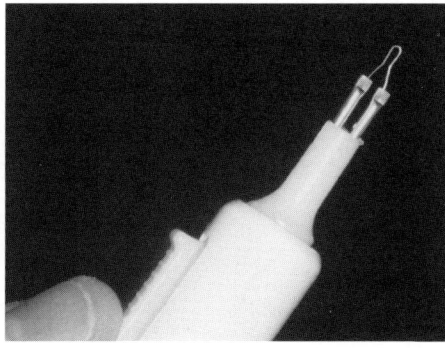

FIGURE 45. Ophthalmic cautery. These disposable units can be used to drain subungual hematomas in the outpatient setting. Activation causes the distal wire to heat until it is red hot.

cautery unit (Figure 45). Heat the cautery for a few seconds until the tip is at its hottest (glowing red), and then firmly press the tip directly through the nail to create a hole through which the hematoma can drain. If the patient is apprehensive about this procedure, offer a digital block, but be sure to inform the patient that placement of the block usually is more painful than the cauterization. If an ophthalmic cautery unit is not available, a hole can be "drilled" into the nail with a large-bore (i.e. 16- or 18-gauge) hypodermic needle. However, this method is much more painful for the patient than ophthalmic cautery, because more pressure has to be applied to the nail. Therefore, a digital block should be placed prior to starting.

FRACTURES IN CHILDREN

The treatment guidelines for children with hand fractures are largely the same as for adults. However, there are some differences that merit discussion. If immobilization is chosen as the treatment for a patient less than 8 years old, the splint should extend above the elbow, with the elbow flexed at 90 degrees. If a standard gauntlet splint is applied, the child probably will toss it aside before exiting your office. Although it may seem like overkill to use a total arm cast for a nondisplaced metacarpal or phalangeal fracture, most chil-

dren of this age will seek to escape from any immobilization. By extending the splint above the elbow, escape is impossible. An important technical point when making this splint is that *the cast padding/wrap must be placed while the elbow is flexed at 90 degrees.* Although this maneuver makes the splint construction more difficult, if the wrap is placed with the arm slightly or fully extended, flexion will cause impingement and compression at the antecubital fossa.

Children may present with a nondisplaced unicortical fracture of the metacarpals or phalanges (also called a "greenstick" fracture). These fractures occur because childrens' bones are incompletely ossified and are more flexible than adults'. They are termed greenstick fractures because the bone bends and fractures at one side, but its flexibility prevents it from completely breaking—like a young (green) tree branch. Greenstick fractures typically are treated with splint immobilization for 3–4 weeks.

Fractures that involve the growth plate can be characterized using the Salter-Harris classification system (Figure 46). Because the growth plate is an area of relative weakness within the bone, fractures in children tend to occur there. Salter-Harris type II fractures are the most common (Figures 47, 48); type V fractures (compressing the growth plate) have the worst prognosis for producing growth deformities.

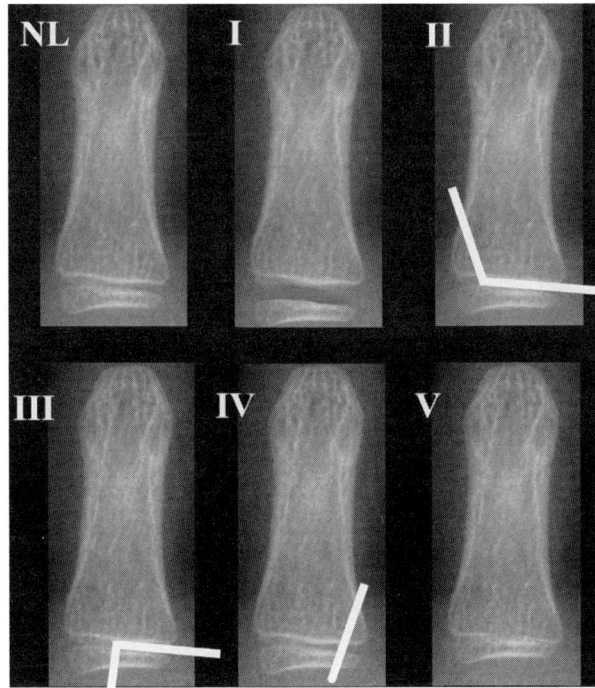

FIGURE 46. Salter-Harris classification of epiphyseal plate fractures. **NL** is a normal proximal phalanx and growth plate in a child. **Type I** is diagnosed by separation of the growth plate. **Type II** involves a fracture as indicated by the *white line.* This is the most common pattern of growth plate fracture. **Types III and IV** are less commonly seen (again, *white line* denotes fracture location). **Type V** involves compression of the growth plate and narrowing of the joint space. This type of growth plate fracture has the worse prognosis for producing growth deformities.

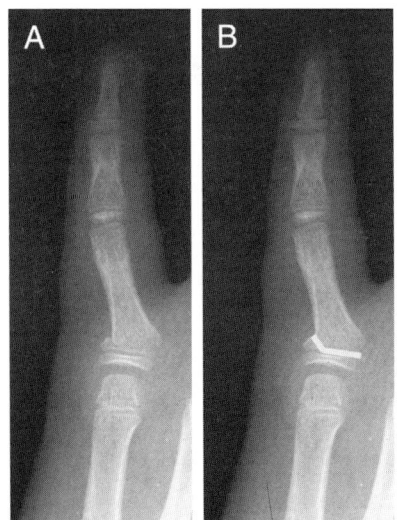

FIGURE 47. **A,** Salter-Harris type II fracture in a 10-year-old girl. **B,** Note the fracture pattern (*white line*).

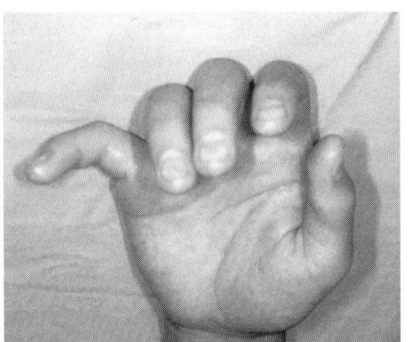
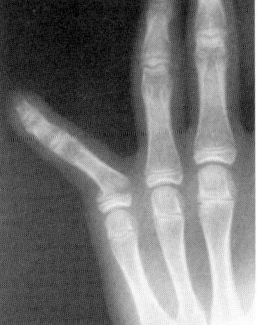

FIGURE 48. Salter Harris type II fracture in a 9-year-old girl.

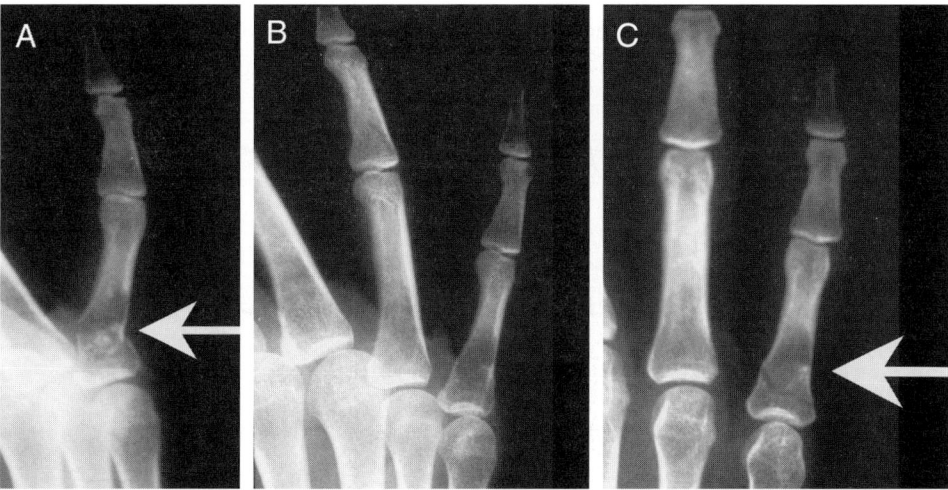

FIGURE 49. Pathologic fractures of the proximal phalanx. **A,** A lytic lesion (*arrow*) in the hand usually is caused by an enchondroma, which is a benign entity that gradually weakens bony cortex, predisposing it to fracture despite minimal or no trauma. **B** and **C,** Lytic lesion (*arrow*) at the base of the fifth proximal phalanx.

Fractures of the growth plate can be difficult to diagnose: a trick for reading these films is to obtain x-rays of the contralateral side for comparison.

PATHOLOGIC FRACTURES

Occasionally, a patient presents with a fracture and a history of minimal or no trauma. Be alert for evidence of an underlying bony lesion on radiographs (Figure 49). Pre-existing conditions (in particular tumors) can weaken the bone, predisposing to ultimate fracture. In the hand, enchondroma frequently is the underlying bony pathology causing pathologic fractures. Enchondroma is a benign tumor of the bone that produces a lytic lesion visible on x-ray. When diagnosed, splinting of the hand and referral to a hand surgeon are necessary for formal treatment of the underlying condition.

Splint Manufacture

The ability to make a comfortable and safe splint is a mandatory skill for taking care of pa-

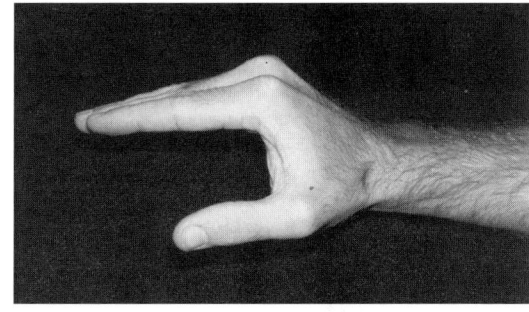

FIGURE 50. The "safe" position for splinting: the wrist is extended approximately 20°, the MCPs are flexed 70–80°, the IP joints are fully extended, and the thumb is abducted away from the palm.

tients with hand injuries. In the acute injury setting, prefabricated splints have little value beyond the treatment of minor wrist strains.

HAND POSITION

The optimum position in which to place the hand and fingers during splinting depends on the type of injury. The position most frequently appropriate (i.e., appropriate for most of the injuries seen) is called the **safe position**: the wrist

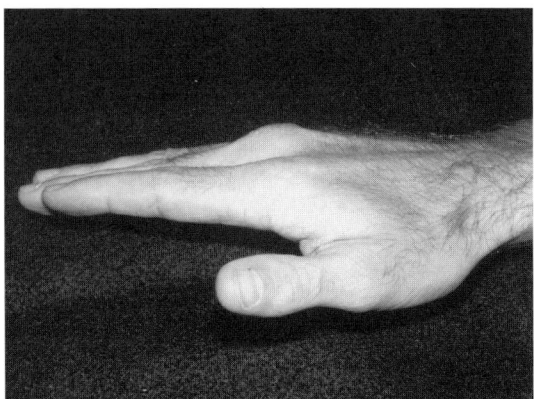

FIGURE 51. The proper hand position for splinting of extensor tendon injuries: the wrist is extended 10–20°, the MCPs are slightly flexed at 10–20°, and the IPs are fully extended.

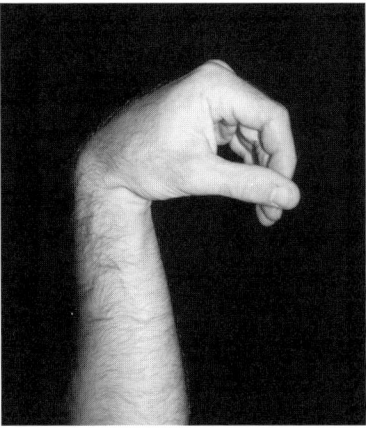

FIGURE 52. Proper positioning for splinting of flexor tendon injuries. The wrist, MCP joints, and IP joints are flexed to decrease tension on the proximal tendon ends. To maintain this position, the splint material is placed on the *dorsal* surface of the hand, rather than the volar surface. The wrist should not be maximally flexed, but placed at about 20° less than full flexion; otherwise the position will be intolerable for an extended period of time.

is placed at approximately 20 degrees of extension with the MCPs at 70–80 degrees of flexion, the IP joints are fully extended, and the thumb is abducted away from the palm (Figure 50). This usually is the best position for stabilizing a patient's hand when there are fractures or other injuries. It is termed safe because moderately

prolonged immobilization will not result in irreversible stiffness.

For **extensor tendon injuries** (repaired or not), the hand is splinted in a more extended posture: the wrist is slightly extended 10–20 degrees, the MCPs are slightly flexed 10–20 degrees, and the IPs are fully extended (Figure 51). This position minimizes tension on the extensor tendons during healing, or minimizes proximal tendon retraction in the prerepair period.

Flexor tendon injuries should be splinted with the wrist, MCPs, and IPs flexed (Figure 52). *The wrist should not be maximally flexed*, or the patient will be unable to tolerate the splint: the wrist position should be 20–25 degrees less than maximal passive flexion. This flexed posture minimizes tension on the proximal flexor tendons prior to repair and prevents excessive retraction into the proximal forearm.

CONSTRUCTION

1. Cut a stockinette and place it on the hand extending from the fingertips to the elbow. Cut a small hole in the side to allow the thumb to come through (Figure 53A). Fashion the stockinette longer than the anticipated splint, to allow folding over of the ends (see step 4).

2. Apply circumferentially several layers of cast padding (Figure 53B). This is particularly important over areas of bony prominence, to provide cushioning and prevent pressure from the splint from injuring the underlying skin and soft tissue.

3. Place the splint material on the volar aspect of the hand and forearm for extensor tendon injuries (dorsal for flexor tendon injuries). The splinting materials used most commonly today are plaster and fiberglass. Fiberglass splint material sets more rapidly and is lighter than plaster; however, it also is more expensive. Both fiberglass and plaster are activated by soaking in water. Stack several layers of splint material (Figure 53C) to ensure that the splint will be strong and rigid enough to prop-

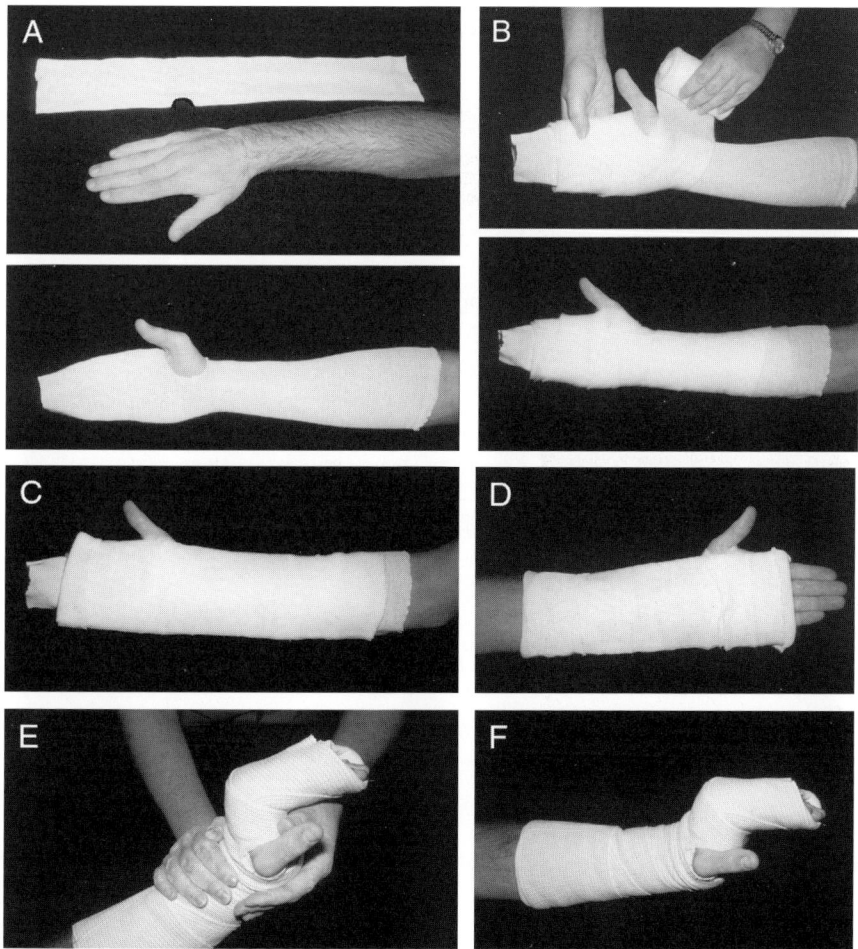

FIGURE 53. Splint manufacture. **A,** Cut a piece of stockinette *longer* than the desired splint, so that the ends can be folded over. Cut a small hole to allow the thumb to protrude. **B,** Apply circumferentially several layers of cast padding to provide cushioning over areas of bony prominence and prevent injury from splint pressure. **C,** Prefold the splint material and check length by placing it over the hand and forearm. After determining correct length and thickness, soak the splint material in water, squeeze excess water out, and replace it in position on the hand and forearm. **D,** Roll the excess proximal and distal stockinette back over the edge of the splint material and cast padding. **E,** Loosely wrap an ace bandage around the entire forearm and hand. While the splint material sets, maintain the hand and fingers in the *precise position* desired. **F,** Completed splint, with the hand in the safe position.

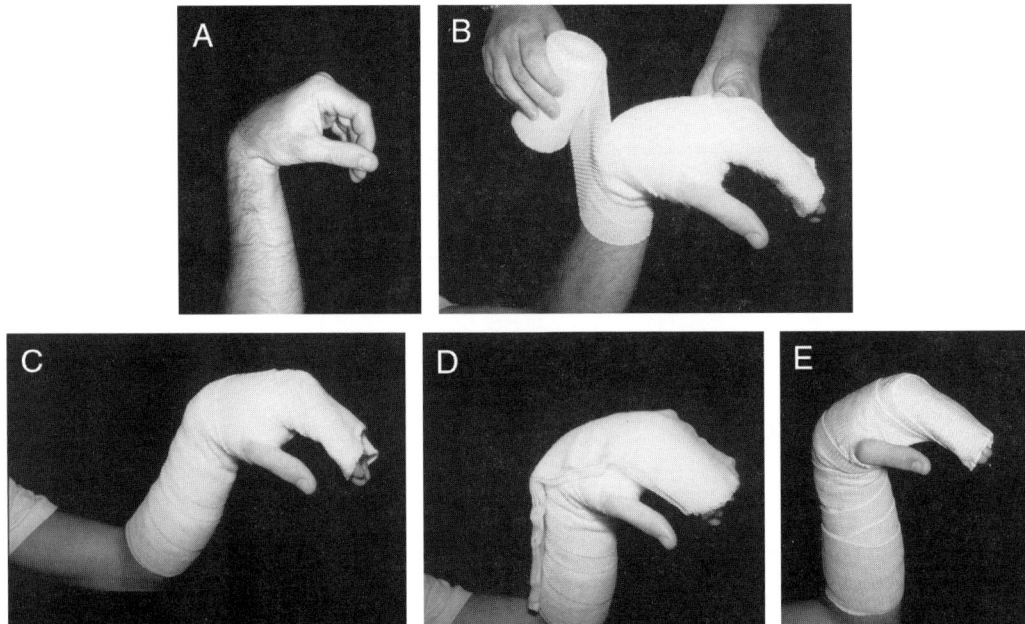

FIGURE 54. Splinting of flexor tendon injuries. **A,** The wrist, MCP joints, and IP joints are maintained in a flexed posture to minimize tension on the tendon ends. **B,** Application of the protective cast padding. It is critical that the wrist joint be in flexion *during* this step. (Similarly, elbow flexion is critical when making a long arm or above-elbow splint). If the joint is fully extended while the cast padding is placed, subsequent flexion may cause compression and impingement. **C,** Hand and upper extremity after application of cast padding. **D,** Place the splint material on the dorsum of the hand and check it for length and thickness. **E,** Wrap the forearm and hand with a bandage. The splint is complete when the splinting material has set.

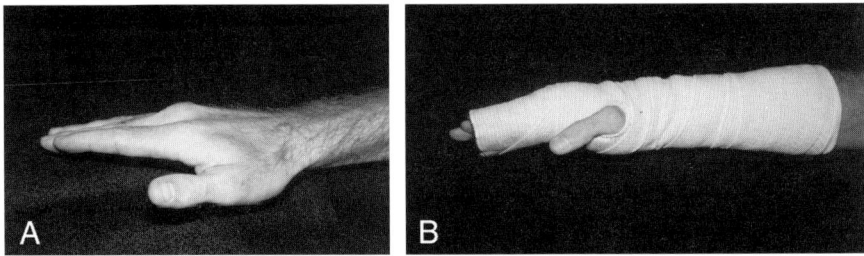

FIGURE 55. Splinting of extensor tendon injuries. **A,** Correct position of hand and wrist. **B,** After application of the cast padding, volar splint material, and ace wrap.

erly immobilize the hand. After selecting and fashioning the correct length of the desired splint, soak it in water, squeeze the excess water out, and then place the material over the cast padding on the hand and forearm. Always wear plastic gloves when working with fiberglass, or you will be left with a residue on your hands that is difficult to remove for a few days.

4. After placing the splint material on the hand and forearm, roll the stockinette back over the ends of the splint proximally and distally (Figure 53D). Then loosely wrap the entire splint (while still malleable) with a 4-inch ace wrap. The stockinette covers the loose edges of the cast padding and splint material and makes the splint look tidy.

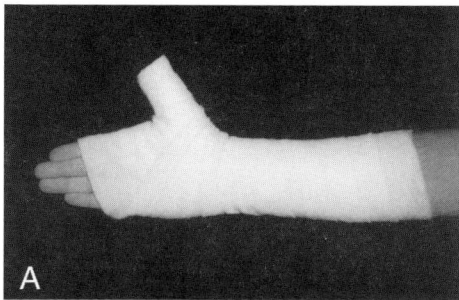

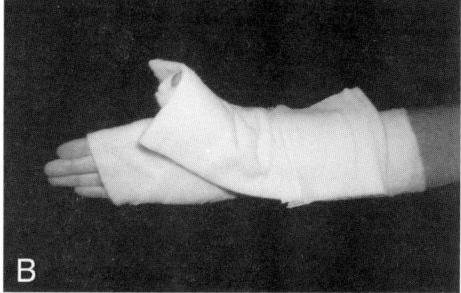

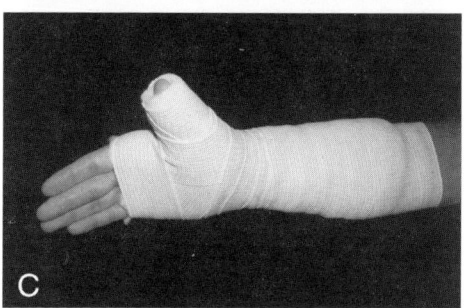

FIGURE 56. Splinting of thumb injuries. **A,** Place the circumferential cast padding over the thumb, hand, and distal forearm. **B,** Apply the splint material (at least 4 inches wide) on the radial aspect of the forearm and thumb, with the two edges at the thumb wrapped volarly to immobilize it completely. **C,** After application of ace wrap.

5. While waiting for the splint to harden, hold the hand and splint in the *precise position* desired until the splint has completely set (Figures 53E and F).

The most common mistake made by individuals with little splinting experience is *too tight* construction. A splint that is too tight can be uncomfortable as well as dangerous; there is risk of ischemic damage to the hand and forearm.

The steps for creation of a splint after flexor tendon injuries are illustrated in Figure 54; for extensor tendon injuries in Figure 55; and for thumb injury in Figure 56.

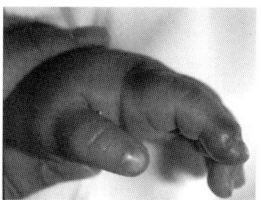

7 Infections of the Hand

The early diagnosis of hand infections and the judicious use of antibiotics has prevented a great deal of hand disability since the advent of the antibiotic era. The cardinal signs and symptoms of infection are: tenderness, local warmth, redness (erythema), and swelling. When evaluating patients with these symptoms and a history of penetrating trauma (i.e., a cut), it is important to ensure that no foreign body is retained (Figure 1). If an infectious process is suspected, determine whether it is a **cellulitis,** or if is there an underlying **abscess** formation. This distinction is critical because the treatment of cellulitis involves antibiotics only, while the presence of an abscess or fluid collection demands drainage in addition to antibiotic therapy. Kanavel (*Infections of the Hand,* Lea & Febiger, 1925) stated that pus is present (even if it can't be seen) if the patient complains of throbbing pain or has lost a night's sleep due to pain. Quite often, patients with serious hand infections do not demonstrate systemic complaints, and do not present with a fever or an elevated white cell count.

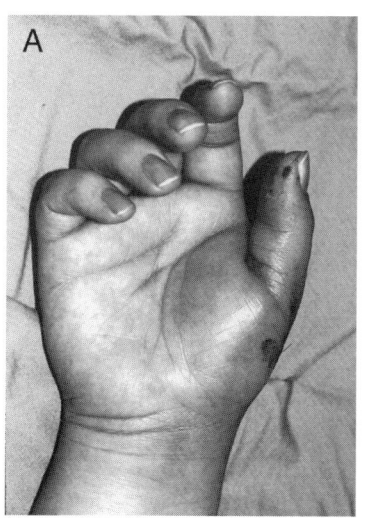
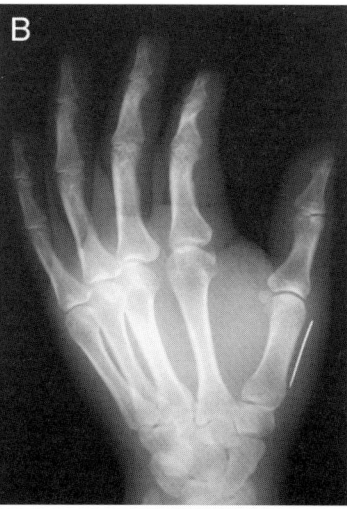

FIGURE 1 **A,** Forty-year-old female with a 3-day history of swelling, erythema, and pain along her thumb and thenar eminence. She denied any history of trauma, but mentioned an episode of pain while dusting a countertop several days prior. **B,** Radiograph demonstrating a retained foreign body (sewing needle) buried deep within the soft tissue of the hand near the first metacarpal. Always check for foreign bodies when evaluating a patient with an infectious process of the hand. While some objects are radiopaque (e.g., metals, types of glass), others may not be visible on radiograph (e.g., thorns, other orgainc material).

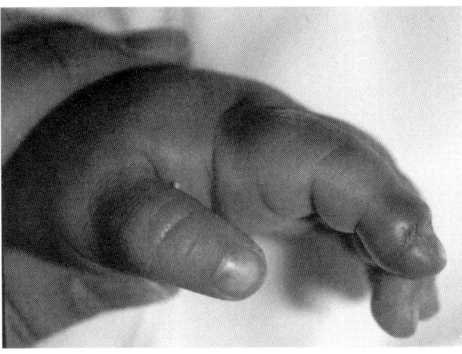 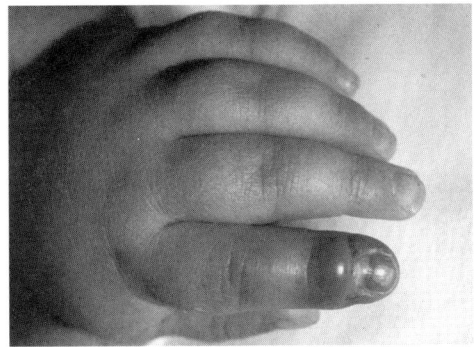

FIGURE 2. Paronychia of the index finger, the most common infection in the hand. Patients complain of pain and demonstrate swelling and erythema around the nail. Treatment involves removal of the offending part of the nail and antibiotics.

Types of Infection

PARONYCHIA

Paronychia is the most common hand infection: the "infected hangnail" (Figure 2). Quite often there is a localized collection of purulence. Drainage of this fluid, removal of the offending part of the nail, and antibiotics usually are sufficient to treat these infections.

When planning a local anesthetic in patients with finger infections, it is best to block the nerves *proximal* to the infection (i.e., with a digital or wrist block). It is *never* a good idea to in-

ject within or near an infected area, because the needle can physically spread the bacteria into uninvolved tissues. When preparing to treat paronychia, a standard digital block at the base of the finger (see Chapter 3) is the most efficacious way to achieve anesthesia, allowing manipulation and drainage.

After the finger is completely anesthetized, elevate the nail from its nail bed by gently sliding a small elevator (Figure 3A) underneath the affected portion (Figure 3B). If the infection is at the proximal nail, the entire nail should be removed (Figure 4). If the infection involves only the ulnar or radial aspect, only that side of the

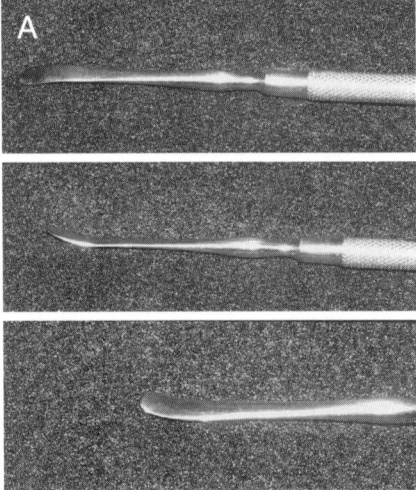 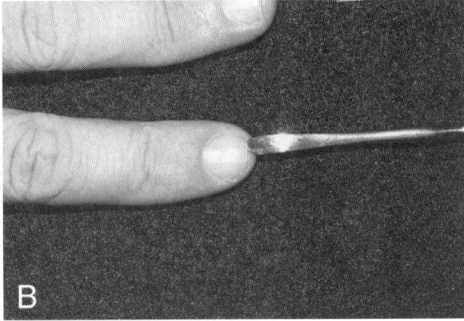

FIGURE 3. Treatment of paronychia. **A,** Use an elevator tool to lift the nail from its underlying nail bed. **B,** Introduce the elevator just under the nail at the hyponychium and advance it proximally.

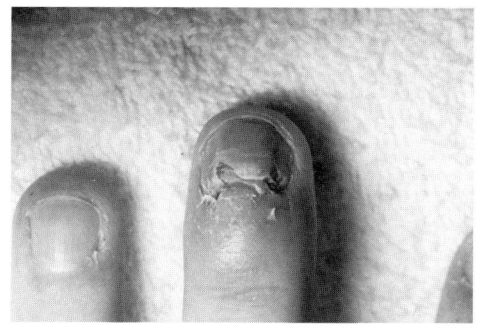

FIGURE 4. Chronic paronychia involving the proximal aspect of the nail bed. In situations such as this, the entire nail should be removed.

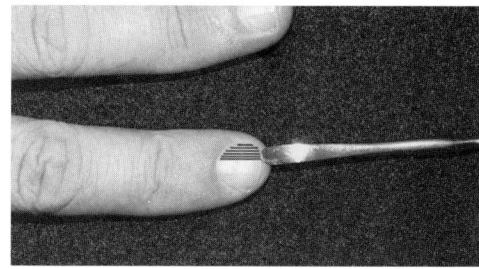

FIGURE 5. Diagrammatic representation of the nail portion that should be removed in ulnar-sided paronychia. In this example, the ulnar aspect of the nail should be elevated from the underlying bed and excised using a scissors. The radial aspect of the nail can be left in place.

nail needs to be removed (Figure 5). Finally, using a scissors directed *away* from the nail bed, open and drain the purulence collection (always remember to send a culture of any fluid encountered when draining abcesses). A small wick of gauze can be placed within the space for 24 hours to maintain drainage; if the entire nail is removed, a thin sheet of silastic or non-adherent gauze should be placed within the eponychial fold (Figure 6). Prescribe an oral-antibiotic with adequate coverage against gram-positive organisms (such as cephalexin) and instruct the patient to start warm soaks of the affected finger several times a day in warm saline.

FELON

A felon is an abscess within the pulp of the volar fingertip and distal phalanx. It usually is exquisitely tender. A felon is a unique type of infection because it is maintained in a small area by the fibrous septae that connect the skin to the underlying bone. Recall that these fibrous connections exist at the palmar hands and at the soles of the feet to prevent shearing off of the skin.

In the past, a "fish mouth" incision was advocated to drain felons (Figure 7). However, this practice has been abandoned due to late problems with scarring. The best approach

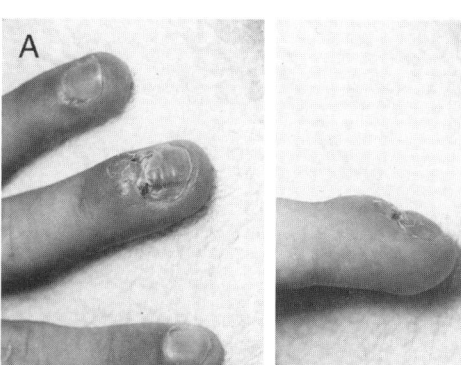
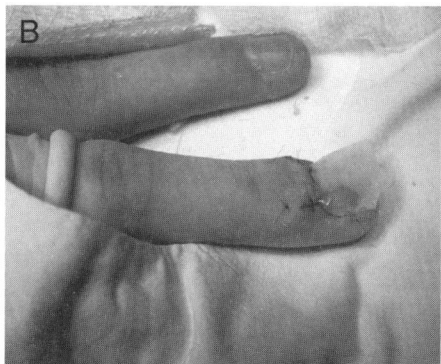

FIGURE 6. **A,** Chronic paronychia involving the proximal aspect of the nail fold. In cases such as this, the entire nail should be removed. **B,** After nail removal, a piece of silicone rubber sheeting is placed within the eponychial fold for several days to maintain the fold during healing.

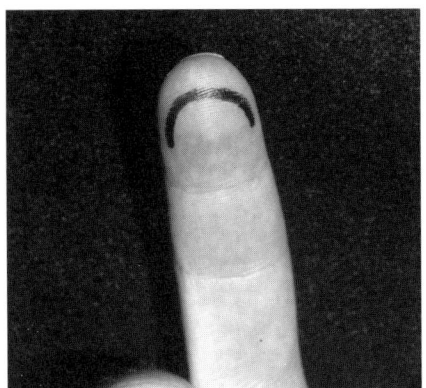

FIGURE 7. "Fish mouth" incision. This incision *should not* be used to drain felons or abscesses of the distal pulp because it often heals poorly, with retraction of the proximal tissue.

when draining these abscesses is a lateral incision on the *noncontact* aspect of the digit, directly overlying the abscess if possible. The noncontact aspect of the finger is the radial side of the ring and fifth fingers and the ulnar side of the index and long fingers (Figures 8, 9). Volar incisions are less desirable because the scar will be in a position of function; however, they may be appropriate if the abscess cannot be reached by a lateral incision. Incise over the point of maximal tenderness.

Note that it is better to make an incision and not discover a fluid collection, than to leave a purulence collection undrained. *Err on the side of aggressive treatment.* Always culture the fluid when an abscess is drained, so that the antibiotic treatment can be confirmed, or corrected if necessary. After drainage, prescribe an oral antibiotic (typically an agent with good staphylococcus coverage, such as cephalexin) and instruct the patient to begin soaks with warm saline several times a day. Whenever an infectious process is drained, the incision should be left open and allowed to heal by secondary intention. It is an error to suture these wounds closed, because the abscess usually will recur.

FLEXOR SHEATH INFECTIONS

Infections within the flexor tendon sheath can be rapidly progressive, resulting in a devastating loss of hand function. They usually occur after a penetrating trauma to the hand during which the flexor sheath is inoculated with bacteria. Early diagnosis and rapid surgical treatment are absolutely mandatory to minimize disability in these patients. Scarring of the flexor tendons of the digit can be so severe that active flexion and extension are blocked. There are several classic signs of this infection (originally outlined by Kanavel):

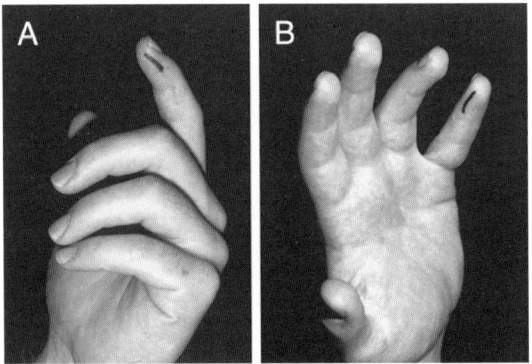

FIGURE 8. Draining incisions are best placed laterally on the noncontact aspect of the finger. **A,** The noncontact aspect of the index finger is the ulnar side. **B,** Of the fifth finger, the radial side.

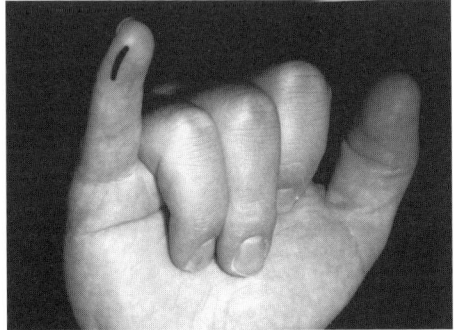

FIGURE 9. Occasionally, the infectious process is located directly over a contact area. In these cases, it is better to incise and drain directly over the fluctuance than to attempt tunneling from the noncontact side to the infected area.

1. The patient holds the finger in a slightly flexed position.
2. The finger has fusiform swelling (acquiring the appearance of an overstuffed sausage).
3. Passive extension of the digit is exquisitely painful for the patient.
4. The patient complains of tenderness proximally on the volar palm along the flexor sheath.

If infection of the flexor tendon sheath is suspected, a hand surgeon should be consulted emergently for irrigation and debridement.

HERPETIC WHITLOW

Herpetic whitlow is caused by the herpes simplex virus and usually presents as vesicular eruptions on the distal finger, with pain and erythema. It is most commonly seen in health care workers, such as dentists, nurses, and anesthesiologists, due to frequent contact with oral secretions. The current climate of increased precautions (to prevent other viral transmission, such as HIV) may have dramatically reduced the incidence of herpetic whitlow in this population.

This viral infection can be confused with a cellulitis, but rupture or unroofing of the vesicles (which can cause a secondary bacterial infection) is not indicated in herpetic whitlow. The diagnosis is made by a combination of physical examination and history. The patient should be reassured that the lesions will resolve within 3–4 weeks. Treatment involves supportive care and antibiotics to protect against secondary bacterial infection.

ONYCHOMYCOSIS

About 50% of patients that present with dystrophic nails (Figures 10, 11) have a fungal infection of the nail bed, while the other 50% suffer from a multitude of other causes (e.g., psoriasis, lichen planus, or trauma). Fungal infections of the nail are much more common in the foot, but when they do occur in the hand they can result in a highly annoying aesthetic and functional deformity. In the past, medical

treatment was problematic, requiring long-term administration of antifungal agents which in turn led to significant toxicity. In addition, recurrence was the rule rather than the exception. Recently, several agents have been developed that appear to be more effective in the treatment of onychomycosis. They require a much shorter treatment period, with less potential toxicity.

Lamisil (terbinafine) is a new antifungal agent that is effective in the treatment of onychomycosis. The dosing schedule is 250 mg orally once a day for 6 weeks. Due to the short treatment period, it is not necessary to obtain liver function tests prior to treatment if the patient is otherwise healthy. If there is a history of hepatitis, liver disease, or heavy alcohol abuse, it may be prudent to obtain liver function tests prior to initiating treatment. Note that the treatment of *toenail* onychomycosis is *not* identical to the treatment in the hand (toe infections require longer dosing schedules); if the patient's toes are affected as well, refer to the dosing information to adjust the treatment. Even though this agent is markedly more effective than prior antifungals for this problem, approximately 30% of patients will have a recurrence after treatment.

An alternative agent for onychomycosis is Sporonox (itraconazole), which can be given orally 200 mg once a day for 6 weeks. An

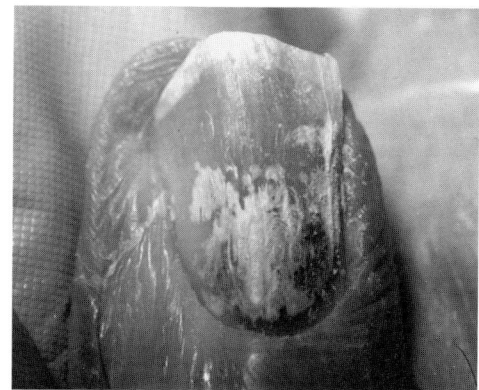

FIGURE 10. Onychomycosis of the nail. This dystrophic nail is the result of an underlying fungal infection. New oral agents feature less hepatic toxicity and are more successful at eliminating these infections than prior options.

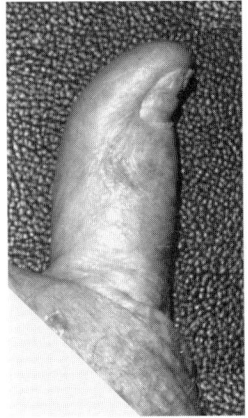
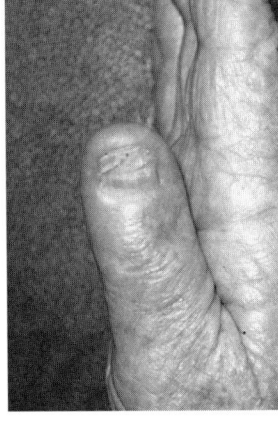

FIGURE 11. Thumb onychomycosis.

alternative method of administering this drug is "pulsed" therapy, in which the patient takes 200 mg twice a day for 1 week and then no drug for 3 weeks; this is repeated thrice, for a total of 3 months. Although this type of dosing is much more convenient for patients (easier to maintain compliance), preliminary reports have indicated that Lamasil is more effective and leads to less recurrence than Sporonox.

WEB SPACE ABSCESS

A web space abscess can occur after penetrating trauma to the distal aspect of the hand. Any sharp instrument can be involved, but often relatively minor lacerations from a knife (e.g., while cooking or preparing food) are the cause. The diagnosis is relatively straightforward because patients present with extreme tenderness, erythema, and swelling over the distal palm at a web space (Figure 12). There often is a subtle separation of the two digits on either side of the abscess, with limited mobility of these digits due to pain. These abscesses must be drained surgically. Drainage is best performed in the operating room suite under loupe magnification because of the close proximity of major structures (digital arteries and nerves, flexor tendons). Urgent referral to a hand surgeon is indicated.

BITES

Animal and human bites to the hand and upper extremity can cause serious infections and often require prompt intervention and the administration of parenteral antibiotics. Refer to Chapter 4 for treatment guidelines.

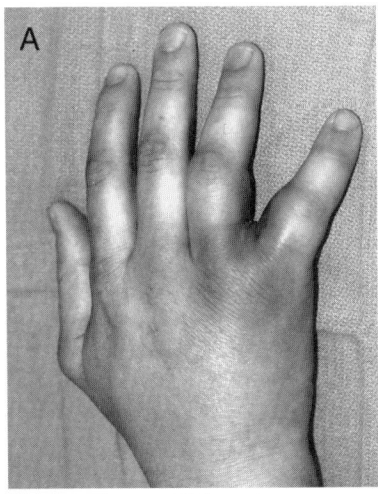
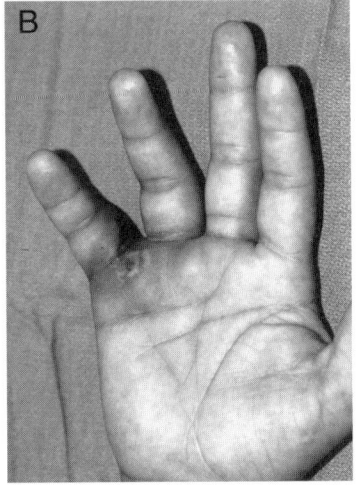

FIGURE 12. Web space abscess. This patient presented with a 3-day history of pain and swelling between the fourth and fifth fingers. **A,** Note the characteristic widening between the fingers and erythema. **B,** The entry point of this stab wound presumably is the cause of the web space abscess. Treatment is operative incision and drainage.

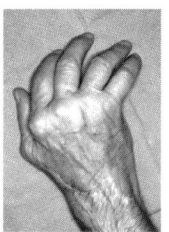

8 Common Hand Problems

Nerve Compression Syndromes

Nerve compression of the upper extremity is a common cause of pain and disability in the general population. It usually occurs via a mechanism of chronic impingement on the nerve by adjacent anatomic structures. Early damage occurs through interruption of the blood supply to the nerve sheath, which makes transmission of nerve signals increasingly difficult to propagate. The degree of nerve injury can be described by the following terms:

Neurapraxia: Characterized by decrease of nerve function and local demyelination, but no peripheral nerve degeneration. After removal of the offending agent, full recovery is the usual outcome.

Axonotmesis: The injury has progressed to the point where axonal degeneration occurs, but the surrounding supporting nerve structures (such as the endoneurium and epineurium) remain intact. Axonal regeneration can occur within these supporting structures, but *complete* regeneration may be limited by scarring and fibrosis.

Neurotmesis: Complete nerve disruption of all elements (i.e., nerve transection).

If corrected early, in the neurapraxia stage, nerve function usually returns after surgical decompression or removal of the compressive force. In nerve injuries that are longstanding, surgical decompression limits further progression of the damage, but the patient may not regain full nerve function. Recovery takes longer when the nerve damage is more severe.

CARPAL TUNNEL SYNDROME

Carpal tunnel syndrome (CTS) is the most common nerve compression syndrome of the upper extremity. Symptoms arise from compression of the median nerve within the carpal tunnel at the wrist. Remember that the carpal tunnel is a rigid structure formed dorsally, radially, and ulnarly by the carpal bones (Figure 1). The "roof" of the carpal tunnel is formed by the volar carpal ligament, which is thick and fibrous (Figure 2). Nine tendons, the flexor pollicis longus, the flexor digitorum superficialis, the flexor digitorum profundus, and the median nerve are all protected within the carpal tunnel, which does not yield to expansion (Figure 3). CTS arises when the pressure within the carpal tunnel increases to the point that the median nerve is compressed, causing nerve injury and symptoms.

The pathogenesis of this injury (like most of the nerve compression syndromes) is related to decreased blood flow to the nerve and its sheath at the level of the carpal tunnel. This process can be caused by a tenosynovitis (swelling of the synovium within the carpal tunnel), which

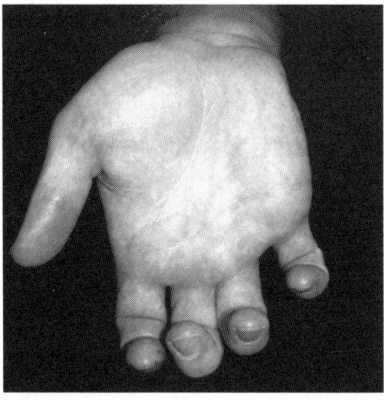

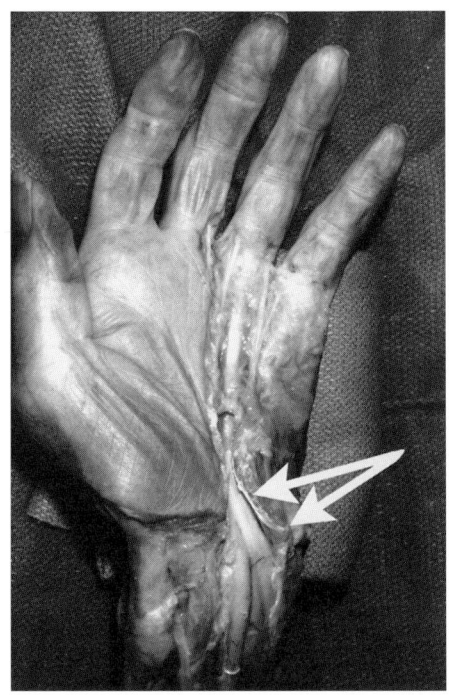

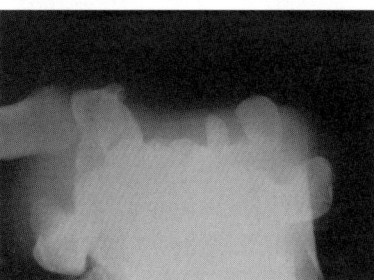

FIGURE 1. Radiographic demonstration of the carpal tunnel (for orientation, the hand is in the same position as the x-ray). The carpal tunnel is formed radially, ulnarly, and dorsally by the carpal bones.

FIGURE 3. Cadaver dissection demonstrating the thick volar carpal ligament (*arrows*). It has been divided, and the flexor tendons can be seen traveling underneath it.

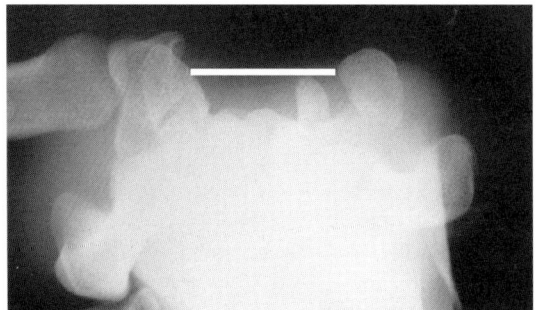

FIGURE 2. The volar carpal ligament (*line*) forms the roof of the carpal tunnel. This thick, fibrous structure does not yield to expansion, and increased pressure within the carpal tunnel can cause impingement of the median nerve.

results in increased pressure within the carpal tunnel. The tenosynovitis can act as a "final common pathway" for CTS development by a number of different etiologies, ultimately resulting in median nerve compression. For ex-

ample, repetitive motion tasks have been implicated in the development of tenosynovitis and resultant CTS. People with certain medical problems, such as diabetes, myxedema, and rheumatoid arthritis, are at an increased risk for developing CTS. Pregnant women have a higher risk of developing temporary CTS, which usually resolves in the postpartum setting.

Presenting Complaints

CTS can be diagnosed reliably by history and physical examination. **Four cardinal signs** are predictive:

1. **Symptoms within the median nerve distribution.** These are manifested primarily as numbness or paraesthesia on the volar aspect of the radial three fingers (Figure 4). Patients may complain of decreased sensation on the radial aspect of the ring finger, with normal sensation on the ulnar aspect. This characteristic reflects

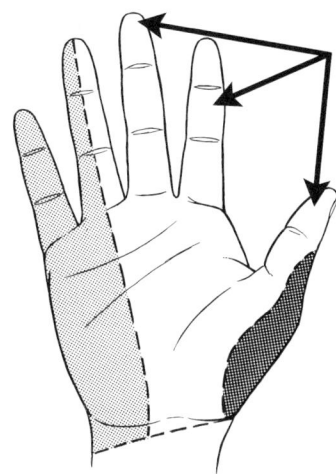

FIGURE 4. Patients with carpal tunnel syndrome complain of numbness or paraesthesia within the median nerve distribution (*white area, arrows*).

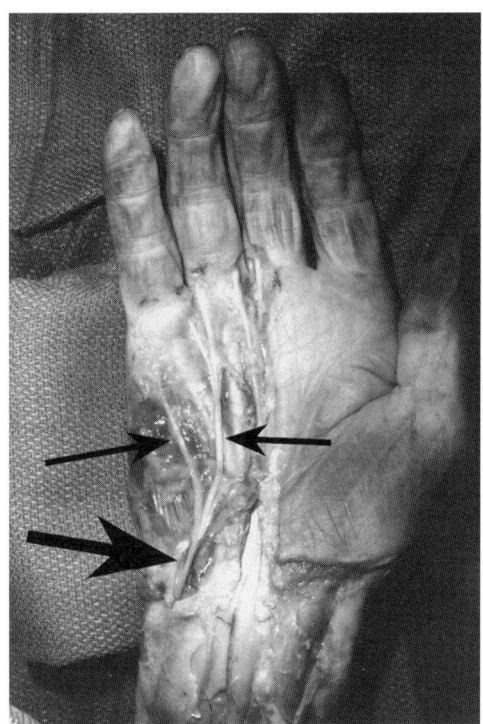

FIGURE 5. Differing innervation to the fingers. The ulnar nerve, shown here emerging from Guyon's canal (*large arrow*), divides into the digital nerves providing sensation to the fifth finger and the ulnar aspect of the ring finger (*small arrows*). The other digital nerves arise from the median nerve.

the differing innervation sources of that finger (Figure 5).

2. **Symptoms that awaken** the patient at night.

3. **A positive Tinel's sign.** A Tinel's sign is elicited by gently tapping the volar wrist at the carpal tunnel with the wrist extended (Figure 6). The test is positive when the patient complains of electrical shocks or "sprangles" that radiate in the median nerve distribution.

4. **A positive Phalen's test.** This test is performed by having the patient maximally flex both wrists against each other and hold the position for 1–2 minutes (Figure 7A). The test is positive if the symptom of paraesthesia or numbness is reproduced. Note how rapidly symptoms develop to quantify the result. For example, if the symptoms start within 20 seconds, the lesion is more severe than in a patient whose symptoms present at 2 minutes. Sometimes a "reversed Phalen's" also can reproduce symptoms (Figure 7B).

These are the *main* signs and symptoms of CTS, but not all patients present with all four. If a patient presents with three of the four symptoms, CTS is probable; if only one of the four symptoms is present, the diagnosis is less likely (but still may exist). In equivocal cases, electro-

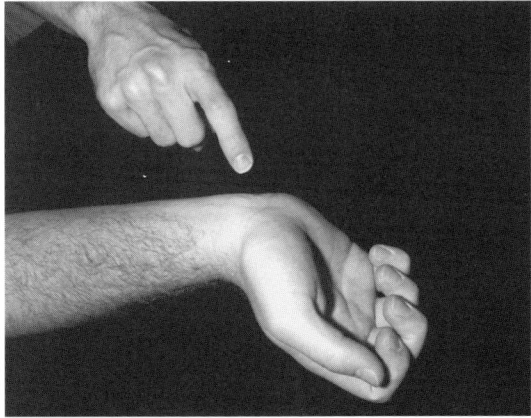

FIGURE 6. Testing for Tinel's sign in CTS. The examiner gently taps the patient's extended wrist directly over the carpal tunnel. The test is positive when the patient complains of electrical shocks or "sprangles" that radiate within the median nerve distribution.

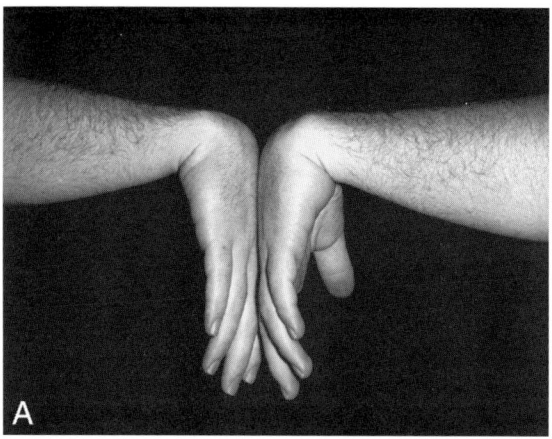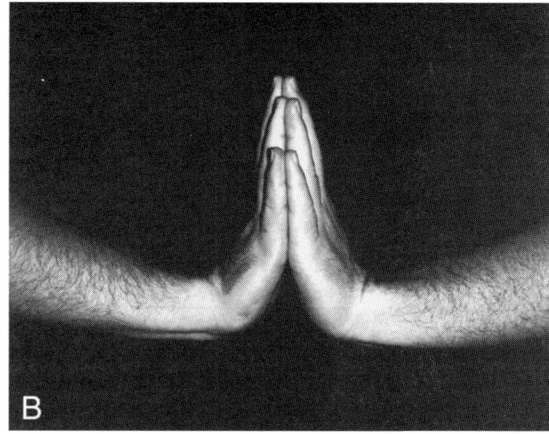

FIGURE 7. **A,** Phalen's test. Patients maximally flex both wrists and hold the position for 1–2 minutes. If symptoms of numbness or paraesthesia within the median nerve distribution are reproduced, the test is positive. **B,** Reversed Phalen's test. Holding the wrists in a hyperextended position occasionally reproduces the symptoms of CTS and provides additional evidence of the presence of the syndrome.

diagnostic testing can be performed to confirm or exclude the diagnosis.

Patients with CTS also may complain of other signs or symptoms, such as hand "clumsiness," weakness of the hand, inability to powerfully flex the fingers, weakness of the forearm, or pain radiating proximally up the forearm. Although these are common complaints, they really do not strengthen the case for carpal tunnel syndrome. They do, however, confuse the clinical picture!

Since the median nerve innervates the muscles of the thenar eminence, a *late finding* in severe CTS is atrophy of the thenar eminence (Figure 8). This atrophy is not normally found in the early stages of CTS; therefore, absence of thenar wasting does not exclude the diagnosis. When present, thenar atrophy indicates severe and longstanding nerve compression, and hand surgical consultation should be expedited.

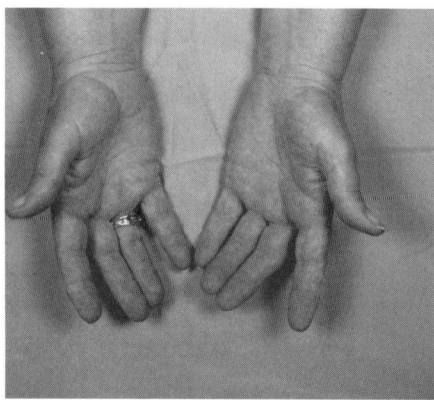

FIGURE 8. Subtle atrophy of the right thenar eminence. Thenar atrophy is a *late* symptom of severe CTS. Since the median nerve provides motor innervation to the muscles of the thenar eminence (i.e., the opponens pollicis, abductor pollicis brevis, and half of the flexor pollicis brevis), severe nerve damage can manifest as atrophy. This tends to be a subtle finding and is usually best appreciated by comparing the patient's hands (assuming unilateral disease).

Electrodiagnostic Studies

In most hospitals and outpatient facilities, electrodiagnostic equipment (electromyograms [EMG] and nerve conduction velocities [NCV]) is available to help with the diagnosis in patients with nerve compression, including CTS. These tests are particularly helpful for confirming or ruling out the diagnosis in equivocal cases. The question arises: Are these tests indicated for every patient with suspected carpal tunnel syndrome? This is an issue that each clinician needs to tailor to his or her particular situation. In my practice, if the diagnosis is relatively straightforward by clinical examination and history, electrodiagnostic testing is not routinely obtained. These tests are best performed when the history and physical examination do not clarify the diagnosis, or when CTS is unlikely but the patient insists that he or she suffers from it. In the latter situation, electrodiagnosic tests can be used as "objective" studies to reassure the patient that this particular disease process is not present.

Treatment

When the diagnosis of carpal tunnel syndrome is first made, the initial treatment choice usually is conservative management. Since compression and resulting nerve injury are caused by increased pressure within the carpal tunnel, which usually is related (at least to some degree) to a tenosynovitis, early conservative management focuses on relieving the tenosynovitis and resultant swelling. To accomplish this, patients are splinted with the wrist at neutral position or in slight extenion for 3–4 weeks. In addition, patients are instructed to take a nonsteroidal antiinflammatory agent (such as ibuprofen) faithfully—*adherence must be consistent even if pain and symptoms are absent.*

If the patient remains symptomatic after 4 weeks of splinting and nonsteroidal antiinflammatory therapy, refer to a hand specialist for consideration of carpal tunnel release. If symptoms *resolve* after conservative management, the patient can resume normal activities without limitation. However, should symptoms recur, the patient should be referred to a hand specialist to discuss possible surgical decompression. It is unrealistic to expect patients to submit to indefinitely prolonged immobilization. When temporary efforts to reduce swelling and tenosynovitis are not successful at relieving symptoms of median nerve compression, long-term conservative measures have no greater impact on the disease process.

Although the carpal tunnel is the most common location for entrapment of the median nerve, patients may present with median nerve compression proximal to the wrist. Nerve conduction tests can provide clues to this situation;

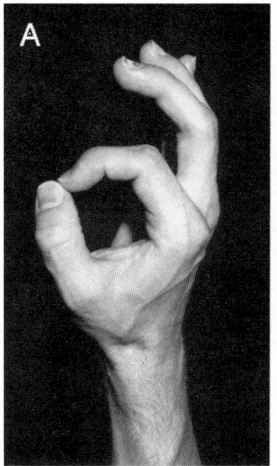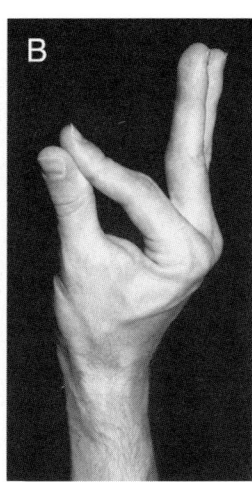

FIGURE 9. The anterior interosseous nerve innervates the flexor pollicis longus, as well as the flexor digitorum profundus to the index and long fingers. **A,** It is responsible for flexion of the thumb interphalangeal (IP) joint and the index finger distal IP joint. **B,** An injury to the median nerve high in the forearm or to the anterior interosseous branch of the median nerve results in the inability to forcefully flex these joints.

other indications are weakness of muscles innervated *proximal* to the carpal tunnel. There is an entrapment syndrome of the anterior interosseous branch of the median nerve, which innervates the flexor pollicis longus, the flexor digitorum profundus to the index and long fingers, and the pronator quadratus. If a patient presents with injury to this nerve, it is evident by weakness of these muscles, with the inability to form a tight pinch between the thumb and index fingertips (Figure 9). Since the anterior interosseous branch of the median nerve does not carry any sensory fibers, this syndrome occurs without sensory loss. A more proximal lesion (for example, of the median nerve near the antecubital fossa) would demonstrate symptoms of muscular weakness as well as sensory loss in the hand.

ULNAR NERVE COMPRESSION

Compression of the ulnar nerve usually occurs at the level of the **cubital tunnel,** although it can occur at Guyon's canal at the wrist

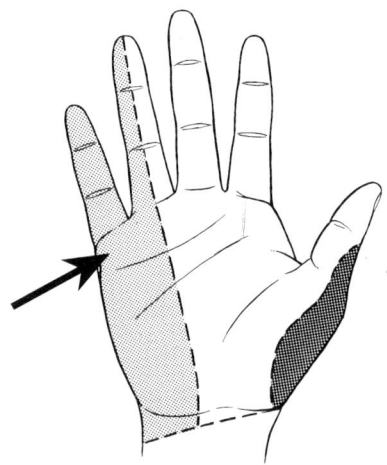

FIGURE 10. Patients with injury or pathology of the ulnar nerve complain of decreased sensation in the ulnar nerve distribution (*light grey area, arrow*). See Figure 5.

(rarely). Patients typically complain of decreased sensation or anesthesia in the ulnar one and a half digits, as well as weakness and "clumsiness" of the hand due to weakness of the hand intrinsic muscles (Figure 10). If a patient presents with symptoms within the ulnar nerve distribution, one way to localize the site of

nerve compression (Guyon's canal versus cubital tunnel) is to specifically check the dorsal-ulnar side of the hand for sensory abnormalities. Since the dorsal sensory branches arise *proximal* to Guyon's canal, if the dorsal-ulnar aspect of the hand is affected, the lesion must be *proximal* to Guyon's canal—in the cubital tunnel (Figures 11, 12).

Patients with ulnar nerve compression often complain that symptoms are worse in certain positions. For example, flexion of the elbow stretches the ulnar nerve and exacerbates the symptoms. If cubital tunnel syndrome is suspected, electrodiagnostic studies may be helpful to confirm the diagnosis. Referral to a hand specialist is indicated, as surgical decompression of the nerve almost always is necessary to resolve these symptoms. Surgical decompression of the ulnar nerve is not as reliably successful as release of the median nerve at the carpal tunnel, but most patients enjoy at least some (if not complete) resolution of their preoperative symptoms. At the very least, progression of the nerve damage is halted by eliminating the offending lesion.

Long-standing compression injury to the ulnar nerve leads to atrophy of the hand intrinsic

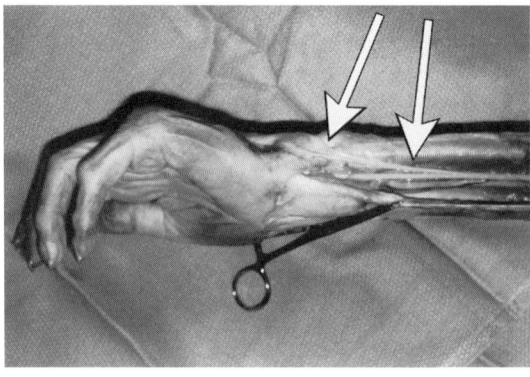

FIGURE 11. Proximal to the wrist, the ulnar nerve gives off dorsal branches to innervate the dorsal-ulnar aspect of the hand (*arrows*). If a patient has signs of ulnar nerve compression that include anesthesia on the dorsal aspect of the hand, it can be inferred that the lesion lies proximal to the wrist (i.e., in the cubital tunnel). If symptoms are within the volar-ulnar nerve distribution, and the dorsal hand is normal, then the lesion probably lies within Guyon's canal.

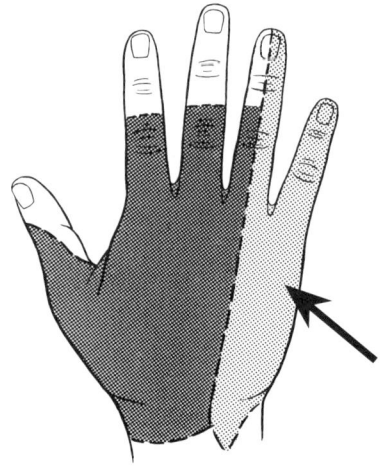

FIGURE 12. Area of innervation (sensation) provided by the dorsal sensory branches of the ulnar nerve (*light gray area, arrow*).

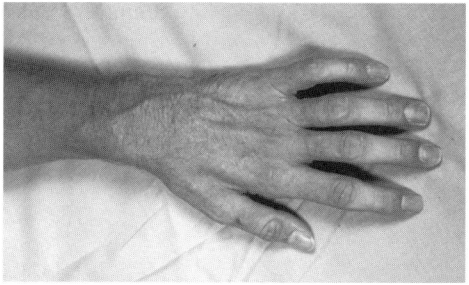

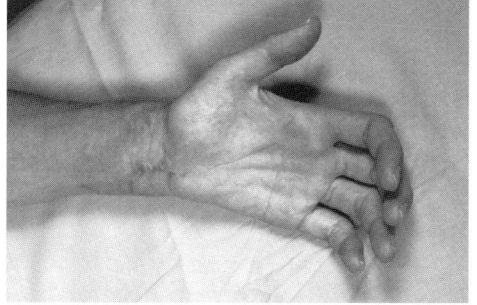

FIGURE 13. Long-standing injuries to the ulnar nerve result in atrophy of the hand intrinsic muscles, with a characteristic "wasting" look. These nerve injuries also may produce a "clawing" posture, particularly at the ring and fifth fingers.

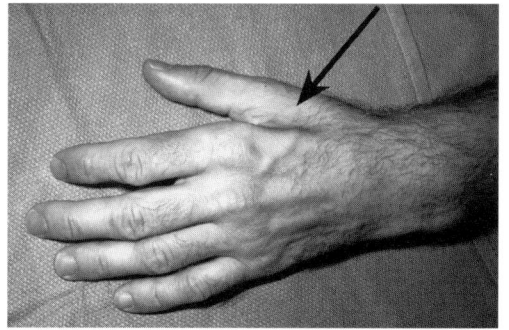

FIGURE 14. It is not unusual for patients with cubital tunnel syndrome to present with signs of muscle atrophy. It is most noticeable at the first web space, where atrophy of the first dorsal interosseous muscle leaves a hollow between the thumb and the index rays (*arrow*).

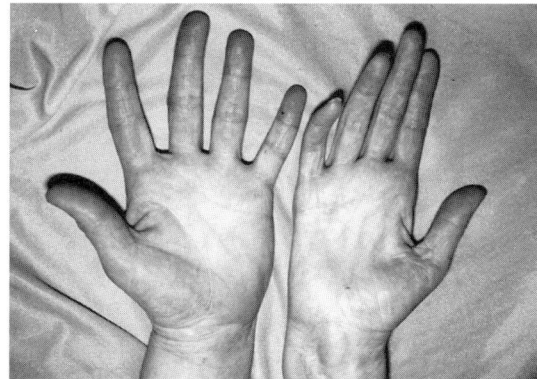

FIGURE 15. When evaluating hand musculature and possible atrophy, it is helpful to compare to the contralateral (uninjured) hand. In comparison, subtle differences may become quite obvious. Here, the atrophy is striking and dramatic.

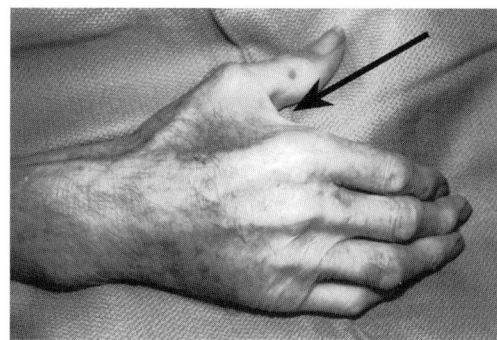

FIGURE 16. Some atrophy of the hand musculature is a normal part of aging. Here, the first dorsal interosseous muscle has atrophied, resulting in hollowing at the first web space. This is a symmetrical finding in this elderly patient, who is asymptomatic. This example reinforces the value of comparing both hands to evaluate for differences.

muscles (Figure 13). It is not unusual for patients with cubital tunnel syndrome to present with some muscle atrophy (Figure 14), in contrast to patients with carpal tunnel syndrome, in whom thenar muscle atrophy is rare. When evaluating the hand musculature it is helpful to compare the affected hand with the normal hand, because the volume loss may not be obvious at first glance (Figure 15). Comparing is especially helpful in elderly patients, who undergo muscle atrophy as a normal consequence of aging; if the atrophic changes are bilateral, they may not be an abnormal finding (Figure 16).

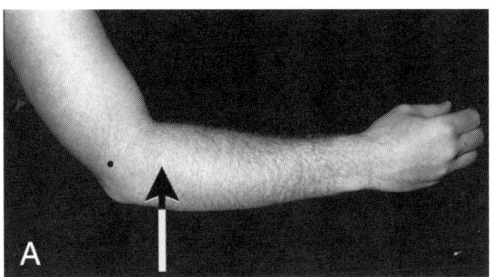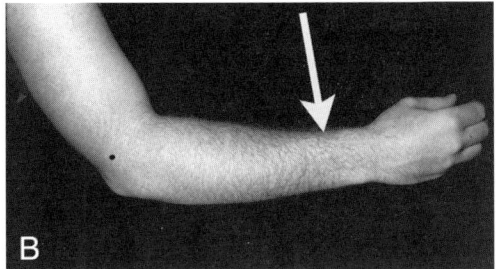

FIGURE 17. **A,** Site of entrapment and maximal tenderness in radial tunnel syndrome (*arrow*). Note the position of the lateral epicondyle (*black dot*). **B,** Area of entrapment and maximal tenderness in Wartenberg's syndrome (*arrow*). This area is where the radial nerve emerges to its most superficial position at the distal forearm.

RADIAL NERVE COMPRESSION

Compression of the radial nerve is less common than compression of the median or ulnar nerves. The two usual sites of radial nerve compression are the radial tunnel immediately distal to the elbow (Figure 17A) and the dorsal wrist (Figure 17B). Patients who have radial nerve entrapment at the radial tunnel (**radial tunnel syndrome**) typically complain of an "aching" pain on the dorsal aspect of the proximal forearm that radiates distally. Radial tunnel syndrome also can involve the distal sensory branches of the radial nerve, causing paraesthesia on the dorsal-radial aspect of the hand (Figure 18). The symptoms may resemble those of lateral epicondylitis (tennis elbow); thus, when patients present with symptoms of lateral forearm/elbow pain, care must be taken to differentiate between the two entities (Table 1).

Electrodiagnostic testing is one way to confirm the diagnosis of radial nerve compression. Additionally, in radial tunnel syndrome the **point of maximal tenderness** is found approx-

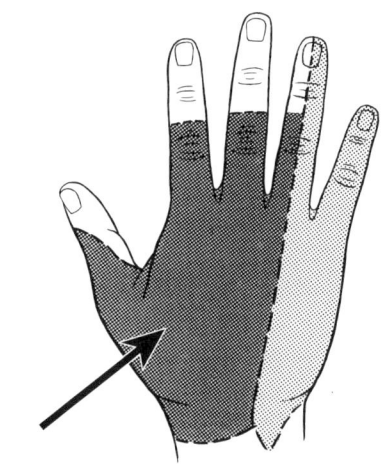

FIGURE 18. Compression or damage to the radial nerve manifests in the area of the radial nerve sensory distribution (*dark gray area, arrow*).

imately 5 centimeters *distal* to the lateral epicondyle, over the extensor musculature. In lateral epicondylitis, maximal tenderness is immediately *adjacent* to the lateral epicondyle (Figure

---

TABLE 1. Differentiating Between Radial Tunnel Syndrome and Lateral Epicondylitis

	Lateral Epicondylitis	**Radial Tunnel Syndrome**
Maximal Tenderness	Lateral epicondyle	5 cm distal to lateral epicondyle
Middle Finger Test (See text)	Negative	Positive
Xylocaine Block	Infiltration at the lateral epicondyle resolves symptoms	Infiltration 5 cm distal to lateral epicondyle; relieves pain but produces radial nerve palsy
Electrodiagnostic Studies	Negative	Evidence of radial nerve compression

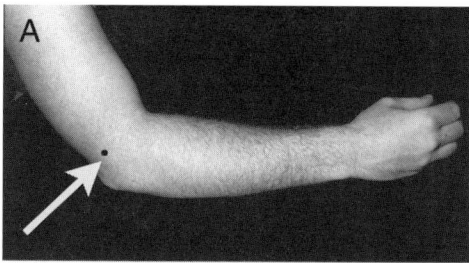

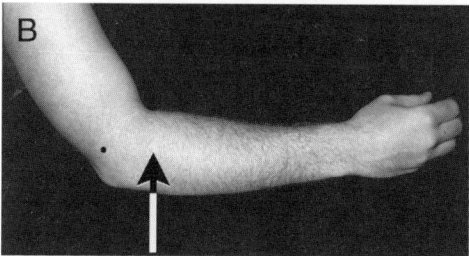

FIGURE 19. It is important to distinguish between radial tunnel syndrome/radial nerve entrapment and lateral epicondylitis in the presence of dorsal-radial forearm pain. **A,** In lateral epicondylitis, maximal tenderness is over the lateral epicondyle (*arrow* and *dot*). **B,** In radial tunnel syndrome, maximal tenderness is approximately 5 cm distal to the epicondyle (*arrow*).

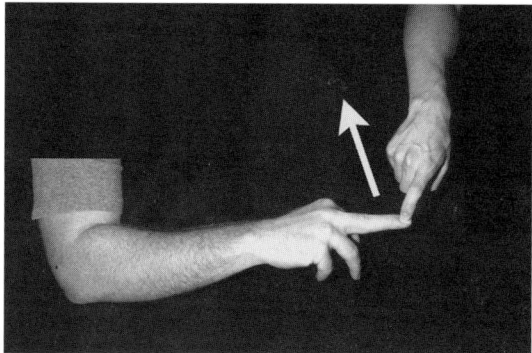

FIGURE 20. The middle finger test. With the elbow flexed to 90° and the wrist in neutral, the patient extends the middle finger (*arrow*) against resistance from the examiner. The test is positive, providing diagnostic evidence of radial tunnel syndrome, if it reproduces the symptoms of pain over the dorsal extensor muscle mass.

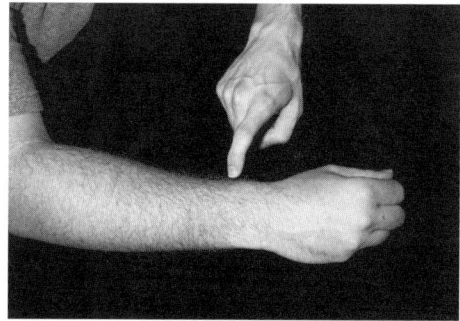

FIGURE 21. Diagnosis of Wartenberg syndrome can be confirmed with a positive Tinel's sign at the distal radial forearm. Gently tap the distal forearm where the nerve arises to its most superficial position. A patient experience of pain and paraesthesia or electrical "sprangles" into the distribution of the radial nerve is evidence of possible radial nerve compression at this level.

19). Another diagnostic study is the "**middle finger" test,** in which the elbow is flexed to approximately 90 degrees, and the wrist is held in a neutral position. The patient then extends the middle finger against resistance. This test is positive if it produces pain over the dorsal extensor muscle mass (Figure 20).

Further examination can include injection of 1% lidocaine at the area of maximal tenderness: if infiltration immediately around the lateral epicondyle relieves the symptoms of pain, the diagnosis of lateral epicondylitis is confirmed. In contrast, if instillation of lidocaine approximately 5 centimeters distal to the lateral epicondyle produces a radial nerve palsy with anesthesia at the dorsal radial hand and *also relieves the symptoms,* radial nerve entrapment is more likely. When radial nerve entrapment is suspected, referral to a hand specialist is indicated for surgical release of the nerve.

Entrapment or compression of the radial nerve at the distal forearm is called **Wartenberg's syndrome.** Since at this level the radial nerve has only a sensory function, patients with this syndrome present with only a sensory loss. They are sensitive to tapping (a positive Tinel's sign) over the radial nerve as it emerges to its more superficial location in the distal forearm (Figure 21), and they may complain of pain or numbness over the dorsal-radial aspect of the distal forearm radiating to the dorsum of the hand (see Figure 18).

There are several potential causes of Wartenberg's syndrome: the nerve may be compressed

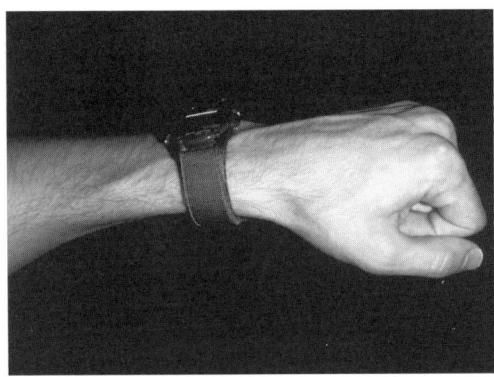

FIGURE 22. Tight-fitting or heavy jewelry may press directly on the radial nerve at its superficial location at the distal forearm, causing symptoms of Wartenberg syndrome.

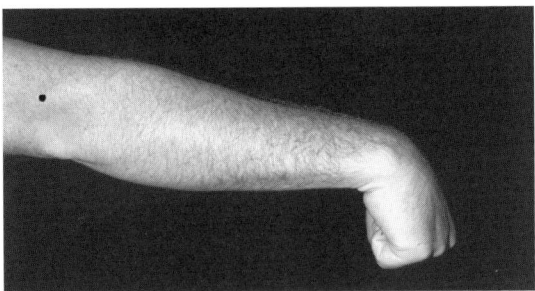

FIGURE 23. In lateral epicondylitis (tennis elbow), the pain can be reproduced by passively flexing the fingers and wrists with the elbow fully extended. Note the position of the lateral epicondyle (*dot*).

by tendons as it emerges to its superficial location at the distal forearm; external items, such as tight-fitting watch bands or jewelry, may be directly pressing on the nerve (Figure 22); or a laceration or severe contusion may have traumatized or injured the radial nerve. Treatment of distal radial nerve compression initially involves conservative management, with removal of the offending external devices (if any), as well as splinting and administration of nonsteroidal anti-inflammatory drugs (NSAIDs). If not successful, referral to a hand specialist is indicated for exploration and release of the sensory branches of the radial nerve.

The radial nerve branches at the distal forearm and hand are susceptible to injury from penetrating trauma due to their superficial location. If lacerated, these branches are prone to exquisitely painful neuroma formation, which can be very troubling to the patient and extremely difficult to treat.

Lateral Epicondylitis (Tennis Elbow)

Lateral epicondylitis is characterized by tenderness and pain at the lateral epicondyle. It is aggravated by wrist and finger extension. This entity is approximately *ten times more common*

than radial tunnel syndrome, which should be included in the differential diagnosis when evaluating patients with lateral arm and elbow pain. The point of maximal tenderness in tennis elbow is the lateral epicondyle, while in radial tunnel syndrome the point of maximal tenderness is approximately 5 centimeters distal to this point, over the dorsal extensor mass (see Table 1 and Figure 21). In radial tunnel syndrome, pain is reproduced by extending the middle finger against resistance; in tennis elbow, pain is reproduced by passively flexing the fingers and wrist with the elbow fully extended (Figure 23). Although electrodiagnostic testing may assist in the confirmation of radial tunnel syndrome, a normal test does not confirm lateral epicondylitis.

Tennis elbow usually responds to nonsurgical (conservative) treatment: an initial period of rest, followed by a program of exercises designed to strengthen the forearm and hand muscles. Exercises are best initiated and overseen by a hand therapist. NSAIDs such as ibuprofen are helpful in this initial period. An injection of a long-acting local anesthetic (such as bupivacaine) mixed with a steroid solution at the lateral epicondyle can relieve symptoms and aid during the resting phase of conservative management. After 2–3 weeks of rest, prescribe a forearm support band for use during any activity that may provoke pain, to prevent subsequent episodes (Figure 24).

Approximately 10% of patients with lateral epicondylitis fail to respond to conservative management. Since the etiology of this disease

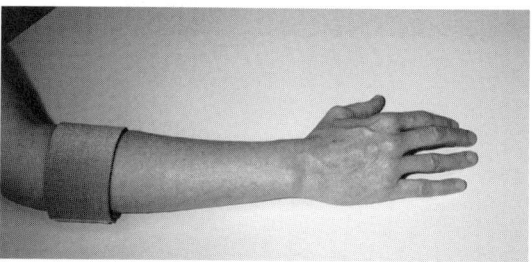

FIGURE 24. A forearm support band is helpful during the convalescent period of lateral epicondylitis. Enlist a hand therapist for supervision of exercises.

process usually involves a minor tear of the common extensor tendon origin at the lateral epicondyle, those patients who do not respond to conservative management require referral to a hand specialist for surgical repair.

Trigger Finger

Trigger finger (stenosing tenosynovitis) is a common entity in which the patient presents complaining of either "triggering" or "snapping" of the finger with attempted flexion or extension. This occurs due to an inability of the flexor tendon to smoothly glide at the start of the fibro-osseous tunnel (at the A-1 pulley; Figure 25). The etiology of this condition involves a vicious cycle that begins with tenosynovitis and inflammation of the tendon and its surrounding sheath at the palmar pulley. The tendon becomes secondarily thickened, further limiting gliding. Digital flexion and motion aggravate the inflammation, and the thickening can progress to a nodular enlargement of the tendon. This nodule blocks movement of the tendon within the pulley system, and the patient eventually is unable to actively extend or flex the tendon past the obstruction.

Trigger finger also can be seen in infants and young children, although in the pediatric population it most commonly involves the thumb. Parents bring the child in noting that the thumb remains flexed within the palm, and there is a history of difficulty in extending the finger past a perceived obstruction or trigger point (Figure 26A). Often a palpable mass is present, representing the nodular enlargement of the tendon ("Notta's node," Figure 26B).

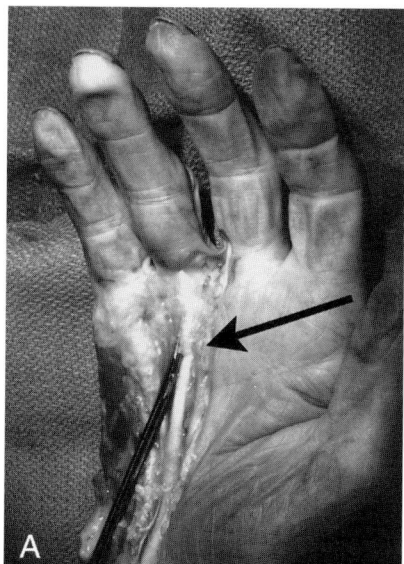
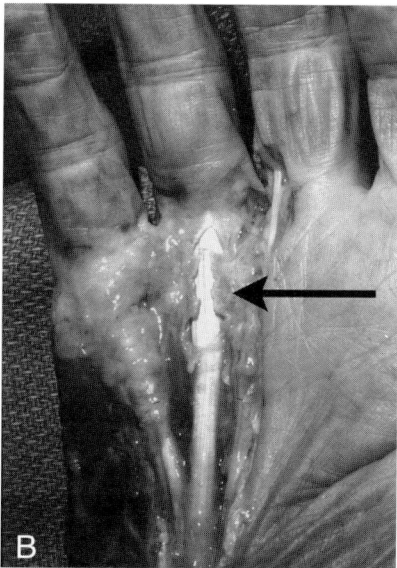

FIGURE 25. **A,** The A-1 pulley marks the start of the fibro-osseous tunnel (*arrow*). The flexor tendons to the ring finger are seen traveling within this tunnel (as is a small probe ulnarly). **B,** The A-1 pulley has been surgically divided in this dissection, exposing the underlying flexor tendons (*arrow*).

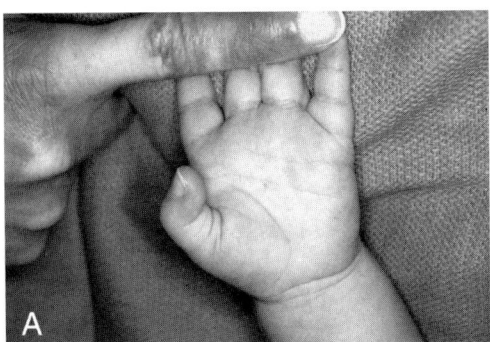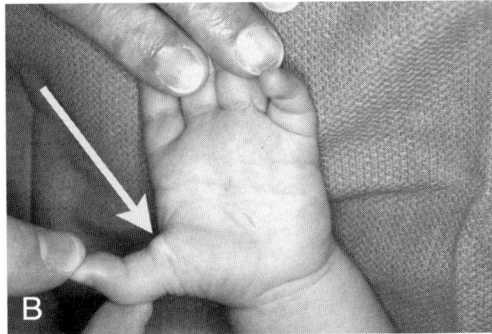

FIGURE 26. **A,** This child cannot actively extend his thumb and it always remains clasped within his hand: the classic presentation of trigger thumb. In infants, the thumb is the most commonly affected digit. **B,** Under a general anesthetic, full passive extension of the thumb still is not possible due to the nodular expansion of the flexor pollicis longus tendon. This nodular enlargement, termed Notta's node, is palpable and visible at the level of the A-1 pulley (*arrow*).

Surgical correction of this entity is straightforward. In an outpatient setting, the hand specialist can divide the offending A-1 pulley, allowing the immediate return of smooth gliding and full range of motion of the finger (Figure 27). Any nodular deformity of the tendon will resolve on its own after removal of the offending pulley.

Some authors have reported success with localized steroid injections in the treatment of triggering. This nonoperative option involves the injection of steroids into the palm at the level of the A-1 pulley. This can be an effective means of addressing this problem in adults, and it is particularly valuable because the patient is spared a surgical procedure. It is not recommended for use in the pediatric population.

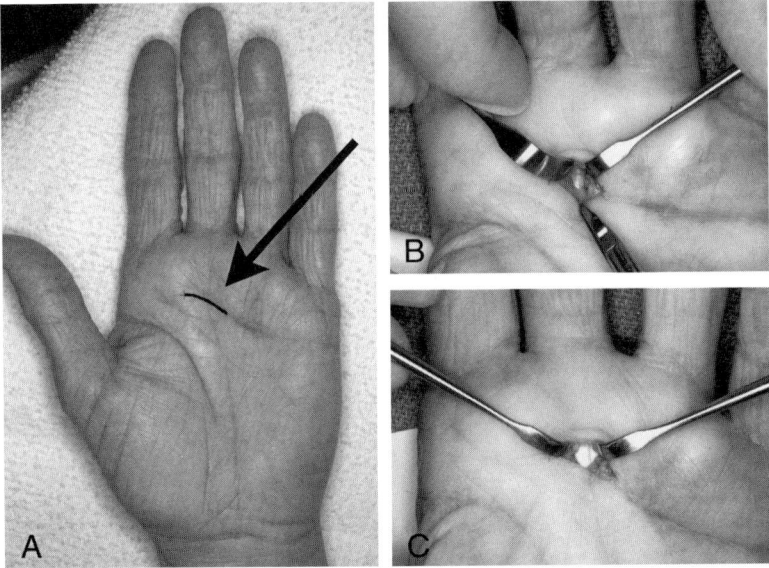

FIGURE 27. **A,** Proposed incision for release of the A-1 pulley of the long finger (*arrow*). **B,** A-1 pulley exposure through the incision. **C,** The underlying flexor tendons are visible after division of the A-1 pulley, which makes full active flexion and extension possible.

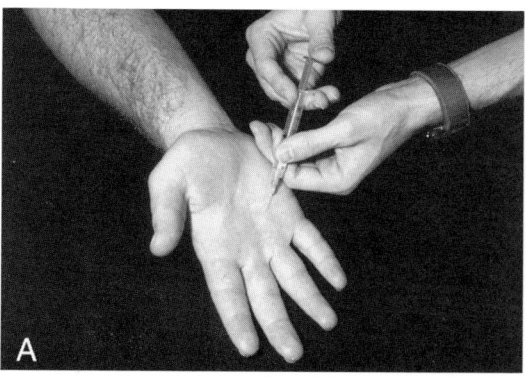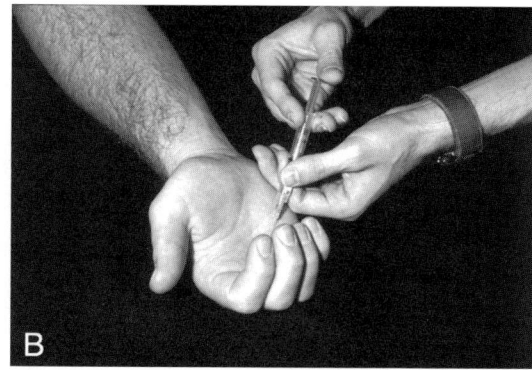

FIGURE 28. Steroid injection for trigger finger. **A,** Infiltrate the steroid mix at the level of the A-1 pulley that corresponds to the proximal palmar crease (see Figure 27A). Do not infiltrate directly into the tendon. **B,** After advancing the needle into the desired position, ask the patient to slowly and gently flex the fingers. If the needle tip moves with flexion, it is embedded within the tendon and must be withdrawn 1–2 ml. Have the patient repeat the flexion to confirm that the needle is outside of the tendon. Once the position is confirmed, infiltration can be performed.

Prepare 0.25 cc of depomethylprednisolone acetate (80 mg/cc) or triamcinolone acetonide (40 mg/cc) diluted with 0.5 cc of 1% lidocaine. Take extreme care to avoid injecting directly into the tendon, because the steroid can irrevocably weaken it and potentially lead to an attritional rupture. One way to avoid this complication is to ask the patient to *gently* flex and extend the fingers after advancing the needle to the desired position (Figure 28). If the needle tip moves with flexion, it is stuck within the tendon. Simply withdraw the needle 1–2 millimeters, and ask the patient to repeat the finger motion. Once the needle does not move with flexion it is safe to infiltrate the steroid.

Steroid injection is *not without risks,* even when extreme caution is exercised. There can be atrophy of the palmar subcutaneous tissue, and thinning of the overlying skin. Because of the risks, multiple steroid injections for trigger finger are not recommended. If the injection is not successful or if the triggering recurs, referral to a hand surgeon for surgical division of the A-1 pulley is indicated.

De Quervain's Tenosynovitis

Stenosing tenosynovitis of the first dorsal compartment of the wrist, or de Quervain's disease, usually presents as pain on the radial aspect of the wrist, particularly with ulnar deviation. Findings include local tenderness and occasionally swelling over the extensor retinaculum on the distal radial aspect of the dorsal forearm (Figure 29). Use of the tendons within this com-

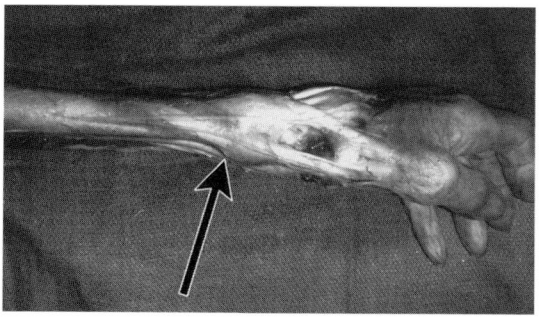

FIGURE 29. Tenosynovitis of the first extensor compartment (*arrow*) within the extensor retinaculum is termed de Quervain's disease. This disorder can be treated with surgical release of the extensor retinaculum.

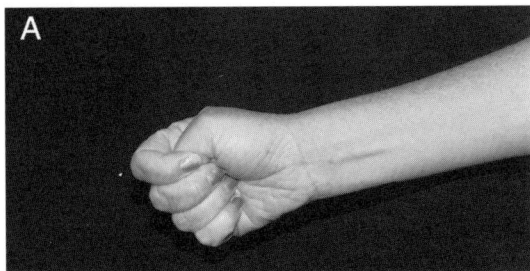

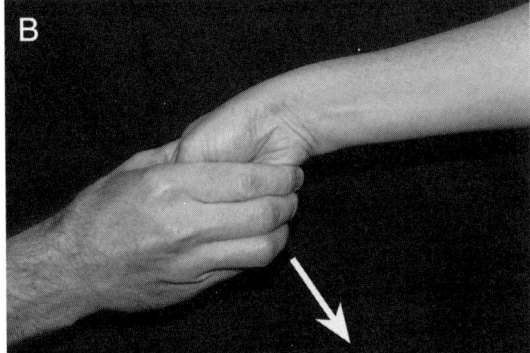

FIGURE 30. Finkelstein's test. **A,** The patient clasps the thumb within the palm. **B,** The examiner then ulnarly deviates the hand (*arrow*). If pain is reproduced, the test is positive and suggestive of de Quervain's disease.

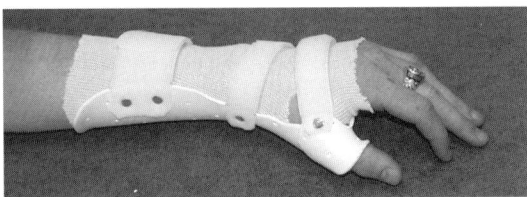

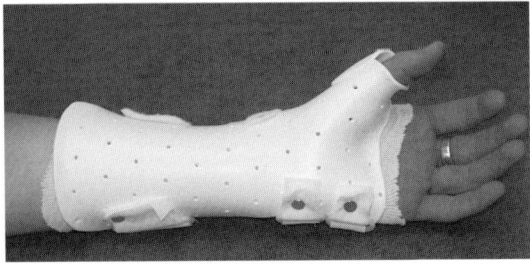

FIGURE 31. Early conservative measures for de Quervain's tenosynovitis include nonsteroidal anti-inflammatory agents and splinting in a thumb spica splint. Patients are instructed to wear the splint faithfully for at least 4 weeks. This splint was manufactured by an occupational therapist using orthoplastic materials. Patients appreciate this type of splint because it is lighter than the traditional plaster or fiberglass and can be removed briefly for showering or other activities.

partment (abductor pollicis longus and extensor pollicis brevis) can result in pain. The diagnosis is easily made using Finkelstein's test: the patient clasps his or her thumb inside a fist, and the examiner ulnarly deviates the wrist, stretching the tendons of the first extensor compartment (Figure 30). If this manuever reproduces the symptoms, the test is positive.

Initial management involves conservative measures such as splinting with a thumb spica splint and administration of NSAIDs (Figure 31). However, this entity is likely to recur even after successful resolution with conservative measures. Referral to a hand specialist then is indicated for surgical release of the first extensor compartment (Figure 32).

Benign Masses

GANGLION CYSTS

Ganglion cysts are the most common masses of the hand and usually present at either the

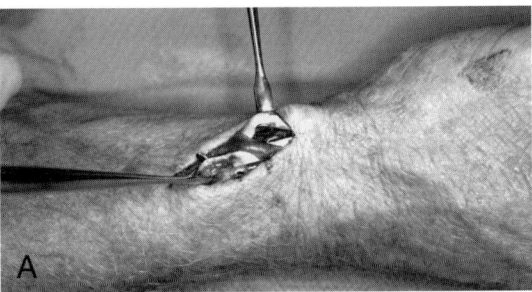

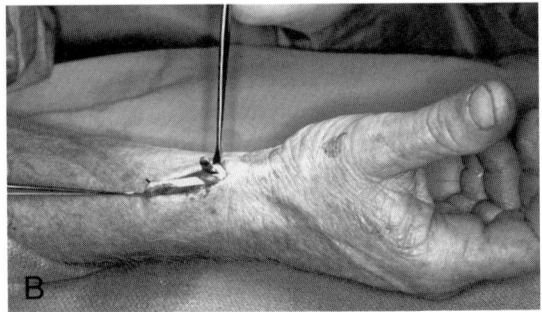

FIGURE 32. **A,** Release of the extensor retinaculum of the first extensor compartment. **B,** The abductor pollicis longus and extensor pollicis brevis are individually identified and full release is confirmed. Proximal pull of these tendons produces thumb abduction.

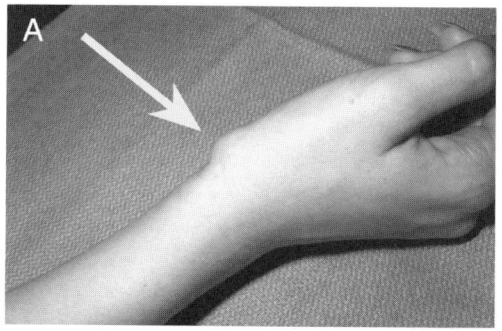

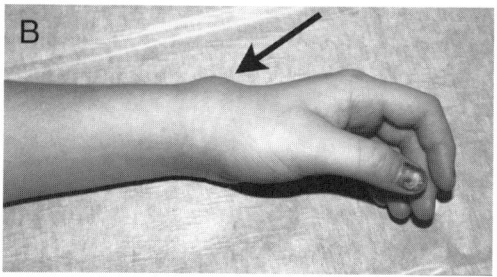

FIGURE 33. **A,** Volar wrist ganglion (*arrow*). **B,** Dorsal wrist ganglion (*arrow*).

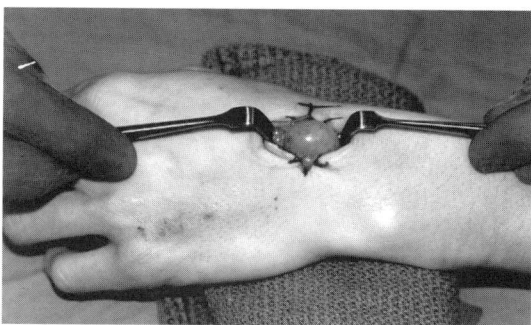

FIGURE 34. Dorsal wrist ganglion at surgical excision. The pseudocysts contain clear, thick, viscous fluid and are connected by a stalk to the underlying wrist capsule.

volar radial or dorsal wrist (Figures 33, 34). They actually are "pseudocysts" that evolve as outpouchings of the underlying wrist joint fluid. Although the pathogenesis of these cysts remains controversial, it is thought that a "one-way valve" (formed after trauma at the wrist joint) allows egress of joint fluid from the joint, but does not allow return. This valvular mechanism is nicely demonstrated by the observation that dye injected at the wrist joint travels into the ganglion cyst, but dye injected into the cyst does not migrate into the wrist joint space. Over time the joint fluid continues to be pushed out, forming a pseudocystic structure ("pseudocystic" because the structure does not have a true epithelial or synovial lining, but rather a lining of compressed collagen fibers). Ganglion cysts contain a clear, thick, viscous fluid high in hyaluronidase. Although the etiology is thought to involve some type of traumatic injury to the underlying joint capsule, if specifically asked, fewer than 20% of patients are able to remember any history of trauma.

Archaic methods for treating ganglion cysts involve rupture of the cyst, typically by slamming a heavy book (such as the family bible) on the resting hand. Rupture disperses the cyst's contents, and the patient becomes asymptomatic—temporarily. (The patient is highly symptomatic during the treatment phase!) *This method of treatment is mentioned only to be condemned.* Recurrence and scarring are the usual outcomes, and definitive surgical treatment after such rough management is more difficult.

If the patient is adamantly opposed to surgical treatment, aspiration of the cyst can be performed in the office with a large-bore needle (*at least* 18 gauge). Aspiration is difficult even with a large-bore needle because the fluid content is thick and viscous. Recurrence rates after aspiration can be as high as 90%, **so patients must be warned that although aspiration *may* work, it probably will not.**

Keep in mind the structures that are susceptible to injury during this procedure. Volar wrist ganglions usually are intimately associated with the radial artery, and care must be taken to avoid inadvertently injuring this vessel (Figure 35). Branches of the dorsal sensory radial nerve are prone to injury with aspiration of dorsal wrist ganglions; traumatic neuromas at this location are difficult to treat and troubling to the patient (Figure 36).

Definitive treatment can be performed on an outpatient basis by a hand surgeon. Treatment entails complete excision of the cyst, as well as obliteration of its stalk at the joint capsule.

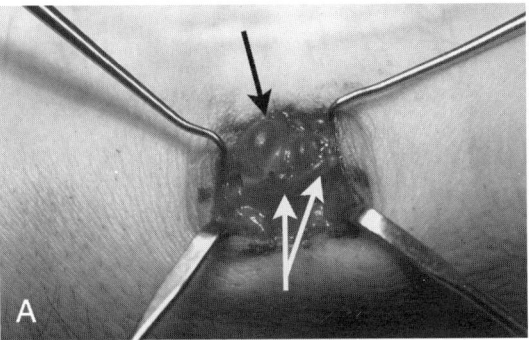

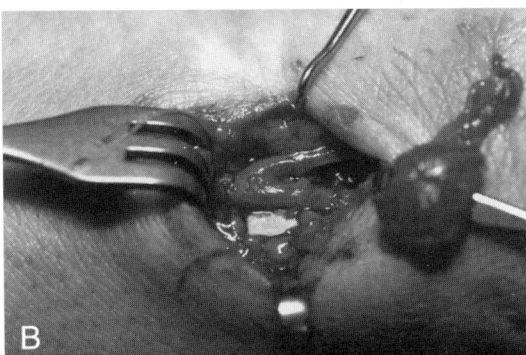

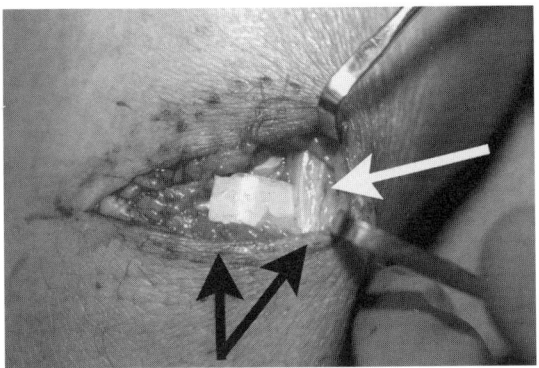

FIGURE 36. Branches of the superficial radial nerve (*white arrow*) are at risk during manipulation or aspiration of dorsal wrist ganglions. Note the location of the ganglion prior to its excision (*black arrows*).

FIGURE 35. Volar wrist ganglions often are intimately associated with the radial artery. **A,** The multiloculated cyst can be seen after initial surgical exposure (*black arrow*). The radial artery is "draped" over the cyst (*white arrows*). **B,** After cyst excision, the radial artery is more apparent within the wound. Inadvertent injury to this artery can cause not only excessive bleeding and/or hematoma but, if there is inadequate perfusion from the ulnar artery, distal finger ischemia and tissue loss.

MUCOUS CYSTS

Mucous cysts occur at the distal dorsal finger and represent a ganglion cyst arising from the distal interphalangeal (DIP) joint (Figure 37A). They are typically small, well-loculated cysts with thin overlying skin, and quite commonly they create a notch in the fingernail due to pressure on the germinal matrix of the nail bed (Figure 37B). Radiographs of the affected hand usually demonstrate osteophytes at the affected DIP joint. Patients with these lesions should be referred to a hand surgeon for debridement of the osteophyte and excision of the mucous cyst, both of which can be performed on an outpatient basis. After resection of the osteocyte and cyst, the nail deformity resolves spontaneously.

INCLUSION CYSTS

Inclusion cysts are the second most common benign tumor of the hand. They almost always arise in a place of prior trauma or injury, developing from a nest of epithelium that has been pushed into the underlying dermis or subcutaneous tissue. The basal layer of the epithelium continues to produce keratinocytes, but the external layer is not sloughed (the normal fate of the outer layers of skin as new layers are produced) because it is trapped by the subcutaneous tissue. As keratinocytes build, a cystic lesion forms. Inclusion cysts usually are softer and more compressible than giant cell tumors (see below), and the diagnosis is suggested if the cyst occurs near on old laceration or puncture wound. Excisional treatment is curative.

GIANT CELL TUMORS

Giant cell tumors are the third most common benign tumor of the hand. They arise from the tendon sheath or from joint synovial tissue, and they typically present as a small, pea-sized nodule on the volar aspect of the hand. Patients may complain of pain, but discomfort usually is due to minor trauma as the mass is bumped during normal daily activities. Giant cell tumors are benign, and excision (including a portion of the underlying tendon sheath) is curative.

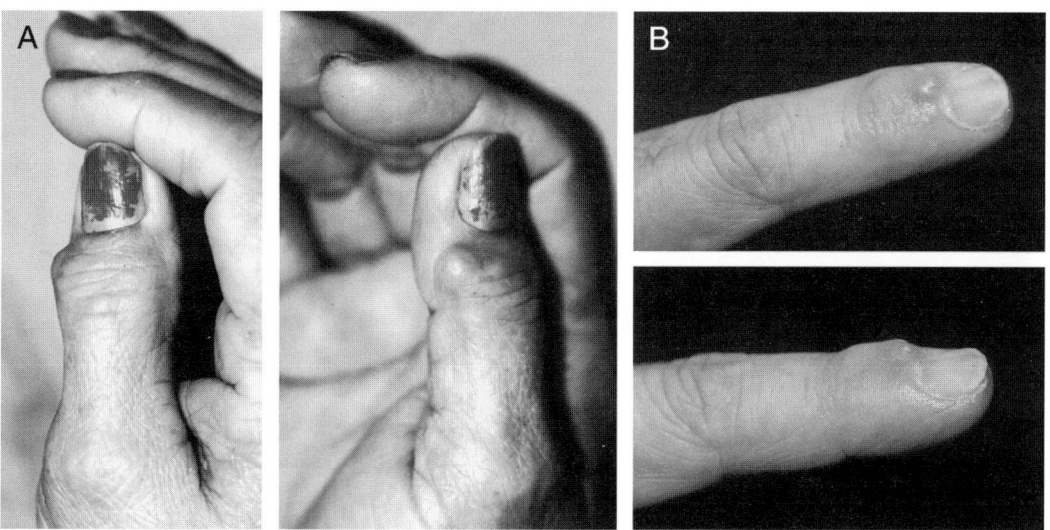

FIGURE 37. **A,** Mucous cyst of the thumb IP joint. These cysts often are small, with thin overlying skin. **B,** Mucous cyst of the index finger that has produced a depression in the distal finger nail. After surgical excision of the cyst and debridement of the osteophyte at the DIP joint, the depression in the nail will resolve spontaneously.

Malignant Masses

The vast majority of malignant tumors encountered on the hand are **squamous cell carcinoma** of the dorsal skin. These tumors are most likely secondary to decades of sun exposure and actinic damage to the dorsal forearm and hand. They present as a raised, sometimes rapidly growing mass that is painless to the patient (Figure 38). Physical examination should specifi-

cally include a check for epitrochlear and axillary lymphadenopathy, although metastasis of these lesions is relatively rare (< 10%). If ignored by the patient for a significant period of time, these lesions can grow to significant size and invade local structures, making resection more difficult to accomplish (Figures 39, 40).

Basal cell carcinoma also can occur on the hand, usually on the dorsal skin. These masses are not as common on the hand as squamous cell

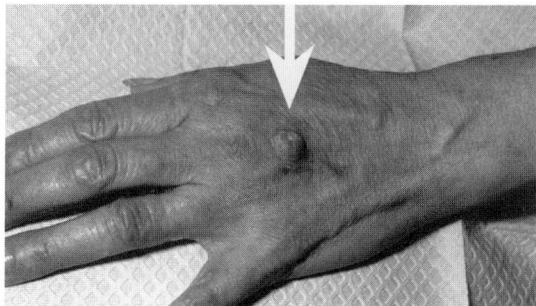

FIGURE 38. Squamous cell carcinoma of the dorsum of the hand (*arrow*). This 56-year-old woman stated that the mass grew rapidly over 6 months. It was 1 cm in diameter and nontender. Excisional biopsy confirmed the diagnosis.

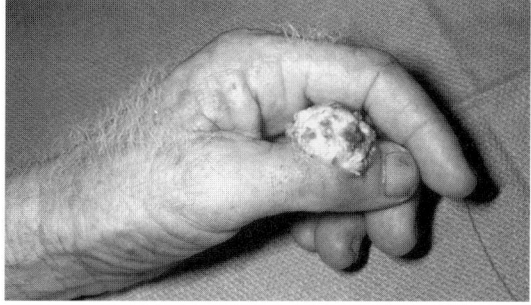

FIGURE 39. Neglected verrucous-type squamous cell carcinoma of the thumb. This patient had this lesion for several years prior to presentation to a physician.

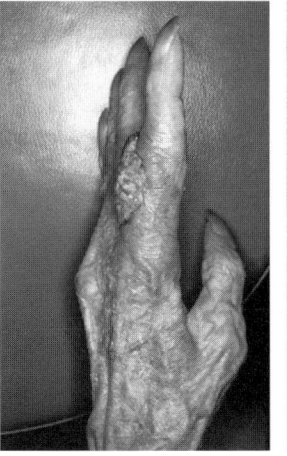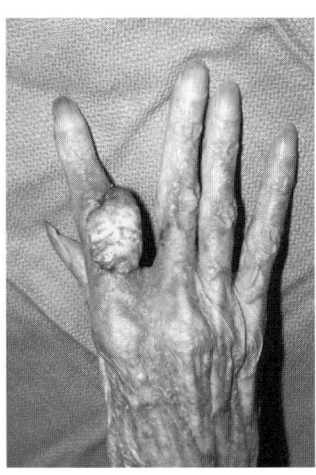

FIGURE 40. Squamous cell carcinoma of the index finger. This 88-year-old man noticed the lesion's growth for 1½ years. Excisional biopsy confirmed squamous cell carcinoma.

carcinoma and tend to grow more slowly; metastasis is rare. Basal cell carcinoma may present as a small nodular mass, pearly white or pink; occasionally it has a central area of depression. Excision is curative.

Malignant melanoma is the least common primary malignant tumor of the hand (skin), but has the most devastating implications for survival. If not diagnosed and resected at an early stage, distant spread and metastatic disease is common. Diagnosis is the same for melanoma at other parts of the body. "Moles" that recently have changed (e.g., enlarged), feature differing

colors (ranging from black to browns and even pink and white), or have irregular borders should be excised for biopsy (Figure 41). Melanomas also can occur at the nail bed (more commonly in dark-pigmented individuals, such as African-Americans) and may present as a brownish spot or linear streak visible on the nail.

Malignant tumors from other parts of the body may metastasize to the hand. The most frequent site of origin is the lung, followed by the kidney. These lesions usually metastasize to the distal phalanx, where a radiograph

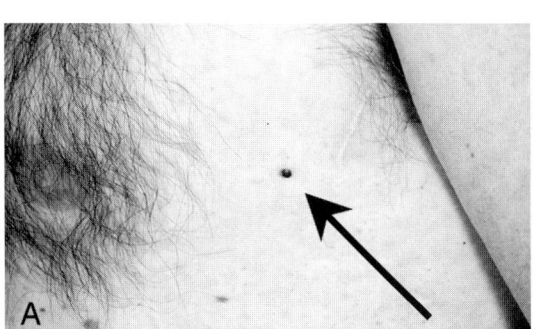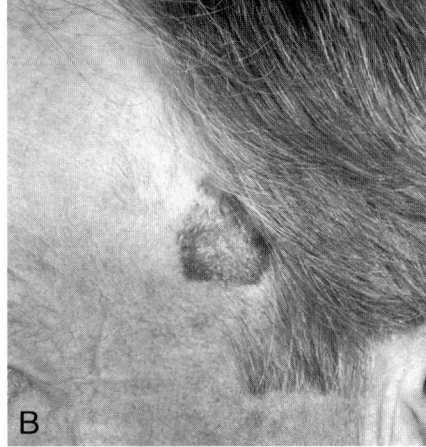

FIGURE 41. **A,** Malignant melanoma on the trunk (nodular type; *arrow*). Note its significantly darker color when compared to the surrounding nevi. **B,** Superficial spreading melanoma on the face. Note the irregular borders.

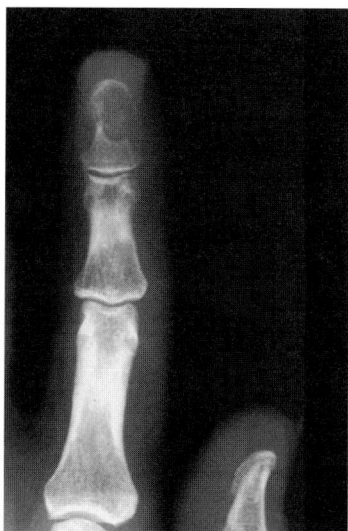

FIGURE 42. Metastatic lung cancer to the distal phalanx, which on x-ray revealed the characteristic finding of a lytic lesion. Lung cancer is the most common metastatic lesion to the hand, followed by kidney. On presentation, the fingers are red, swollen, and tender, and these symptoms can be confused with an infectious process.

demonstrates a lytic lesion (Figure 42). Patients present with pain and swelling of the affected digit, which can be confused with an infectious process. Treatment involves amputation for palliation.

Extensor Tendon Derangements

SWAN NECK DEFORMITY

The swan neck deformity is caused by an extensor tendon derangement that allows the lateral bands of the finger to migrate dorsally. The posture of this deformity is flexion of the distal phalanx, with hyperextension of the proximal interphalangeal (PIP) joint (Figure 43). Active extension of the DIP joint is not possible because the lateral bands of the extensor mechanism (largely responsible for this action) have migrated *dorsally* and cannot contract enough to make up this mechanical disadvantage. This derangement can be caused by many different etiologies, such as a chronic untreated mallet finger, rheumatoid arthritis, or trauma. Surgical consultation is recommended to attempt to restore normal function to these patients.

BOUTONNIÉRE DEFORMITY

The boutonniére deformity also is the result of an extensor tendon derangement, but the characteristic position of the finger is different than recurvatum (swan neck): the PIP joint is flexed, and the DIP joint is hyperextended (Figure 44). In these patients, the lateral bands of the extensor mechanism have migrated *volar* to their normal

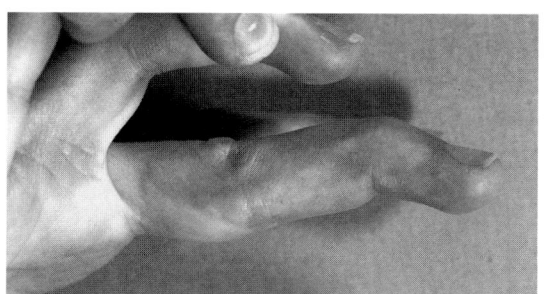

FIGURE 43. The swan neck deformity (recurvatum) involves hyperextension of the PIP joint with flexion of the DIP joint. This is caused by a derangement in the extensor mechanism, with a dorsal migration of the lateral bands.

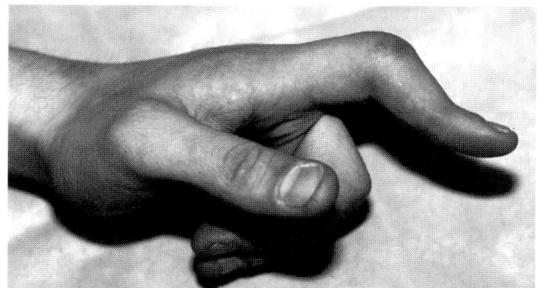

FIGURE 44. The boutonniére deformity, involving hyperextension of the DIP joint with flexion of the PIP joint, also is caused by a derangement of the extensor mechanism—typically a rupture of the central extensor tendon at its insertion in the middle phalanx. Early diagnosis and prolonged splinting of the PIP in extension are necessary for successful treatment of this difficult injury.

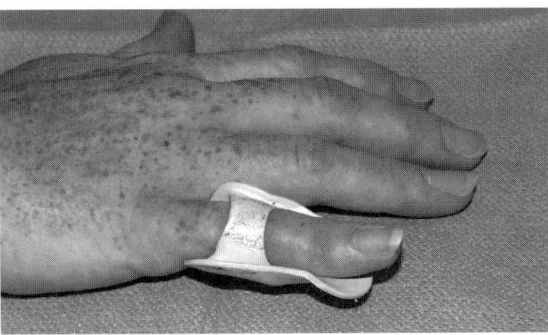
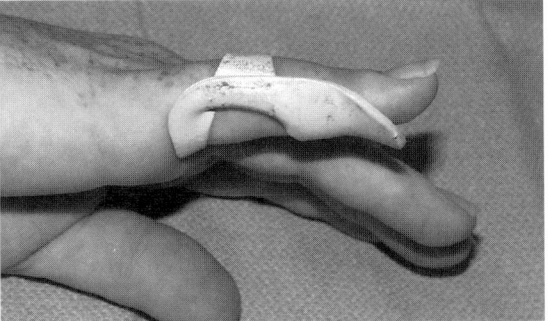

FIGURE 45. Splint for treating the closed boutonniére deformity. The PIP joint is maintained in extension, while the DIP and MCP joints are left free. Closed injuries are treated with splinting alone, because the disrupted central slip of the extensor tendon usually is frayed and attenuated, making direct repair impossible. If the deformity arises from a clean laceration, referral to a hand surgeon for direct repair of the extensor tendon should be considered.

positions. This deformity usually is caused by rupture or transection of the central slip of the extensor mechanism (the attachment of the tendon to the base of the middle phalanx). When the injury occurs, quite often the classic position of the finger is not manifested acutely. Weeks later, as the lateral bands shift volarly, the finger begins to demonstrate PIP flexion and DIP hyperextension.

The most important component in successful treatment of boutonniére deformity is early diagnosis. If a patient begins to manifest the characteristic posture, splinting of the PIP joint in full extension—leaving the DIP joint free—is indicated (Figure 45). Similar to treatment of the mallet deformity, prolonged immobilization (12 weeks or more) may be neccessary. If early splinting is not instituted, fixed flexion contracture of the PIP joint makes correction difficult, if not impossible, to achieve.

SYNDACTYLY

Myriad congenital hand deformities have been described; fortunately, they are relatively

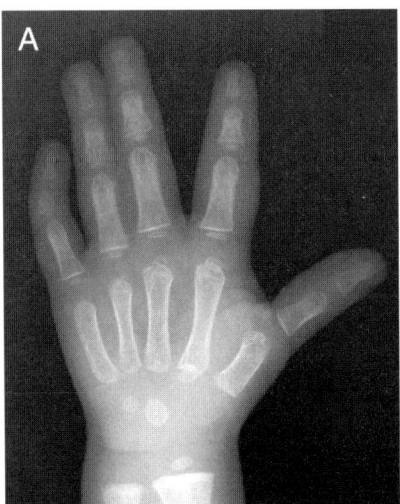
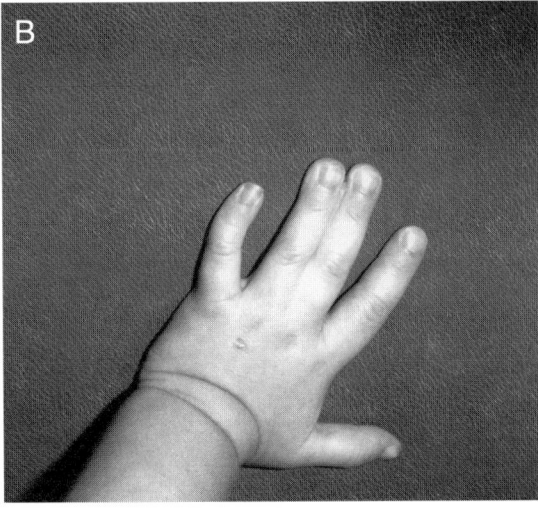

FIGURE 46. Simple, complete syndactyly of the third web space, between the ring and long fingers. This is the typical location of syndactyly. **A,** In this case it is "simple" because there is no bony connection between the adjacent phalanges. **B,** It is "complete" because the soft tissue attachment involves the entire length of the fingers.

rare. The one most commonly encountered in the typical practice is syndactyly: the connection of adjacent fingers by skin or bone. In a **simple** syndactyly, only soft tissue connects the fingers (Figure 46A). In a **complex** syndactyly, there is bony fusion between adjacent phalanges. A **complete** syndactyly is fusion along the entire length of the finger (Figure 46B); **partial** syndactyly features a connection only along a portion of the proximal finger. The most commonly affected web space is the third, connecting the ring and long fingers.

Surgical separation of the digits usually can be deferred until the child is 18–24 months old. Preservation of important structures (such as the digital nerves) is technically easier when the child (and the hand) has grown a bit. If the connection between the two digits begins to alter growth of one of them—typically manifested by tethering and lateral deviation of the longer digit—then earlier separation is indicated.

DUPUYTREN'S CONTRACTURE

Dupuytren's contracture is a disease process that involves contracture of the palmar fascia of

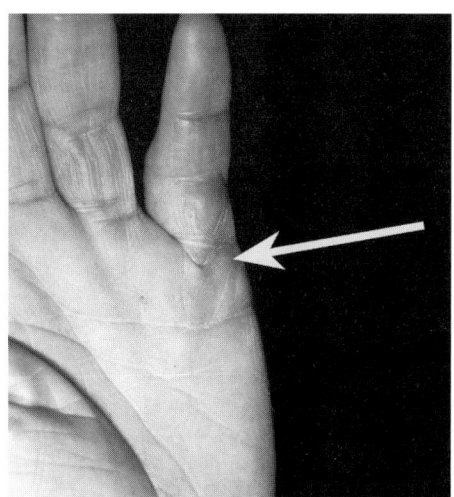

FIGURE 47. Early Dupuytren's contracture. The first manifestation may be a nodule or pit formation at the palm (*arrow*).

the hand. The earliest stage usually is heralded by a nodule or pit formation in the palm (Figure 47). As the disease progresses, fibrous bands of the palmar fascia can cause flexion contractures at the metacarpophalangeal (MCP) and PIP joints (Figure 48). These contractures may

FIGURE 48. As Dupuytren's contracture progresses, fibrous bands of diseased palmar fascia can contract to pull the finger into flexion. **A,** The fibrous band can be seen at the level of the proximal palmar crease of the ring finger. **B,** Early Dupuytren's contracture producing flexion of the fifth finger.

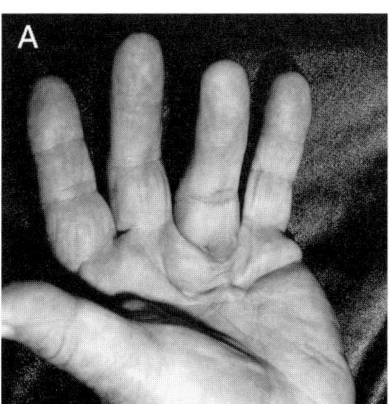

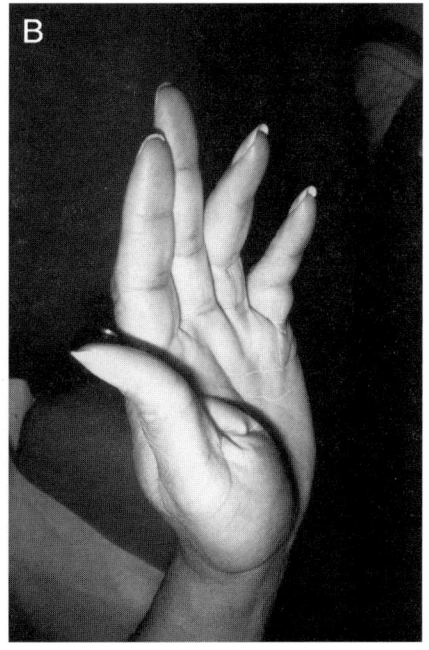

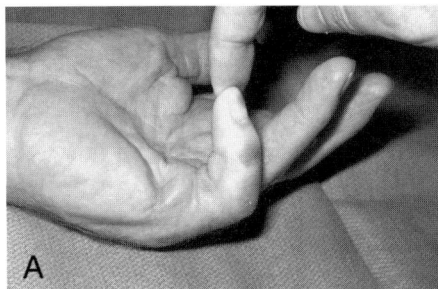
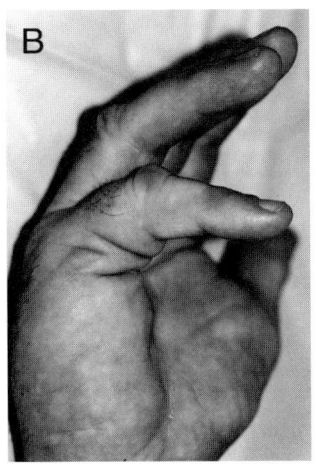

FIGURE 49. **A,** Severe Dupuytren's contracture with an inability to extend the PIP beyond 90° of flexion. Flexion contractures this severe interfere with normal daily activities. **B,** Severe Dupuytren's contracture of the fifth finger with flexion of the MCP and PIP joints.

progress to the point that patients are unable to fit their hands into gloves, and the flexed digits interfere with normal activities (Figure 49). Although Dupuytren's contracture can affect any of the digits, it most commonly affects the ring and fifth fingers.

The pathogenesis of this disease process is unclear. Although a higher risk has been noted in people of Celtic origin, alcoholics, people with seizure disorders, and diabetics, no cause and effect association between these risk factors and the disease process has been established.

Treatment involves surgical excision of the nodules and the underlying diseased fascia and release of the volar contracture, allowing the fingers to extend. *Any* flexion contracture of the PIP joint or 20 degrees of flexion of the MCP joint is an indication for surgery. Occasionally, patients may complain of pain from the palmar nodules before finger contractures have occurred. Symptomatic disease such as this (even without contracture formation) also can be an indication for elective surgical excision. If a patient is asymptomatic, surgery is not mandated until contractures of the PIP or MCP joints begin.

Arthritis

Patients present to the primary care physician with various types of arthritis for evaluation and treatment. The most common in the hand is osteoarthritis (degenerative joint disease). Rheumatoid arthritis and its variants is the next most common; least commonly encountered is gouty arthritis.

OSTEOARTHRITIS

Degenerative joint disease is not a systemic disease, and it typically affects only the heavily stressed or weight-bearing joints. In the hand, it usually affects the **DIP and PIP joints,** but spares the MCP joints. Quite often it affects the basilar joint of the thumb (the carpometacarpal joint; Figure 50). Osteoarthritis also can occur in any previously injured joint—particularly if cartilaginous disruption has occurred. Any incongruity of the joint surface, such as may occur after trauma, can gradually wear away the overlying articular cartilage, producing the symptoms of arthritis.

At the DIP joints, Heberden's nodes and loss of cartilage thickness can result in deformity with angulation (Figures 51, 52). The osteophytes typically are not painful, but the loss of articular cartilage results in pain with motion. The mainstay of conservative treatment in degenerative joint disease is NSAIDs. If a patient remains symptomatic, has pain at the DIP joints on motion, and is no longer helped by NSAIDs, referral to a hand specialist should be

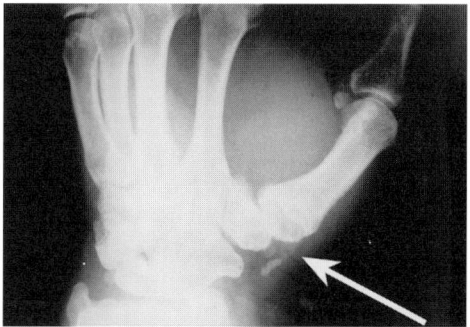

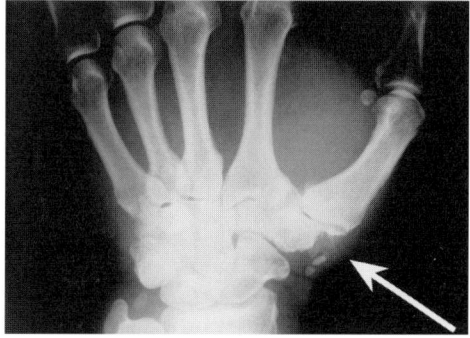

FIGURE 50. Severe arthritis of the basilar joint of the thumb (*arrow*). This is a common location of joint disease in osteoarthritis, perhaps because of the heavy stresses to which this joint is subject.

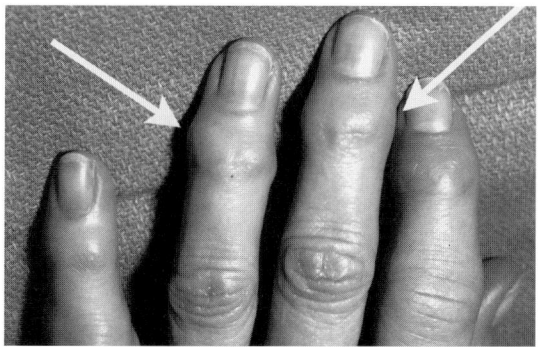

FIGURE 51. Patients with degenerative joint disease of the hands can present with Heberden's nodes (*arrows*). These nodules represent osteophytes at the DIP joint.

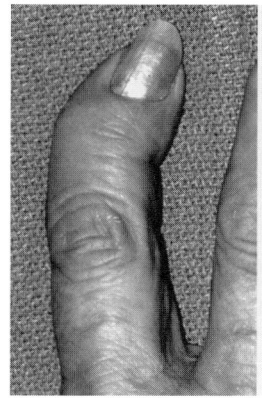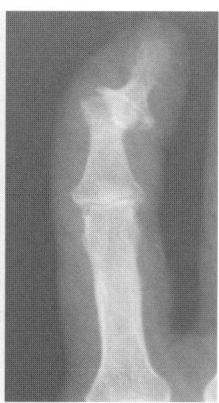

FIGURE 52. Severe osteoarthritis at the DIP joint of the fifth finger. Osteophyte formation, joint destruction, and angulation are demonstrated.

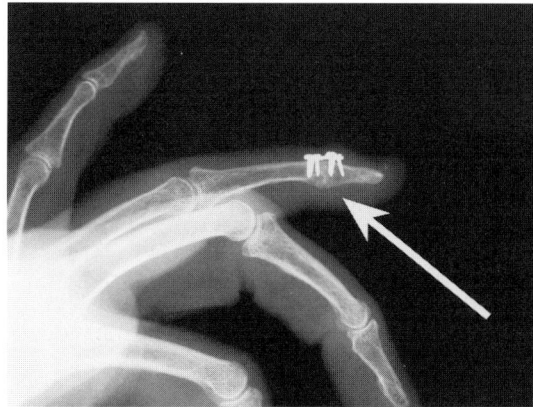

FIGURE 53. Fusion of the DIP joint can be accomplished via several different techniques. In general, the remaining cartilage of the joint is resected, and the distal and middle phalanges are fixed into position to heal like a fracture. Bone fixation can be done with small screws and plates (as here). Note the healed bone (*arrow*); the joint space has been replaced with a smooth cortical surface.

considered for fusion of the joint (Figure 53). Joint fusion eliminates pain and allows the joint to be placed in a position of function. Ironically, joint fusion usually *increases* hand function—despite the loss of motion at the DIP joint—because of significant pain relief.

Similar options exist for degenerative joint disease at the PIP joints. Due to the high mechanical stresses that are placed at this joint (particularly radially and ulnarly directed forces), artificial joint replacement rarely is successful. If the patient's symptoms are not controlled with NSAIDs, fusion remains an option to reduce pain and increase hand function.

Patients with osteoarthritis of the **basilar, or carpometacarpal (CMC), joint** present with

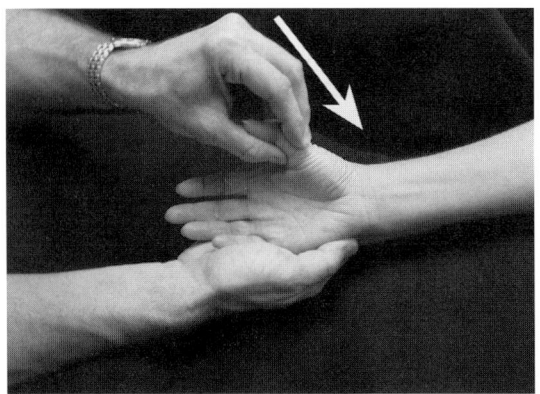

FIGURE 54. The grind test is positive in patients with degenerative joint disease of the basilar joint (the CMC joint of the thumb). The examiner holds the proximal phalanx of the thumb and gently pushes downward (*arrow*). Pain is confirmatory.

pain at the base of the thumb, particularly with activity. Subluxation of the first metacarpal may develop, with contracture into the palm. The diagnosis generally is established by radiographic evidence of degeneration at the CMC joint and a positive "grind test" (Figure 54). The examiner performs this test by placing an axial load on the patient's thumb, gently pushing

down towards the base of the first metacarpal. The test is positive if the patient complains of pain.

Early conservative measures include NSAIDs and supportive splinting in a thumb spica splint (see Figure 31). Surgical treatment of basilar joint arthritis involves resection of the diseased trapezium bone with tendon rebalancing, which can provide dramatic pain relief for these patients.

RHEUMATOID ARTHRITIS

Rheumatoid arthritis is a systemic autoimmune disease whose major target organ (as viewed by the hand surgeon) is the **synovium.** Any area in which the synovium resides can be affected by this disease process. The synovium becomes boggy and hypertrophic and can invade ligaments, tendons, cartilage, and even bone. Ligaments not destroyed by the synovium can be stretched, weakened, and rendered unstable by its expansion. This can then lead to joint subluxation, further destroying the architecture and balance of the hand. The synovium's invasion into the tendon can cause it to weaken and rupture. If the synovial-lined glid-

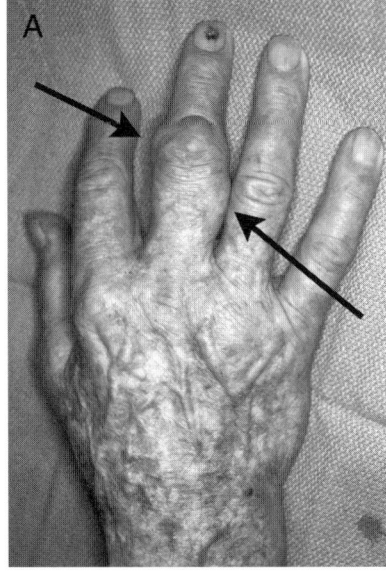

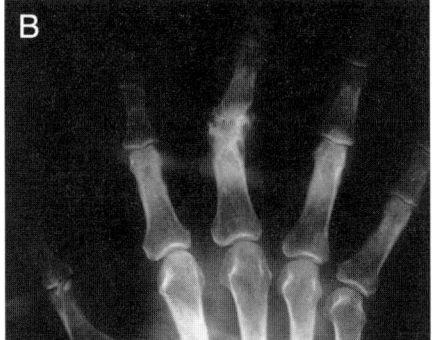

FIGURE 55. **A,** Patient with rheumatoid arthritis and a large mass of boggy, hypertrophic synovium over the proximal phalanx of the long finger (*arrow*). **B,** Note the destruction of the PIP joint. Excisional biopsy confirmed the diagnosis. Typically the DIP and PIP joints are spared in this disease process.

ing surfaces of the tendon are lost, rough bony protuberances (such as Lister's tubercle at the distal radius) can erode and weaken the tendons, also leading to rupture.

The diagnosis of rheumatoid arthritis usually is made before significant hand deformities present. Typically, these patients require the management of a specialist, such as a rheumatologist, to treat and follow the systemic manifestations of this progressive disease. At what point should patients with rheumatoid arthritis be referred? It appears that many aspects of this disease can be improved or prevented with **early, aggressive synovectomy.** As soon as there is a noticeable, palpable pannus of synovium (demonstrated by persistant soft tissue swelling), it can be surgically excised, preventing the subsequent invasion into and destruction of surrounding tendons and ligamentous structures (Figure 55A). Unfortunately, many patients who could have benefitted from preemptive synovectomy ultimately progress to tendon rupture, joint subluxation, and contractures prior to referral. Once disruption and deformity occur, recapturing hand function is more difficult.

In contrast to osteoarthritis, rheumatoid arthritis typically affects the MCP joints, sparing the DIP and PIP joints (although not universally; Figure 55B). Patients also may have severe disease in the wrist, with advanced cases progressing to carpal collapse requiring wrist fusion.

Tendon Rupture

The diagnosis of tendon rupture generally is straightforward. The patient complains of inability to perform a certain action, such as thumb extension or finger flexion, and typically remembers an audible "pop" that he or she can relate temporally to the loss of function. The sound is caused by acute rupture after the gradual wearing down of a tendon by constant abrasion over a bony surface.

Lost function usually can be recaptured operatively, although direct repair of the ruptured tendon rarely is possible, due to the frayed and attenuated nature of the tendon ends. Repair of

the distal tendon end to an adjacent (uninjured) tendon with similar function may be an option, or tendon grafts may be used to reconstruct the ruptured tendon. Tendon transfer, in which a different tendon motor replaces the action of the lost motor, also can be helpful in this situation. An example is rerouting the extensor indicis proprius to motor a ruptured extensor pollicis longus (EPL) tendon. The EPL is a commonly ruptured tendon in patients with rheumatoid arthritis, due to abrasion over the distal radius at Lister's tubercle. Remember that *prevention* of this deformity (via synovectomy) has a much better result than treatment of an established attritional rupture.

The classic, end-stage, disabled rheumatic hand displays destruction of the MCP joints, with volar subluxation, ulnar deviation of the digits at the MCP joints, wrist dislocation, and loss of most hand function (Figure 56). At this point, the MCP joints can be replaced with artificial implants, the extensor tendons can be rebalanced, and synovectomy can be performed. These treatments decrease pain and dramatically improve function (Figure 57).

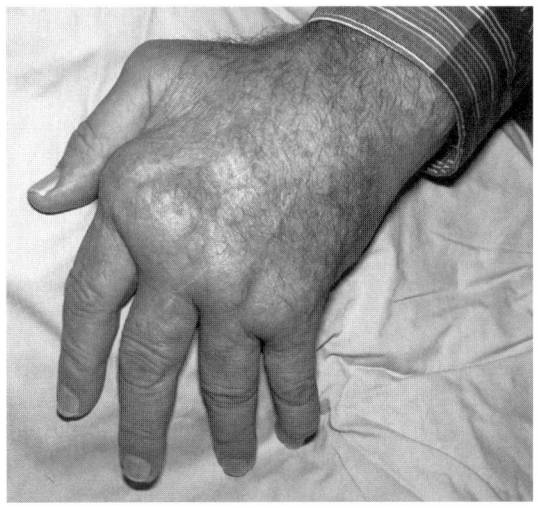

FIGURE 56. Classic, end-stage rheumatoid hand deformity. This patient has volar subluxation of the MCP joints; ulnar deviation of the digits; and hypertrophic, boggy synovium along the dorsum of the hand, particularly over the MCP joints.

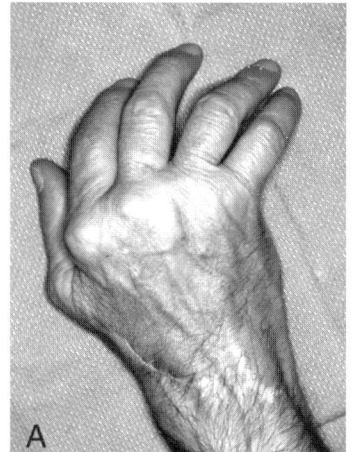
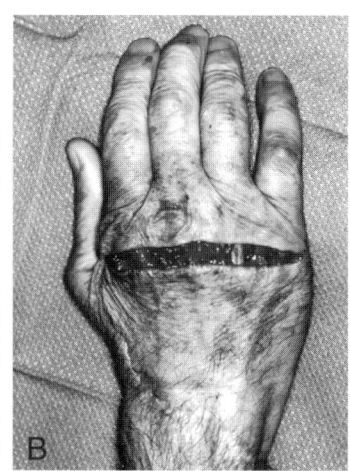

FIGURE 57. Rheumatoid hand reconstruction. **A,** Preoperatively, the patient exhibited subluxation and destruction of the MCP joints, attenuation and dislocation of the extensor tendons to the fingers, and significant hypertrophic synovium on the dorsum. **B,** Postoperatively, note the position of the fingers prior to skin closure. Synovial resection, MCP joint replacement with silastic implants, and rebalancing of the extensor mechanism for each finger were performed.

GOUT

Gouty arthritis is rare and usually presents as an acute exacerbation in the emergency room department. Typically the patient has a single affected joint or digit that is swollen, red, and exquisitely tender—symptoms that are easily confused with an infectious process such as cellulitis or abscess. The pathogenesis of this disease involves an excess of uric acid, which precipitates throughout the body, with a predilection for the joints of the hand and feet. These precipitated deposits are called **tophi** (Figure 58).

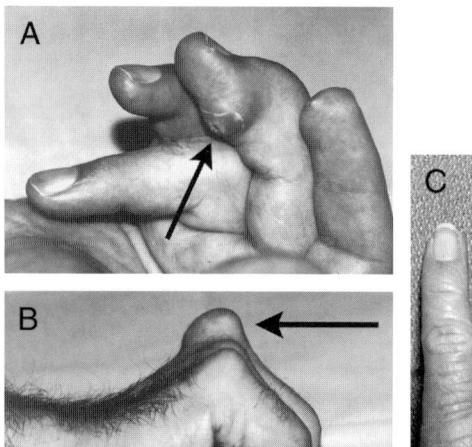
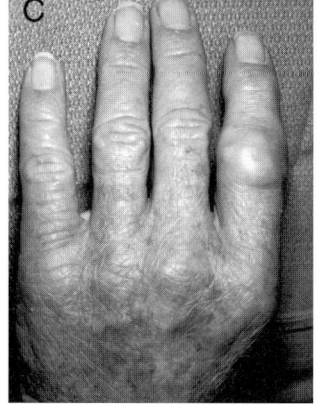

FIGURE 58. **A,** Gouty tophus deposition on the volar aspect of the long finger (*arrow*). This patient has severe gouty arthritis with multiple tophaceous deposits, resistant to medical management. **B,** Same patient as Figure 55, demonstrating a large tophus over the MCP joint of the dorsal long finger (*arrow*). **C,** Symptomatic gouty tophus at the PIP joint of the index finger.

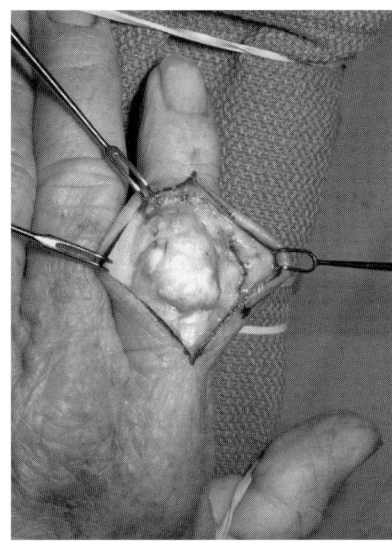

FIGURE 59. Same patient as Figure 58C: after retraction of the skin, the tophaceous deposit invading through the extensor mechanism of the digit is evident.

The mainstay of treatment for gouty arthritis is medical management, controlling uric acid levels to prevent tophus formation. Patients with acute symptoms:

1. are affected by severe forms of gout (resistant to medical management), *or*

2. have become symptomatic because of noncompliance with medication, *or*

3. have not been diagnosed yet.

Treat an acute exacerbation with 2 milligrams of colchicine administered via slow IV push. If the patient remains symptomatic, give additional colchicine (0.5 milligrams every 6 hours). Due to potential serious toxicity, do not administer more than 4 milligrams in a 24-hour period, and after a full course of IV therapy (4 milligrams maximum) no further colchicine is recommended for at least 7 days. After the acute attack has resolved, chronic medical management (using allopurinol, probenecid, and/or colchicine) can be started or resumed. Antibiotics are unnecessary during an acute gouty attack. If the patient has tophi that do not resolve with medical management, referral to a hand surgeon is indicated for excision on an outpatient basis (Figure 59).

An elevated serum uric acid level does not confirm the diagnosis of gout. During an acute exacerbation, the diagnosis is made by microscopic examination (under polarized light) of fluid aspirated from the affected area: the presence of shiny white, needle-shaped, birefringent crystals is confirmatory.

Burns

The following discussion assumes that the patient has only an isolated burn of the hand or arm. If the burn is more extensive, the patient should be referred promptly to a burn center for fluid resuscitation and inpatient management. Deep burns—even if isolated only to the hand—also should be referred to a burn center or hand surgeon, due to the potentially devastating effects of late scarring if adequate debridement and grafting (if needed) is not performed (Figure 60).

THERMAL BURNS

Diagnosis

The diagnosis is easily made from the patient's history. However, an understanding of the depth of the burn is more problematic, and

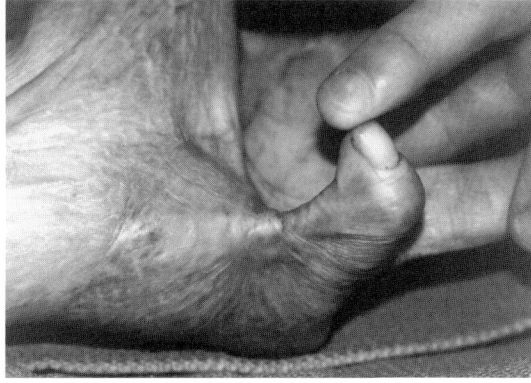

FIGURE 60. Severe burn contracture from a thermal injury to the volar hand. No medical treatment was obtained. Early and aggressive medical management is required to prevent flexion contracture of the hand. Rigorous attention to splinting and occupational therapy also are important.

accurate assessment is critical because treatment options *(after initial first aid is applied)* are based on burn depth. If there is any doubt as to the depth of burn, referral to a burn center or hand surgeon is prudent.

First-degree burns are the most superficial, involving only the surface epidermis. They are characterized by intense pain, marked erythema, and, occasionally, edema. First-degree burns are somewhat analogous to a severe sunburn.

Second-degree burns extend deeper than first-degree burns, into the dermis, and are characterized by blistering and bullae formation. Burned areas may appear whitish and are difficult to distinguish from third-degree burns.

Third-degree burns extend completely through the epidermis and dermis and are characterized (ironically) by lack of pain and sensation in the affected areas. This anesthesia is one of the ways to diagnose third-degree burns, but it is not foolproof. *Burn depth can increase after the initial injury,* if proper therapeutic measures to prevent secondary infection and dessication are not taken.

Treatment

The initial treatment of all thermal burns, *regardless of the depth,* is the same. The area should be cooled with chilled water (but not ice), particularly during the first hour post-burn. Analgesia can be given as required to make the patient more comfortable. After these measures, assess the burn depth for guidance in decision making about treatment and surgical referral. Dress all burns with an antibacterial ointment such as Silvadene (silver sulfadiazine) twice a day, to prevent burn dessication and secondary bacterial infection, both of which can increase the area and depth of the injured tissue.

For first-degree burns and superficial second-degree burns, topical Silvadene dressings are the only treatment required. First-degree burns typically heal within 72 hours, heralded by a significant decrease in pain as reported by the patient.

If blisters are present in second-degree burns, rupture them sterilely, but leave the blis-

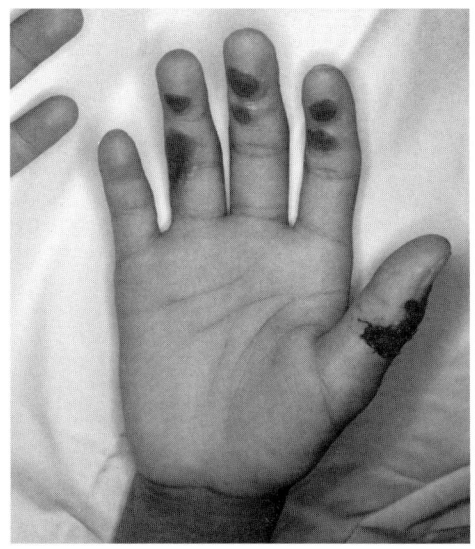

FIGURE 61. Skin grafts on the volar hand of an African-American child. These burns resulted from an electrocution injury.

tered skin in place. This membrane covering makes dessication of the underlying dermis and epidermis less likely. Liberally apply a topical antibacterial cream (such as Silvadene) over the burned and blistered skin. Rupturing the blister is advantageous because the fluid has been shown to contain potentially damaging factors, such as thromboxane A_2, which could impede wound healing and increase burn depth.

Deeper second-degree and third-degree burns must be treated surgically, and referral should be expedited within 24–48 hours, but the initial treatment (i.e., cooling, topical antibiotic ointment) is the same as for the more superficial injuries. The advent of early burn debridement and skin grafting has revolutionized the care and outcome of burn victims (Figure 61). Early debridement (if required) should occur within 72 hours of the injury.

CHEMICAL BURNS

There are many caustic agents that can cause a cutaneous injury after exposure to the skin or mucous membranes (Table 2).

TABLE 2.   Burns From Chemical Agents

Chemical Agent	Comments	Treatment
Alkyl mercuric agents	Typically present with erythema, blisters. Debride blister and liberally irrigate with saline (mercury left within blister fluid may cause further tissue injury and deepening of burn). Cutaneous absorption of mercury can be fatal. If significant skin exposure, refer to burn center.	Copious water irrigation (after blister debridement, if necessary)
Ammonia (NH_4)	A strong alkali. Watch for possible respiratory problems from prolonged fume exposure.	Copious water lavage. Pay attention to respiratory injuries, if present.
Asphalt and/or tar	Adheres to skin; difficult to remove. Burns due to prolonged contact with hot tar.	Cool with cold water, then remove tar using petroleum-based compound (e.g., bacitracin, neosporin ointment).
Calcium hydroxide	A strong alkali	Copious water lavage
Chromic acid (CrO_3)	Yellow viscous liquid used in metal cleaning; can cause ulceration and blister formation after skin contact	Copious water lavage
Cantharide	Used in past as veterinary aphrodisiac (Spanish fly); can cause papules ≤ 1 cm in diameter and produce severe histamine (allergic-type) response	Copious water lavage
Cement	A strong alkali, which may cause burns after prolonged contact	Copious water lavage
Creosol, creosote	Related substances, used as disinfectants and in wood preservatives; may cause severe dermatitis with exposure. Depth and severity of injury related to **phenol** content.	Since phenol present, water contraindicated (see section on phenol). Apply polyethylene glycol to burned area (if unavailable, use a mixture of propylene glycol and glycerol.)
Dichromate salts	Used in metal electroplating; highly corrosive to skin. Also highly toxic if ingested: lethal dose may be as low as 500 mg. Death from cutaneous absorption has been reported.	Smaller burns: copious water lavage. Larger exposures: consider immediate excision to avoid lethal toxicity.
Formic acid	Used in tanning. Skin may appear green, with late formation of blisters.	Copious water lavage
Freon	Fluorocarbon once widely used as refrigerant; still used in manufacture of Teflon. Cutaneous exposure results in frostbite-type burns.	Treat as for frostbite: rapid rewarming, aspirin (for its antiprostaglandin activity)
Gasoline and hydrocarbons	Primarily skin irritants. Prolonged exposure may result in skin burn.	Copious water lavage
Hydrofluoric acid	Intense, deep pain that may be delayed in onset for several hours. Progressive tissue destruction can cause bony erosion. Death can result due to severe **hypocalcemia.** Pain is related to concentration of hydrofluoric acid: fluoride ion binds to intracellular calcium and magnesium, resulting in cell death. Then fluoride ion is released into surrounding tissue, causing further cellular destruction.	Copious water lavage and application of calcium gluconate gel to induce fluoride binding. If unavailable, use calcium-carbonate mixture. Inject 10% calcium gluconate subeschar. Pain relief is end point of therapy, allowing titration of calcium gluconate for injection. For this reason, **anesthesia and analgesia are contraindicated.** Due to danger of life-threatening hypocalcemia, patients should be admitted to intensive care and closely observed.
Hydrochloric acid (muriatic acid)	Extremely strong acid; severe scarring may occur.	Copious water lavage

(Continued)

TABLE 2. Burns From Chemical Agents (*Cont.*)

Chemical Agent	Comments	Treatment
Lithium	Strong, corrosive alkali; found most commonly in batteries	Water lavage ≥ 1 hr. Remaining lithium fragments must be removed or covered with mineral oil before irrigation, to prevent serious deep burns.
Lye	General term for very corrosive alkali agents (e.g., sodium hydroxide, calcium hydroxide, potassium hydroxide)	Copious water lavage
Nitric acid	Skin may be stained bright yellow after exposure.	Copious water lavage
Phenol	When absorbed through skin, arrhythmias, convulsions, and cardiovascular collapse can result. Monitor patients for at least 24 hr after exposure.	Most effective: direct application of poly-ethylene glycol to burned area. If unavailable, use mixture of propylene glycol and glycerol. Water is **contra-indicated** because it dilutes concentration of phenol. Dilute phenol allows deeper penetration with higher toxicity; concen-trated phenol denatures superficial skin proteins, which then act as barrier to phenol, preventing further absorption.
Phosphorous	In presence of air, is rapidly oxidized in extreme exothermic reaction. Fire can be extinguished by immersion into water. However, re-exposure to air reignites particles.	Remaining phosphorous particles must be removed under water to prevent reignition. Particles best seen with Woods lamp. Use mineral oil to coat burn and particles to prevent air exposure prior to removal.
Elemental potassium	Reacts explosively in presence of water; **water lavage contraindicated.**	Apply mineral oil to burned areas. Dispose of potassium fragments by placing in pure tertbutyl alcohol.
Potassium hydroxide	A very corrosive alkali	Copious water lavage
Potassium permanganate	Causes coagulative necrosis with surround-ing deep-purple staining of skin	Copious water lavage
Providone-iodine	Extended exposure can cause burns.	Copious water lavage
Propane (liquid)	May produce massive deep-tissue edema and cutaneous burns. Fasciotomy may be required for compartment syndrome caused by swelling.	Treat like frostbite injuries: rapid rewarming, aspirin for antiprostaglandin effects
Sodium (elemental)	Like potassium, reacts explosively with water	Remove particles and cover with mineral oil to prevent water exposure (even to mois-ture in air). Surgical debridement may be required. Dispose of elemental sodium particles in pure isopropyl alcohol (con-taining less than 2% water).
Sodium hypochlorite	A corrosive alkali used in bleaches and medicine (Dakin's solution). Can result in cutaneous liquifactive necrosis if solution is concentrated enough.	Copious water lavage
Sodium hydroxide	A severely caustic alkali used in drain cleaners	Copious water lavage
Sulfuric acid	Found in common batteries and household cleaners. Burns range from 1st degree with erythema and blistering to deeply penetrating ulcers.	Copious water lavage
Trichloroacetic acid (TCA)	Burn depth dependent on TCA concentration	Copious water lavage

Adapted from Concannon MJ, Chick LR, Lister GD: Emergency Management of Thermal, Electrical, and Chemical Burns. In Kasdan ML (ed): Occupational Hand & Upper Extremity Injuries & Diseases, 2nd ed. Philadelphia, Hanley & Belfus, Inc., 1998, pp 361–371.

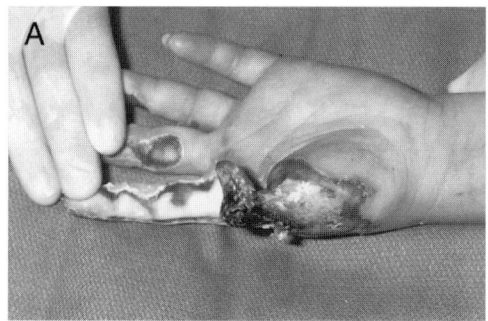

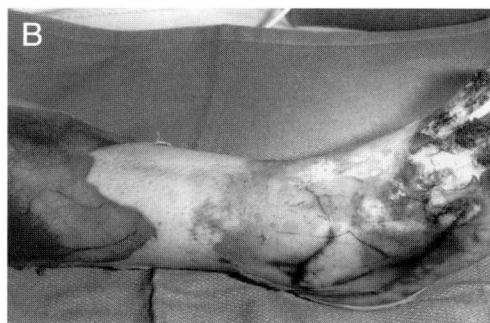

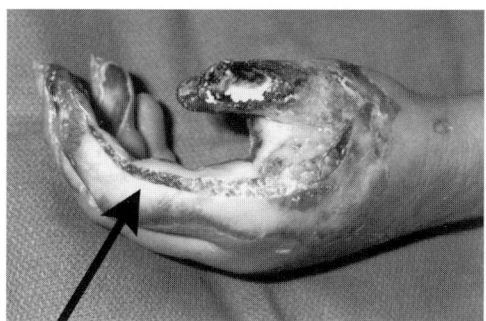

FIGURE 62. Severe electrocution injury. **A,** This patient touched a high-voltage electrical wire and suffered severe damage to the thumb, index, and long fingers. Note the lateral escharotomy performed by the burn team (*arrow*). When circumferential burns are present in the digits or forearm, an escharotomy is required to prevent critical ischemia due to secondary swelling underneath unyielding burned skin. **B,** The entire foot was lost due to the exit wound. The extremities frequently are damaged in electrocution injuries because they often function as entrance and exit points.

ELECTRICAL BURNS

Electrocution commonly involves at least one of the upper limbs, either as a contact point (e.g., touching a power line) or as an exit (Figure 62). Electrocution injuries may appear trivial on cursory exam, but the entrance and exit points frequently are only the "tip of the iceberg" as far as tissue damage is concerned (Figure 63). Cardiac monitoring and intravenous fluid resuscitation should be promptly instituted, and these patients should be emergently referred to a critical care or burn specialist for evaluation and observation.

FROSTBITE

Because of their peripheral positions, the hands and feet are at most risk for frostbite injury. Treatment of suspected or confirmed frostbite involves rapid rewarming of the affected part for 15–30 minutes in water that is precisely 104–108 degrees. This stops any further ice crystal formation and reverses the potent vasoconstriction induced by the cold. Blisters (similar to the treatment of second-degree burns) should be incised sterilely to remove the fluid, but leave the blister skin intact to help prevent subsequent dessication. Instead of an antibacterial ointment, an aloe vera ointment is suggested as a dressing due to its antiprostaglandin activities. Give ibuprofen, also for its antiprostaglandin activity (12 mg/kg/day). Administer penicillin for the first 3 days after injury to reduce the risk of gram-positive infection; in the absence of infection, no antibiotics are required after that time.

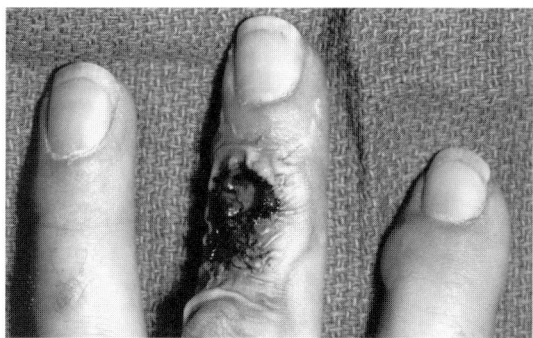

FIGURE 63. Electrical wound of the dorsal aspect of the long finger. Although this particular wound may appear trivial in comparison to other electrical wounds, a thorough physical examination should be performed to rule out occult damage, as the visible cutaneous damage may be only the "tip of the iceberg."

Index

Abduction, 1, 2
Abductor digiti quinti, anatomy, function, and innervation of, 19, 22
Abductor pollicis brevis
　anatomy, function, and innervation of, 15, 18, 43
Abductor pollicis longus
　anatomy, function, and innervation of, 11
　in Bennett's fractures, 115
　in de Quervain's disease, 145–146
　function testing of, 37, 38, 39
　transection of, 66
Abraded skin, re-epithelization of, 67
Abrasions, case example of, 48
Abscess. See also Infections
　differentiated from cellulitis, 127
Adduction, 1
Adductor digiti minimi, anatomy, function, and innervation of, 21
Adductor pollicis
　anatomy, function, and innervation of, 19, 22, 23
　function testing of, 45, 48
Allen's test, 7, 32, 33
Amputations, **77–97**
　conservative management of, 88–89
　of multiple digits, 78–79, 80–81
　replantation techniques for, 77–87
　　preservation of amputated parts, 83–85
　　relative indications and contraindications to, 77–83, 84, 85
　　revision, 77, 81, 86–87
　skin grafts for, 88, 89–92
　　distant, 96–97
　　grafting methods for, 92–96, 97
　　local, 92–96, 97
　subtotal, 85–86
Analgesics. See also Nonsteroidal anti-inflammatory drugs
　for laceration patients, 68, 69, 70
Anatomic snuff box
　anatomy of, 11, 12, 13
　palpation of, 13
　scaphoid fracture-related tenderness of, 110
Anatomy and function, of the hand, **1–25**
　bony anatomy, 4–6, 7. See also specific bones

Anatomy and function, of the hand (*Cont.*)
　innervation of muscles and tendons, 8–25
　　by median nerve, 7, 8, 9, 10, 15–18, 21, 33, 34, 35–36, 37, 133
　　by radial nerve, 10–14, 37–71, 42, 58, 59, 61
　　by ulnar nerve, 8, 9, 10, 18–25, 58, 59, 61, 62, 135
　　of juncturae tendinum, 25
　　terminology of, 1–4
　　vascular anatomy, 6–8
Anesthesia. See Local anesthesia
Angular deformities, of the fingers, 28
Antecubital fossa, 15
Antibiotic prophylaxis/therapy
　for bite wounds, 73, 74
　for felons, 130
　for infections, 127
　for lacerations, 68–69, 72–73
　for paronychia, 129
Arterial anatomy, of the hand, 6–8. See also Radial artery; Ulnar artery
Arterial injuries
　avulsion injury-related, 80
　laceration-related, 72
Arteriography, of radial and ulnar arteries, 8
Arthritis, 154–159
　gouty, 154, 158–159
　osteoarthritis, 155–156
　pyogenic, 75
　rheumatoid, 156–158, 159
　　as carpal tunnel risk factor, 134
　　as swan neck deformity risk factor, 151
　　of the wrist, scaphoid fracture nonunion-related, 110–111
Aspiration, of ganglion cysts, 147
Atrophy, muscular, 28, 29, 139
Avulsion injuries
　of the dorsum, 49–51
　as replantation contraindication, 79–80, 84
　ring, 79–80, 84
Axonotmesis, 133

Bacitracin, 65–66
Basal cell carcinoma, 149–150
Basilar joint, osteoarthritis of, 154, 155–156

Bennett's fractures, 114–115
  reverse, 115
Betadine, 65
Bier blocks, 63–64, 65
Bite wounds, 73–75
  animal, 73–74, 132
  human, 74–75, 132
  infection of, 132
Blisters
  burn-related, 160
  frostbite-related, 163
Blood supply, of the hand. *See* Vascular anatomy, of the
        hand
Bone rongeurs, 86–87
Bones, of the hand and wrist. *See also* Capitate bone; Hamate
        bone; Lunate bone; Pisiform bone; Radius bone;
        Scaphoid bone; Sesamoid bone; Trapezium bone;
        Trapezoid bone; Triquetrum bone; Ulna bone
  anatomy of, 4–6, 7
  ossification of, 4
Bony chip, gamekeeper's thumb-associated, 107–108
Bony injuries. *See* Fractures
Boutonniere deformity, 151–152
Buddy-taping, of interphalangeal joint dislocations, 102, 103,
        105
Burns, 159–163
  chemical, 160–162
  as contracture cause, 89, 159
  electrical, 160, 163
  thermal, 150–160

Calipers, use in sensory testing, 34
Cancer, 149–151
Capitate bone, radiographic visualization of, 6
Cardiovascular disease, as replantation contraindication, 82
Carpal bones. *See also* Capitate bone; Hamate bone; Lunate
        bone; Pisiform bone; Scaphoid bone; Sesamoid
        bone; Trapezium bone; Trapezoid bone; Triquetrum
        bone
  anatomy of, 4, 6
  fractures of, 109–111
  radiographic visualization of, 4, 6
Carpal ligaments, 4
  volar, 133, 134
Carpal tunnel
  anatomy of, 17, 133, 134
  in median nerve block, 60–61
Carpal tunnel syndrome, 17–18, 133–137
  muscle atrophy associated with, 28, 139
Carpometacarpal joint, osteoarthritis of, 154, 155–156
Cascade position, of the fingers, 28
Casting, of metacarpal fractures, 113, 114
Caustic agents, as burn cause, 160–163
Cautery units, ophthalmic, use in subungual hematoma
        drainage, 118–119
Cellulitis
  cat bite-related, 73, 74
  differentiated from abscess, 127

Children
  amputations in
    conservative management of, 88
    replantation techniques for, 78, 79
  fractures in, 119–121
  hand evaluation in, 29
  open epiphyses in, 4, 7
  syndactyly in, 152–153
  trigger finger in, 143–144
Collateral ligaments
  anatomy and function of, 99
  in proximal interphalangeal joint dislocations, 99, 100
    buddy-taping of, 102, 103
    radial, tears of, 104, 105
  ulnar
    disruption of, 106–107
    tears of, 104, 105
Common hand problems, **133–163**
  arthritis, 154–159
    gout, 154, 158–159
    osteoarthritis, 134, 151, 154–156
    rheumatoid arthritis, 156–158
  benign masses, 146–148, 149
  burns, 159–163
    chemical, 160–162
    electrical, 160, 163
    thermal, 159–160
  de Quervain's tenosynovitis, 145–146
  Dupuytren's contracture, 153–154
  extensor tendon derangements, 151–152
  lateral epicondylitis, 140–141, 142–143
  malignant masses, 149–151
  nerve compression syndromes, 133–142
    carpal tunnel syndrome, 17–18, 133–137
    radial nerve compression, 140–142
    ulnar nerve compression, 137–139
  syndactyly, 152–153
  trigger finger, 143–145
Contractures
  boutonniere deformity of, 152
  burn-related, 89, 159
  Dupuytren's, 153–154
  osteoarthritis-related, 156
Contusions, case example of, 48
Coordination, as ulnar nerve function, 10
Creases, of volar aspect of the hand, 3
Crossfinger flap, 93–94, 95, 97
Crush injuries
  case example of, 48–49
  physical examination of, 27, 28
  as replantation contraindication, 79
Cubital tunnel, as ulnar nerve site, 19, 20
Cubital tunnel syndrome, 137–139
  muscle atrophy associated with, 28, 29
Cyst
  ganglion, 146–148
  inclusion, 148
  mucous, 148, 149

Debridement, 67
  of bite wounds, 75
  of burns, 159, 160
  of open fractures, 71–72
Decompression
  of median nerve, as carpal tunnel syndrome treatment, 137
  of ulnar nerve, as cubital tunnel syndrome treatment, 138
De Quervain's tenosynovitis, 145–146
Diabetes
  as carpal tunnel syndrome risk factor, 134
  as replantation contraindication, 82
Digital artery, anatomy of, 7, 9
Digital nerve blocks, 57–59
Digital nerves
  anatomy of, 9, 135
  entrapment of, within fingertip scars, 87
Dislocations
  of distal interphalangeal joints, reduction failure of, 106
  of metacarpophalangeal joints, 106–109
    gamekeeper's thumb, 106–108
    mallet finger, 105–106, 108–109, 151
  perilunate, 110, 111
  of proximal interphalangeal joints, 99–106
    buddy taping of, 102, 103, 105
    dorsal, 99–104
    lateral, 99, 104–105
    with overlying lacerations, 101
    reduction failure of, 102–103, 104
    reduction of, 101–104
    volar, 99, 100, 105
Distal, definitioon of, 4
Distal interphalangeal joint
  anatomy of, 4, 5
  boutonniere deformity of, 151–152
  mallet finger of, 105–106, 108–109, 151
  mucous cysts of, 148, 149
  osteoarthritis of, 154, 155
  swan neck deformity of, 151
Distal phalanx, fractures of, 105, 117–118
"Dog ears" deformity, 86, 87
Doppler probes, 32
Dorsal aspect
  of the forearm. *See* Forearm, dorsal
  of the hand. *See* Dorsum
Dorsum, 2–3
  anatomy of, 5
  injuries to
    avulsion injuries, 49–51
    lacerations of, 49–51
    local anesthesia for, 57
    tendon injuries associated with, 39–40
  interosseuous muscles of
    anatomy, function, and innervation of, 19, 21–22, 23, 24
    function testing of, 36, 45, 47
  musculotendinous unit examination of, 37–41
  radial nerve innervation of, 10–14
  vascular anatomy of, 6

Drainage
  of felon, 129–130
  of paronychia, 129
  of subungual hematoma, 117, 118–119
  of web space abscess, 132
Dressings
  for burns, 160
  for lacerations, 69
Dupuytren's contracture, 153–154

Ecchymosis, crush injury-related, 28
Elderly patients, muscle atrophy in, 28, 29, 139
Electrodiagnostic studies
  for carpal tunnel syndrome diagnosis, 136–137
  for cubital tunnel syndrome diagnosis, 138
  for radial tunnel syndrome diagnosis, 140, 142
Electromyography, for carpal tunnel syndrome diagnosis, 136–137
Enchondroma, 121
Epicondylitis, lateral, 142–143
  differentiated from radial tunnel syndrome, 140–141, 142
Epinephrine, as ischemia cause, 57
Epiphyseal plates
  fractures of, 119–121
    Salter-Harris classification of, 119–120
  open, 4, 7
  radiographic visualization of, 29, 31
Examination, of the hand, **27–55**
  history, 27
    case examples of, 48, 49, 51, 52, 54
  physical examination, 27–48
    case examples of, 48, 49–50, 51, 52–53, 54
    of lacerations, 65
    musculotendinous unit examination, 37–48
    neural examination, 33–37
    vascular examination, 32–33, 48, 50, 51, 52, 54
    visual examination, 27–32
Extension, as radial nerve function, 10
Extensor carpi radialis brevis
  anatomy, function, and innervation of, 11, 12, 13, 14
  function testing of, 37, 38, 39
Extensor carpi radialis longus
  anatomy, function, and innervation of, 11, 12, 13, 14
  transection of, 66
  function testing of, 37, 38, 39
Extensor carpi ulnaris
  anatomy, function, and innervation of, 11, 14
  function testing of, 40, 42, 42
Extensor digiti quinti
  anatomy, function, and innervation of, 11, 14, 23
  function testing of, 37, 41
Extensor digitorum communis
  anatomy, function, and innervation of, 11, 12, 13, 14, 23, 24
  function testing of, 37, 39–40
  occult transection of, 39
Extensor indicis proprius
  anatomy, function, and innervation of, 11, 12, 14, 23
  function testing of, 40, 41

Extensor mechanism, of the hand, anatomy and function of, 22–24
Extensor pollicis brevis
    anatomy, function, and innervation of, 11, 13, 11, 13
    in de Quervain's disease, 145–146
    transection of, 66
Extensor pollicis longus
    anatomy, function, and innervation of, 11–12, 13
    rheumatoid arthritis-related rupture of, 157
Extensor retinaculum
    anatomy and function of, 10–11, 12
    in de Quervain's disease, 145
Extensor tendons. *See also* specific extensor tendons
    derangements of, 151–152
    extrinsic, 23, 24
    injuries to
        laceration-related, 70–71
        as lateral epicondylitis cause, 142–143
        splinting of, 122, 124, 125
        tears/transections of, 49–51, 142–143
    juncturae tendinum of, 25
    in revision amputations, 87
    splinting of
        for injuries, 122, 124, 125
        prior to surgical repair, 70–71

Felons, 129–130
Fibro-osseous tunnel ("no man's land"), 17, 18
Fingers
    cascade position of, 28
    multiple injuries to, wrist blocks for, 57, 60–61
    nomenclature of, 3, 4
Fingertips, amputation of, 86–87
Finkelstein's test, 146
Fish mouth incision, 129, 130
Flaps. *See* Grafts, skin
Flexion, as median nerve function, 10
Flexor carpi radialis
    anatomy, function, and innervation of, 15, 16
    function testing of, 43, 44
    transection of, 66
Flexor carpi ulnaris
    anatomy, function, and innervation of, 19, 20, 21
    function testing of, 45, 46
    palpation of, 61
    in ulnar nerve blocks, 61–62
Flexor digiti quinti
    anatomy, function, and innervation of, 19, 22
Flexor digitorum profundus
    anatomy, function, and innervation of, 15, 17, 18, 19, 19, 21, 22
    function testing of, 37, 45
    location within carpal tunnel, 133
    transection of, 28
        case example of, 52–55
        implication for finger replantation, 81–82
Flexor digitorum superficialis
    amputations distal to, 79, 82, 83

Flexor digitorum superficialis (*Cont.*)
    anatomy, function, and innervation of, 15, 17, 18, 21
    function testing of, 41, 43
    location within carpal tunnel, 133
    transection of, 28
        case example of, 52–55
        implication for finger replantation, 81, 82
Flexor pollicis brevis
    anatomy, function, and innervation of, 15, 18
    function testing of, 43
Flexor pollicis longus
    anatomy, function, and innervation of, 15, 17, 19
    function testing of, 35, 37, 43, 44
    location within carpal tunnel, 133
Flexor sheath, infections of, 130–131
Flexor tendons. *See also* specific flexor tendons
    injuries to
        laceration-related, 69–70, 71
        splinting of, 71, 72, 122, 124, 125
        transections, 69–70, 71, 72
    in revision amputations, 87
    in stenosing tenosynovitis, 143
Forearm
    dorsal
        innervation of, 10–14, 11, 37–41
        muscles of, 10
        musculotendinous unit examination of, 37–41
    incomplete arterial transection of, 72
    lacerations of, local anesthesia for, 57
    physical examination of, 28–29
    volar
        median nerve innervation of, 15–18
        musculotendinous unit examination of, 41–48
        ulnar nerve innervation of, 18–25
Forearm support band, as lateral epicondylitis therapy, 142, 143
Foreign bodies, as infection cause, 127
Fractures, 109–125
    in children, 119–121
    comminuted
        distal phalangeal, 117–119
        metacarpal, 113–114
        proximal phalangeal, 116
    of distal radius, 109–110
    of epiphyseal plate, 119–121
        Salter-Harris classification of, 119–120
    metacarpal, 111–115
        Bennett's, 114–115
        boxer's, 111–113
        in children, 119
        comminuted, 113–114
        greenstick, 119
        spiral, 112, 113–114
    open, 71–72
    with overlying lacerations, 71–72
    pathologic, 121
    phalangeal
        as angular deviation cause, 28

Fractures (*Cont.*)
distal, 117–119
proximal and middle, 51–52, 101, 115–117, 121
radiographic evaluation of, 29–32, 49–51
splinting of
hand positioning for, 121–122
splint manufacture for, 121, 122–125
tuft, 117
of wrist (carpal), 109–111
Frostbite, 163, 163
of amputated parts, 83
Fungal infection, of the nail bed, 131–132
"Funny bone," 20

Gamekeeper's thumb, 106–108
Ganglion, 146–148
Gauze sponge, use in joint dislocation reduction, 101–102, 106
Giant cell tumors, 148
Gout, 158–159
Grafts
skin, 88, 89–92
for burn wounds, 159, 160
distant, 96–97
grafting methods for, 89–92
local, 92–96, 97
revascularization of, 92, 96
venous, 80
Grind test, 156
Guyon's canal
as ulnar nerve compression site, 137–138
as ulnar nerve site, 10, 19, 20

Hamate bone, radiographic visualization of, 6
Hammer head deformity, 86, 87
Hand
dorsal. *See* Dorsum
radiographic visualization of, 29–32
volar. *See* Volar aspect, of the hand
Heberden's nodes, 154, 155
Hematoma
as skin graft failure cause, 92
subungual, 117, 118–119
Hematoma nerve blocks, 62–63
of boxer's fractures, 111
Hook of hamate, radiographic visualization of, 6
Hypothenar flap, 95, 96, 97

Iatrogenic injuries, local anesthesia-related, 57, 60–61
Immobilization. *See also* Splinting
for pain management, 57
Incisions, for felon drainage, 129–130
Infections, of the hand, **127–132**
bite-related, 132
felon, 129–130
of the flexor sheath, 130–131
herpetic whitlow, 131
onychomycosis, 131–132
paronychia, 128–129

Infections, of the hand (*Cont.*)
web space abscess, 132
Interosseous muscles
dorsal
anatomy, function, and innervation of, 19, 21–22, 23, 24
function testing of, 36, 45, 47
volar
anatomy, function, and innervation of, 19, 21–22, 23, 24
function testing of, 45, 47
Interosseous nerve
anterior, 17
compression of, 137
posterior, 10, 11, 14
Interphalangeal joints
anatomy of, 4
distal. *See* Distal interphalangeal joints
proximal. *See* Proximal interphalangeal joints
Interrupted sutures, 68, 73
Irrigation
of bite wounds, 73, 74, 74–75
devices for, 65, 66
of lacerations, 65, 66
of open fractures, 71–72
Ischemia
epinephrine-related, 57
physical appearance of, 28
radial artery injury-related, 6–7
as replantation contraindication, 82
vascular examination of, 32

Joint stiffness, proximal interphalangeal joint dislocation-related, 102, 103–104
Juncturae tendinum, 25

Kidney cancer, metastatic, 150, 151
K-wire fixation
of boxer's fractures, 113
of mallet fingers, 109
of phalangeal fractures, 116

Lacerations, **65–75**
anesthesia for, 65
antibiotic therapy/prophylaxis for, 68–69, 72–73
arterial damage associated with, 72
bite wound-related, 73–75
deep structures involved in, 69–70
of the dorsal hand, 49–51
dressings and post-care for, 69
fractures associated with, 71–72
nerve blocks for, 57–59
neural damage associated with, 72
with overlying dislocations, 101, 101
physical examination of, 65
as subtotal amputation, 85
sutures and suturing methods for, 67–68, 69
as tendon damage cause, 70–71
at ulnar wrist, case example of, 54–55
wound preparation of, 65–67

Lidocaine
    as Bier block, 63–64
    as digital block, 57–59
    as hematoma block, 62–63
    maximum dosage of, 57
    as wrist block, 60–62
Ligaments
    as carpal bone support, 4
    collateral. *See* Collateral ligaments
    volar, 133, 134
Local anesthesia, **57–64.** *See also* Lidocaine
    implication for physical examination, 65
    for lacerations, 65
    neurovascular bundles and, 7, 8
    for proximal interphalangeal joint dislocation treatment, 101
    techniques of, **57–64**
        Bier blocks, 63–64, 65
        digital blocks, 57–59
        hematoma blocks, 62–63, 111
        wrist blocks, 57, 60–62
Lumbrical muscles, anatomy, function, and innervation of, 15, 19, 22, 23
Lunate bone
    radiographic visualization of, 6
    volar displacement of, 111
Lung cancer, metastatic, 150–151
Lytic lesions, enchondroma-related, 121

Malignant masses, 149–151
Malignant melanoma, 150–151
Mallet finger, 105–106, 108–109
    untreated, 151
Malpractice, local anesthesia-related, 57
Mattress sutures, 67–68
Median nerve
    anatomy and function of, 7, 8, 15–18, 21
    compression of. *See also* Carpal tunnel syndrome
        of anterior interosseous branch, 137
    function testing of, 33, 34, 35–36, 37
    location within carpal tunnel, 133
    overlap with ulnar nerve, 21
    sensory distribution of, 9, 10, 15–18
Median nerve block, 60–61
Medical history, 27
    case examples of, 48, 49, 51, 52, 54
Metacarpals
    anatomy of, 4
    fractures of, 111–115
        chronic nonunion of, 30
        radiographic visualization of, 49–51
        reduction of, local anesthesia for, 62–63
        spiral, 29
        transverse, 30
    nomenclature of, 3, 4
Metacarpophalangeal joints
    anatomy of, 4, 5
    Dupuytren's contracture of, 153–154

Metacarpophalangeal joints (*Cont.*)
    dislocations of, 106–109
        gamekeeper's thumb, 106–108
        mallet finger, 108–109
    extension of, 10
    human bite wounds of, 74–75
    hypertension of, folowing fracture healing, 112–113
    in radial nerve testing, 36
    rheumatoid arthritis of, 157, 158
Metastatic disease, 149, 150–151
Microscrew fixation
    of mallet finger, 109
    of proximal phalangeal fractures, 116–117
Middle finger test, 141
Middle phalanges, fractures of, 115–117
Motor tests, 35. *See also* function testing under individual muscles and tendons
Muscles. *See also* specific muscles
    atrophy of, 28, 29, 138–139
    innervation of, 9–25
        by median nerve, 7, 8, 9, 10, 15–18, 21, 33, 34, 35–36, 37, 133
        by radial nerve, 8–9, 10–14, 33, 34, 36–61, 42, 58, 59, 61
        by ulnar nerve, 8, 9, 10, 18–25, 58, 59, 61, 62, 135, 137–139
    intrinsic
        atrophy of, 138–139
        innervation of, 18–19, 20, 21–25
        position of maximum function of, 24
        ulnar nerve compression-related atrophy of, 138–139
    physical examination of, 28
Musculotendinous units, examination of, 35, 37–48
    case examples of, 48, 50, 51, 52–53, 54
Myxedema, as carpal tunnel syndrome risk factor, 134

Nail bed
    distal phalangeal fracture-associated injuries to, 117–119
    melanoma of, 150
    onychomycosis of, 131–132
    paronychia of, 128–129
Nail fold, paronychia of, 129
Nerve(s), of the hand, 8–25, 58, 59. *See also* Interosseous nerves; Median nerve; Radial nerve; Ulnar nerve
    examination of, 33–37
        case examples of, 48, 50, 51, 52, 54
    laceration-related injuries to, 72
Nerve blocks, 57–64
    Bier, 63–64
    digital, 57–59
    effect on diagnostic accuracy, 57
    hematoma, 62–63, 111
    implication for physical examination, 65
    wrist, 60–62
Nerve compression syndromes, 133–142
    carpal tunnel syndrome, 17–18, 28, 133–137, 139
    radial nerve compression, 140–142
    ulnar nerve compression, 137–139
Nerve conduction studies, for carpal tunnel syndrome diagnosis, 136–137

Neurapraxia, 133
Neuroma, of radial nerve, 147
Neurotmesis, 133
Neurovascular bundles, 7–8, 9, 58
"No man's land" (fibro-osseous tunnel), 17, 18
Nonsteroidal anti-inflammatory drugs
  as carpal tunnel syndrome therapy, 137
  as de Quervain's tenosynovitis therapy, 146
  as osteoarthritis therapy, 154–155, 156
Notta's node, 143, 144

Occupational history, 27
Onychomycosis, 131–132
"Open joints," 101
Open reduction and fixation
  of metacarpal fractures, 113–114
  of proximal phalangeal fractures, 116–117
Opponens digiti quinti, anatomy, function, and innervation
  of, 19
Opponens pollicis
  anatomy, function, and innervation of, 15, 18, 19
  function testing of, 43
Opposition, 2
Osteoarthritis, 134, 151, 154–156
Osteophytes, 148, 154, 155

Pain management. *See also* Analgesics; Nonsteroidal anti-
  inflammatory drugs
  for temporary pain alleviation, 57
Palmar arch, superficial, anatomy of, 7, 9
Palmar aspect, of the hand. *See* Volar aspect, of the hand
Palmar creases, 3
Palmaris longus
  absence of, 16
  anatomy, function, and innervation of, 15, 16
  function testing of, 43, 44
Paresthesia, carpal tunnel syndrome-related, 134–135
Paronychia, 128–129
Parrot beak deformity, 88, 89
Phalanges
  distal, fractures of, 105, 117–118
  nomenclature of, 4
  proximal
    bony chip in, 107, 108
    fractures of, 51–52, 115–117
Phalen's test, 135–136
Physical examination, of the hand, 27–48
  case examples of, 48, 49–50, 51, 52–53, 54
  of lacerations, 65
  musculotendinous unit examination in, 35, 37–48
  nerve examination in, 33–37
  vascular examination in, 32–33
  visual examination in, 27–32
Pinprick test, 32
Pisiform bone, radiographic visualization of, 6
Plate and screw fixation
  of metacarpal fractures, 113–114
  of proximal phalangeal fractures, 116–117

Pregnancy, as carpal tunnel syndrome risk factor, 134
Probes, Doppler, 32
Pronation, 1, 2
Pronator quadratus
  anatomy, function, and innervation of, 15, 16m, 17
  function testing of, 43, 45
Pronator teres
  anatomy, function, and innervation of, 15, 16
  function testing of, 41, 42
Proximal, definition of, 4
Proximal injuries, neural examination of, 35–37
Proximal interphalangeal joints
  anatomy of, 4, 5
  boutonniere deformity of, 151–152
  dislocations of, 99–106
    dorsal, 99–104
    lateral, 99, 104–105
    reduction of, 101–104
    volar, 99, 100, 105
  Dupuytrens' contracture of, 153–154
  osteoarthritis of, 154, 155
  swan neck deformity of, 151
Proximal phalanges
  bony chips in, 51–52, 107, 108
  fractures of, 115–117
Pseudocysts, 147
Pulleys, 18
  A-1, 17, 143, 144
Pulmonary disease, as replantation contraindication, 82
Pus, 127

Radial artery
  anatomy of, 6–7, 8
  arteriography of, 8
  collateral relationship with ulnar artery, 6–7, 8
  examination of, 32, 33
  injuries to, as ischemia cause, 6–7
  sensory distribution of, 9, 10
  thrombosis of, 6–7, 72
  volar wrist ganglions associated with, 147, 148
Radial aspect, of the hand, 3
Radial nerve
  anatomy and function of, 10–14, 58, 59, 61
  function testing of, 8–9, 33, 34
  involvement in dorsal wrist ganglions, 147, 148
  muscles of, 36–37
  musculotendinous unit examination of, 37–41, 42
  neuroma of, 147
  sensory distribution of, 10–14
Radial nerve block, 61
Radial tunnel syndrome, 140–142
  differentiated from lateral epicondylitis, 140–141, 142
Radiographic evaluation
  of bony injuries, 29–32
  of carpal bones, 6
  of fractures
    in children, 120
    metacarpal, 111, 112, 113, 114, 115

Radiographic evaluation (*Cont.*)
    phalangeal, 116, 117, 118
      scaphoid, 6
  of gamekeeper's thumb, 107
  multiple views in, 49–51
  of normal hand bony anatomy, 5
  of proximal interphalangeal joint dislocations, 100, 101,
    102
Radius bone
  distal, fractures of, 109–110
  radiographic visualization of, 6
Reduction
  of boxer's fractures, 111, 113–114
  of proximal phalangeal fractures, 116
Replantation, of amputated parts, 77–83
  preservation of amputated parts for, 83–85
  relative indications and contraindidcations to, 77–83, 84, 85
  revision, 77, 81, 86–87
Revascularization, of skin grafts, 92, 96
Rheumatoid arthritis, 156–158, 159
  as carpal tunnel syndrome risk factor, 134
  as swan neck deformity cause, 151
Ring blocks, 58, 59
Rongeurs, bone, 86–87
Rotational deformities, of the fingers, 28
Running sutures, 68, 69

Salter-Harris classification, of epiphyseal plate fractures,
    119–120
Scaphoid bone
  fractures of, 31–32, 109–111
    nonunion of, 110–111
  radiographic visualization of, 6
Scissoring, fracture-related, 112, 113, 115
Screw fixation,
  of mallet finger, 109
  of proximal phalangeal fractures, 116–117
Sensory tests, 33, 34. *See also* function testing under specific
    muscles; nerves, and tendons
Seroma, as skin graft failure cause, 92, 93
Sesamoid bones, 4, 5
Skier's thumb. *See* Gamekeeper's thumb
Skin
  abraded, re-epithelization of, 67
  grafts of. *See* Grafts, skin
  physical examination of, 27
Skin cancer, 149–151
Smoking, as replantation contraindication, 82
Soft-tissue injuries
  conservative management of, 88–89
  open fracture-associated, 71–72
  skin grafts for, 88, 89–92
    for burn wounds, 159, 160
    distant, 96–97
    grafting methods for, 89–92
    local, 92–96, 97
    revascularization of, 92, 96
  tissue loss, 87

Splinting
  of arthritic basilar joint, 156
  of boutonniere deformity, 152
  as carpal tunnel syndrome therapy, 137
  as de Quervain's tenosynovitis therapy, 146
  of distal phalangeal injuries, 118
  of extensor tendon injuries, 70–71, 122, 124, 125
  of flexor tendon injuries, 71, 72, 122, 124, 125
  of fractures
    in children, 119
    metacarpal, 111–112, 113, 114
    pathologic, 121
    phalangeal, 117
    scaphoid, 31–32, 110
  of gamekeeper's thumb, 107–108
  hand positioning for, 70, 71
  of laceration injuries, 69, 70–71, 72
  of mallet finger, 108–109
  for pain management, 57
  of proximal interphalangeal joint dislocations, 102, 105
  of thumb injuries, 125
Squamous cell carcinoma, 149–150
Stab wounds
  examination of, 52–54
  skin grafts for, 89, 91
  as web space abscess cause, 132
Stener lesions, 107–108
Steroid injections, as trigger finger therapy, 144–145
Supination, 1–2
Sutures and suturing methods
  for bite wounds, 73, 74
  for wound closure, 67–68, 69
Swan neck deformity, 151
Syndactyly, 152–153
Synovectomy, as rheumatoid arthritis treatment, 157
Synovium, in rheumatoid arthritis, 156–157

Tar, as wound contaminant, 65–66
Tendons. *See also* specific tendons
  iatrogenic injuries to, 60–61
  lacerations of, 66, 67
  in replantations, 81–82, 83, 84
  rupture of, rheumatoid arthritis-related, 156–157, 158
Tennis elbow. *See* Epicondylitis, lateral
Tenosynovitis
  as carpal tunnel syndrome cause, 133–134, 137
  de Quervain's, 145–146
  stenosing
    of first dorsal compartment. *See* Tenosynovitis, de
      Quervain's
    trigger finger, 143–145
Tetanus immunization, 65, 66
Thenar crease, 3
Thenar eminence, muscles of
  anatomy, function, and innervation of, 18, 19
  atrophy of, carpal tunnel syndrome-related, 136
  function testing of, 36, 43, 46
Thrombosis, of radial artery, 6–7, 72

Thumb
  abduction of, 1, 2, 11
  amputation of, 80
  basilar joint of, osteoarthritis of, 154, 155–156
  Bennet's fractures of, 114–115
  bony anatomy of, 4
  digital nerve blocks of, 58, 59
  dislocations of, 104
  extension of, 10, 11
  gamekeeper's, 106–108
  neurovascular bundles of, 7–8, 9
  opposition of, 2
  replantation of, 78, 79
  splinting of, 125
  trigger finger of, 143, 144
Tinel's sign
  in carpal tunnel syndrome, 135
  in Wartenberg's syndrome, 141
Toenails, onychomycosis of, 131
Tophi, 158, 159
Tourniquets, double pneumatic, use in Bier blocks, 63–64
Trapezium bone, radiographic visualization of, 6
Trapezoid bone, radiographic visualization of, 6
Trigger finger, 17, 143–145, 143–1456
Triquetrum bone, radiographic visualization of, 6
Tumors
  benign, 146–148, 149
  malignant, 149–151
Two-point discrimination test, 34

Ulna bone, radiographic visualization of, 6
Ulnar artery
  anatomy of, 6–7
  arteriography of, 8
  collateral relationship with radial artery, 6–7, 8
  examination of, 32, 33
  transections of, case example of, 52–54
Ulnar aspect, of the hand, 3
Ulnar nerve
  anatomy and function of, 8, 9, 10, 18–25, 35, 36, 58, 59,
    61, 62, 135, 137–139
  compression of, 137–139
  function testing of, 35, 36
  injuries to
    as muscle atrophy cause, 28, 29
    painful trauma ("funny bone"), 20
    transections, case example of, 52–54
  overlap with median nerve, 21

Ulnar nerve (*Cont.*)
  sensory distribution of, 9, 10, 18–25
Ulnar nerve block, 61–62
Uric acid, as gouty arthritis marker, 158

Vascular anatomy, of the hand, 6–8
Vascular examination, of the hand, 32–33
  case examples of, 48, 50, 51, 52, 54
Vascular injuries, occult, case example of, 52–54
Vascularity, tests of, 67
Vasospasm
  arterial transection-related, 72
  local anesthesia-related, 57
Veins, grafts of, 80
Venous congestion, examination of, 32
Visual examination, of the hand, 27–32
Volar aspect
  of the forearm. *See* Forearm, volar
  of the hand, 2–3
    anatomy of, 58
    creases, 3
    innervation of, 15–25
    local anesthesia for, 57
    musculotendinous unit examination of, 41–48
    neurovascular bundles of, 58
Volar carpal ligament, 133, 134
Volar plate
  anatomy and function of, 99
  in proximal interphalangeal joint dislocations, 99, 100, 104
    buddy-taping of, 102, 103
V-Y advancement flap, 93, 94, 95

Wartenberg's syndrome, 141–142
Web spaces
  abscess of, 132
  muscle atrophy of, 28, 29
Whitlows, herpetic, 131
Wounds. *See also* Lacerations
  closure of, 67–69
  debridement of, 67
  preparation of, 65–67
  physical examination of, 27–28
Wrist
  arthritis of, scaphoid fracture nonunion-related, 110–111
  fractures of, 109–111
Wrist nerve blocks, 57, 60–62

X-rays. *See* Radiogaphic evaluation